THE MRI MANUAL

The MRI Manual

ROBERT B. LUFKIN, M.D.

Associate Professor
Department of Radiology
UCLA School of Medicine
Los Angeles, California

YEAR BOOK MEDICAL PUBLISHERS, INC.
CHICAGO • LONDON • BOCA RATON • LITTLETON, MASS.

1 2 3 4 5 6 7 8 9 0 M R 94 93 92 91 90

Library of Congress Cataloging-in-Publication Data

Lufkin, Robert B.
    The MRI manual / Robert B. Lufkin.
        p.   cm.
    Includes bibliographical references.
    ISBN 0-8151-5593-X
    1. Magnetic resonance imaging—Handbooks, manuals, etc.
  I. Title.
    [DNLM: 1. Magnetic resonance imaging.   WN 445 L949m]
    RC78.7.N83L84   1990
    616.07'548—dc20   89-22486
    DNLM/DLC   CIP
    for Library of Congress

Sponsoring Editor: James D. Ryan
Associate Managing Editor, Manuscript Services: Deborah Thorp
Production Project Coordinator: Gayle Paprocki
Proofroom Supervisor: Barbara M. Kelly

This book is dedicated to my parents.

Life's but a walking shadow, a poor player
That struts and frets his hour upon the stage
And then is heard no more; it is a tale
Told by an idiot, full of sound and fury,
Signifying nothing.

Macbeth
William Shakespeare

CONTRIBUTORS

ZORAN L. BARBARIC, M.D.
Professor, Department of Radiology
UCLA School of Medicine
Vice Chairman
Department of Radiology
Chief, Abdominal Division
UCLA Medical Center
Los Angeles, California

LAWRENCE W. BASSETT, M.D.
Professor of Radiological Sciences
UCLA School of Medicine
Vice Chairman
Department of Radiological Sciences
UCLA Medical Center
Los Angeles, California

POONAM BATRA, M.D.
Associate Clinical Professor
UCLA School of Medicine
Department of Radiological Sciences
UCLA Medical Center
Los Angeles, California

JOHN R. BENTSON, M.D.
Professor of Radiological Sciences
UCLA School of Medicine
Chief of Neuroradiology
UCLA Medical Center
Los Angeles, California

M. INES BOECHAT, M.D.
Assistant Professor of Radiology
UCLA School of Medicine
Section Chief
Pediatric Radiology
UCLA Medical Center
Los Angeles, California

LEE C. CHIU, M.D.
Clinical Professor
Department of Radiological Science
UCLA School of Medicine
Chief, MRI Division
St. Joseph Medical Center
Los Angeles, California

ROSALIND B. DIETRICH, M.B., Ch.B.
Assistant Professor in Residence
UCLA School of Medicine
Los Angeles, California

ANTOINETTE S. GOMES, M.D.
Associate Professor of Radiology and
  Medicine
Department of Radiological Sciences
UCLA Medical Center
Los Angeles, California

THEODORE R. HALL, M.D.
Assistant Professor-in-Residence
UCLA School of Medicine
Attending Radiologist
UCLA Medical Center
Los Angeles, California

WILLIAM N. HANAFEE, M.D.
Professor of Radiology
UCLA School of Medicine
Los Angeles, California

HOOSHANG KANGARLOO, M.D.
Professor of Pediatrics
Professor of Radiology
UCLA School of Medicine
Chairman, Department of Radiological
  Sciences
UCLA Medical Center
Los Angeles, California

JUAN F. LOIS, M.D.
Assistant Clinical Professor
Department of Radiological Sciences
UCLA Medical Center
Los Angeles, California

ROBERT B. LUFKIN, M.D.
Associate Professor
Department of Radiology
UCLA School of Medicine
Los Angeles, California

LEANNE L. SEEGER, M.D.
Chief, Musculoskeletal Radiology
Assistant Professor
Department of Radiological Sciences
UCLA School of Medicine
Los Angeles, California

ERIC SPICKLER, M.D.
Staff Neuroradiologist
Henry Ford Hospital
Detroit, Michigan

FOREWORD

Members of the faculty of the UCLA Department of Radiology have been conducting a visiting fellowship program in MRI since 1984. Many physicians have requested that we provide a consolidated book of the material covered during the course. The "students" are particularly interested in atomic diagrams, pulsing sequence routines, and unusual MR manifestations of disease. This book provides a condensation of the presentations made at this program over the years and reflects the state of the art of clinical magnetic resonance imaging.

The full-time faculty and guest faculty of the course have provided chapters covering their individual subspecialties in radiology: orthopedics, chest, cardiovascular, neurology, head and neck. The monthly fellowship program is a week long, which allows ample time to correlate the basic physics of MR to the clinical examination. Dr. Lufkin and his fellow faculty members do this in an exemplary manner.

This manual is intended to provide the beginning practitioner in MRI with a foundation that can later be altered to suit their individual needs. It may also prove handy to the individual who is embarking on an examination of a body region with which he is not thoroughly familiar.

We sincerely hope that the readers of this manual will enjoy using it as much as we have enjoyed putting the material together. The intellectual exchanges of our fellowship program have been immensely stimulating to both faculty and participants. We hope that the reader will share in the fruits of this labor.

William N. Hanafee, M.D.
Professor of Radiology
UCLA Medical School
Los Angeles, California

PREFACE

In a relatively brief period of time, MRI has progressed from an experimental technique to a powerful clinical tool that has displaced CT, plain x-rays, arthrography, myelography, and even angiography, as the imaging study of choice for a growing number of diseases. As the applications of MR have increased, more and more physicians have become interested in this powerful imaging modality

This text has been prepared in order to facilitate the understanding and interpretation of MR images. It has been developed and has been used along with the UCLA magnetic resonance imaging visiting fellowship. Both the fellowship and this text have been in a constant state of evolution over the last 6 years, reflecting the remarkable advances made in MR technology.

The manual is intended to be used with all MRI units operating at all current field strengths. It was developed using MR instruments operating at field strengths from 0.3 to 1.5 T. All major magnet types including superconductive, permanent, and iron core resistive (hybrid), were used in the development of this manual.

The chosen format allows the reader to master the basic fundamentals of MRI in the first chapters, and to apply this knowledge to the specific anatomic areas or disease processes that are covered in subsequent chapters. Detailed discussions of pathology, differential diagnoses, or pathophysiology have been minimized to allow coverage of clinically important issues of MRI. This is intended to be a manual of MRI rather than a textbook. We hope that the informal, practical, and nonintimidating presentation style and associated discussions will provide the reader with stimulating challenges and the knowledge needed to better utilize and interpret MR images in clinical medicine.

Robert B. Lufkin, M.D.

ACKNOWLEDGMENTS

Preparation of this book required the time, effort, and talent of many individuals. We wish to acknowledge and thank those who have helped so much on this project.

First, we thank John Robert, Loris Hirokawa, Bobby Keen, and Julien Keesing whose cheerful attitudes and tireless efforts have made this project manageable. Their work has added immensely to the quality of this book. We also thank our MR technologists, Valerie Gausche, Maria Warner, Sharon Chandler, and Sandy Eldredge, for the care and concern they gave our patients and the MR examinations. We extend a special note of thanks to Mike Anselmo, M.D., Usha Sinha, Ph.D., Shantanu Sinha, Ph.D., and Melody Duran for their suggestions and critical review of the manuscript. Jim Ryan, Gayle Paprocki, and Deborah Thorp at Year Book Medical Publishers provided enthusiastic support and editorial advice. We also acknowledge the extremely important role played by Dr. Hooshang Kangarloo, Chairman of the Department of Radiological Sciences at UCLA, in making this project possible.

Finally, and most important, thanks are also due to all the fellows attending the UCLA MRI visiting fellowship over the last six years. Their probing questions and helpful criticisms of early versions of this text are largely responsible for the current form of the manual.

Robert B. Lufkin, M.D.

CONTENTS

PART I

Basic Principles

Chapter 1

Nuclear Magnetic Resonance Physics

Robert B. Lufkin, M.D.

Magnetic resonance imaging (MRI) is one of the most significant advances in medical imaging in this century. The physical principles on which this amazing technology is based are complex. A complete discussion of the physics of nuclear magnetic resonance (NMR) is beyond the scope of this chapter. For more explicit details the interested reader is referred to several excellent works on this topic.[1-18] However, anyone can appreciate the basic principles of NMR as applied to MRI just by remembering the letters NMR.

NUCLEUS OF THE ATOM

The letter *N* in NMR stands for nuclear. Unlike x-ray images which are produced by attenuation of x-ray photons by outer orbital electrons, the NMR signal arises in the very center of the atom known as the *nucleus*. Although the chemical properties of an atom depend on its electron structure, the physical properties depend largely on the nucleus which accounts for almost all of the atom's mass.

The nuclei of all atoms except hydrogen contain two basic types of particles or nucleons— protons and neutrons. These two particles along with the planetary electrons make up the atom. Although the number of positively charged protons and negatively charged orbiting electrons are usually the same in order to maintain electrical neutrality, the number of protons and neutrons are often unequal.

The concept of the balance between the number of protons and/or neutrons in an atom determines the *angular momentum* of the nucleus. If a nucleus contains either unpaired protons or neutrons or both, then it has net spin and angular momentum. If there are no unpaired nucleons, the nuclear angular momentum is zero. Any other combination of un-balanced nucleons results in a nonzero nuclear angular momentum. (Although a neutron is electrically neutral, its component charges are not uniformly distributed and thus may have net spin if not balanced with a partner.)

Only the subset of atoms with unpaired protons and/or neutrons (such as hydrogen, sodium-23, phosphorus-31, carbon-13, and others) may be used to produce a signal in NMR. Although roughly one third of the almost 300 stable nuclei have unpaired nuclei and, there-fore, have angular momentum, only a select subset of these are of interest for biological systems.

TABLE 1–1.

Magnetic Resonance Properties of Selected Nuclei

Nucleus	Spin	Relative Abundance	Relative Sensitivity
^{1}H	$^1/_2$	99.98	1.0
^{2}H	1	0.015	0.0096
^{13}C	$^1/_2$	1.11	0.016
^{23}Na	$^3/_2$	100	0.093
^{31}P	$^1/_2$	100	0.066
^{19}F	$^1/_2$	100	0.830

Angular momentum is a term which describes the rotational motion of a body and must be nonzero in order for the NMR phenomenon to occur. Without angular momentum, a nucleus will not precess or wobble when placed in a magnetic field. Without precession, there will be no resonance and no NMR signal.

Of all the atoms with unpaired nucleons, hydrogen is the simplest because it has only one nucleon—a proton. The most important atom for medical MRI today, hydrogen is a particularly good material to look at with MR in humans because it makes up two thirds of all atoms in human beings. In addition to its large relative and isotopic abundance in the human body, it is also highly magnetic which yields a high MR sensitivity (Table 1–1).

MRI with nuclei other than hydrogen is possible in humans but produces images with at least an order of magnitude poorer signal because of the lower abundance and sensitivity. Although the word *nuclear* has been dropped from the name for medical NMR imaging, the vast majority of all human MRI studies are based on the nucleus of the hydrogen atom. Therefore, the remainder of the text will concentrate on proton or hydrogen MR. Unless otherwise mentioned the word *proton* or spin will refer to the nucleus of the hydrogen atom from now on.

MAGNETIC PROPERTIES OF THE NUCLEUS

The letter *M* in NMR stands for magnetic. As has been discussed, the nucleus of the hydrogen atom is a proton which is a small positively charged particle with associated angular momentum or spin.

This situation represents a current loop and results in the formation of a magnetic field (or moment) with two poles (north and south). This is also referred to as a magnetic dipole moment (Fig 1–1). All nuclei used in MRI imaging must have this property.

A material with a magnetic dipole moment tends to align with externally applied magnetic fields. These protons may be thought of as acting like small bar magnets. An arrow or "vector" is often used to describe the orientation and magnitude of the north and south poles of the magnetic dipole moment. In the absence of any great externally applied magnetic field the vectors of the magnetic dipole moments of our protons are oriented randomly (Fig 1–2).

In order to produce an MR image the first step is to place the patient in a large, powerful, uniform magnetic field. Magnetic field strength is measured in units of Tesla [in the International System of units (SI) or MKS system]. Field strength is also sometimes given in the older units of gauss (from the CHS system). The tesla (T) is the preferred unit for medical magnetic resonance imaging applications. One tesla is equal to 10,000 gauss.

The magnetic field strength for most systems for medical MRI ranges from 2 T (20,000 gauss) to 0.02 T (200 gauss) in strength. Interestingly, MR images have recently been produced

A   B

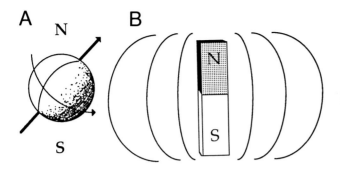

FIG 1–1.
Magnetic dipole moment of the spinning proton (**A**) is similar to the fields produced by the bar magnet (**B**).

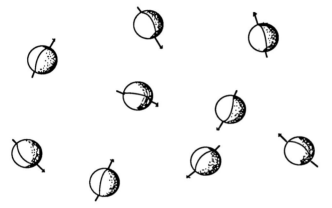

FIG 1–2.
Proton dipole moments in random orientations in the absence of an applied magnetic field.

using only the earth's magnetic field.[19] This is undoubtedly the lowest field strength used for MRI since the earth's magnetic field in the United States is approximately 0.00005 T (or 0.5 gauss). This figure varies around the world from 0.3 gauss at the equator to 0.7 gauss at the poles depending on the latitude.

When the protons are initially placed in a large external magnetic field, they will tend to align with the applied field like tiny bar magnets or compasses (Fig 1–3). The vector representing this large external magnetic field is called B_0. Since protons are extremely small they do not exactly follow the same rules of classical *newtonian physics* that describe the behavior of objects the size of bar magnets and compasses in our everyday world.[20] Rather, objects the size of protons and electrons must follow the rules of *quantum mechanics*.[21]

Unlike newtonian bar magnets or compasses which may align precisely with the applied magnetic field, quantum theory limits the possibilities of orientation of the spinning nuclei. Protons can have only one of two discrete orientations or states, either parallel or antiparallel to the applied field.

The protons oriented parallel to the applied field are in the low-energy condition which is called the *ground state*. The orientation antiparallel to the applied field is the high-energy condition and is referred to as the *excited state*. When placed in the magnetic field approximately half of the protons align in each direction. Actually slightly more are in the ground state parallel to B_0 due to the effect of the applied field.

The difference depends on the strength of the applied magnetic field but is small in all cases. In a population of 10^6 protons, approximately one out of a million more will be in the parallel rather than the antiparallel position. Although incredibly small, the difference is still sufficient to produce an MR signal.

The actual total number of protons in a given patient or sample is of course much greater. Every cubic centimeter of water has approximately 10^{23} protons. Because of these extremely large numbers the sum of all the spin magnetic orientations may be thought of as a single arrow or vector known as the *net magnetic field vector* (M_0). It is easier to conceptualize a single arrow rather than 10^{23} separate arrows. The population of protons placed in the static magnetic field would thus have a net magnetic field vector whose direction would be parallel to the applied field (B_0) due to the slightly greater number of protons in the parallel orientation.

The degree to which a material responds to the applied magnetic field is called its *magnetic susceptibility*. While most soft tissues of the body have similar susceptibilities, certain substances with unpaired *electrons* which are said to be paramagnetic or ferromagnetic have significantly different susceptibilities. For example, a stronger local field may be induced in tissues containing some forms of iron rather than in surrounding tissues. This concept of susceptibility will be useful later when paramagnetism, ferromagnetism, MR contrast agents, and certain MR image artifacts are covered.

RESONANCE OF THE NUCLEUS

The letter R in NMR stands for *resonance*. Resonance is a common phenomenon that occurs throughout nature. In order to understand resonance, it is necessary to discuss precession. In addition to their spinning action, protons also wobble or precess about the axis of the applied magnetic field B_0. The protons thus do not line up precisely with the axis of the applied magnetic field but actually wobble a few degrees off the central axis (Figs 1–4 and 1–5).

In order to combine the concepts of the two energy states and proton precession in one drawing, it may be clearer to adopt an "hourglass" display convention shown in Figure 1–5. The sum of this energy and precessional information is represented by the net magnetization vector (M_0).

This precession may be thought of as analogous to how a spinning gyroscope or top wobbles in the earth's gravitational field. The frequency of precession is known as the resonant or Larmor frequency, after the British physicist Sir Joseph Larmor. The frequency is proportional to the strength of the applied magnetic field.

FIG 1–3.
After the protons are placed in the magnetic field, alignment occurs. The net magnetic field vector (M_0) is parallel to the applied field (B_0).

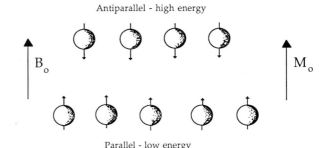

Antiparallel - high energy

Parallel - low energy

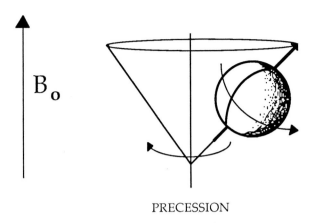

B_O

FIG 1–4.
Precession of spinning proton about the axis of the applied field (B$_0$).

PRECESSION

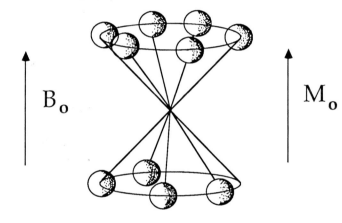

B$_O$

M$_O$

FIG 1–5.
Hourglass representation of precession of protons combines the concepts of Figs 1–3 and 1–4. Slightly more protons are in the lower energy position and thus the magnetization vector (M$_0$) is directly parallel to the main field vector, B$_0$. Because the protons are out of phase or spread all around their orbital path, no component of the magnetization occurs in the transverse plane. Note that the protons are only allowed two possible orientations (high or low).

This fundamental relationship is the basis for spatial encoding of the NMR signal that makes all MR imaging possible:

$$W = B_0 \times \text{gyromagnetic ratio}$$

where W = precessional frequency, B$_0$ = static magnetic field strength, and gyromagnetic ratio = constant for given nucleus.

The gyromagnetic (or magnetogyric) ratio relates static magnetic field to the precessional frequency and varies for different nuclei (i.e., sodium has a different gyromagnetic ratio than hydrogen). The value for hydrogen (protons) is 42.58 MHz/T. MHz means megahertz (or hertz $\times 10^6$) which is equal to one million cycles per second.

Each MR instrument will thus have a characteristic Larmor frequency based on its static magnetic field strength. From the equation, the Larmor frequency for any MR instrument can be calculated from its field strength. The resonant frequency of an MRI system thus varies directly with the operating field strength. Protons precess faster with a higher magnetic field affecting them. For a 1-T system the protons will resonate at 42.58 MHz. At 0.3 T the protons will resonate at approximately 12.8 MHz.

The location of NMR in the *electromagnetic spectrum* is shown in Figure 1–6. High-energy and high-frequency radiation is shown above. This group includes x-rays and various other forms of ionizing radiation. Radiation of this sort is often used for cross-sectional medical imaging because the body is transparent to it. The drawback of course is the potential harm to the living cell from ionizing effects.

Lower energy and lower-frequency radiation in the range of visible, infrared, and ultraviolet light is safer to use because it is no longer ionizing. However, this range of radiation is less useful for cross-sectional medical imaging because the human body is not transparent to light in this portion of the spectrum. Finally, at very low frequency, low-energy, nonionizing radiation in the radiowave range, the body once again becomes transparent to radiation in this part of the spectrum. *This is the NMR window.*

In order to produce the MR signal that may be detected and processed to make an image, the net magnetization vector must be moved into the transverse plane where it will cause a signal in the radio frequency (RF) receiver coils. The transverse plane is the plane which is transverse relative to the main longitudinal axis of the system. To move the vector into the transverse plane it is necessary to apply a second magnetic field. This will push the net magnetization vector from the equilibrium longitudinal position (parallel with the main magnetic field) into the transverse plane (Fig 1–7).

In addition, it is also necessary to bring the protons into phase (or all spinning together). In quantum mechanical terms energy is being added to the system and moving some of the nuclei to the higher energy state. The effect is the same, and the net magnetization (M_0) is now in the transverse plane for detection by RF coils.

To accomplish this, the applied second magnetic field must be synchronized with the resonant frequency of the precessing protons. This is analogous to pushing a child on a swing. A swing has a natural resonant frequency of oscillation based on its weight and length and other factors. In order to effectively add energy and increase the amplitude of the swinging

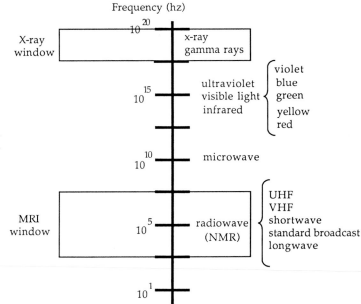

FIG 1–6.
The electromagnetic spectrum. *Abbreviations:* UHF, ultrahigh frequency; VHF, very high frequency.

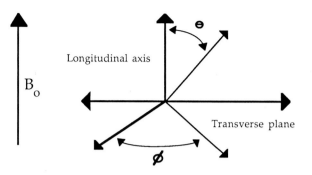

FIG 1-7.
Diagram of longitudinal axis and transverse plane and magnetization vector.

motion, the frequency of pushing must be the same (or in resonance) with the natural resonant frequency of the system.

The oscillating second magnetic field which is applied is the same as a RF pulse. In order for resonance to occur the frequency of the oscillation is thus the resonant frequency of the system. The RF pulse in NMR changes the direction of the net magnetization to the transverse plane. This is necessary because only the component of magnetization vector in the transverse plane may be detected by receiver RF coils.

The amplitude and duration of the RF may be controlled to produce a variety of amounts of angulation of the vector toward the transverse plane. The amount of tip of the magnetization vector following the RF pulse from the longitudinal axis toward the transverse plane is referred to as the *tip* or *flip angle* [θ (theta)] (Fig 1-7).

The amount of angulation of the vector may be varied by using different amounts and durations of RF energy. A 180 degree RF pulse causes the magnetization to move 180 degrees. A 90 degree RF pulse moves the longitudinal magnetization into the transverse plane. RF pulses with flip angles of less than 90 degrees result in a smaller magnetization vector in the transverse plane but are sometimes useful for fast scanning applications with gradient refocusing or field echoes (FAST, GRASS, FLASH, FISP, etc.).

In addition to moving some of the spins to the higher energy level, the RF pulse also rephases the protons so that they are in coherence. This has the effect of moving the net magnetization vector into the transverse plane (Fig 1-8). *Only when the protons are precessing in phase is it possible to detect a signal with the RF receiver coils.*

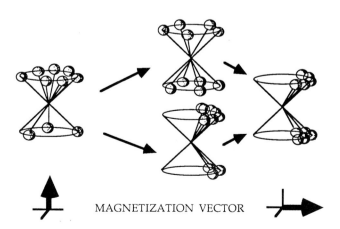

MAGNETIZATION VECTOR

FIG 1-8.
Following a 90 degree RF pulse the net magnetization vector nutates to the transverse plane. In order for this to occur, two processes must take place simultaneously. First, protons are moved to the higher energy state until there is an equal number of protons in the higher and lower energy states. Second, the protons are brought into coherence (all protons are precessing in phase). Again note that although the protons can be in only one of two orientations, the resulting magnetization vector may be in a variety of directions.

TRANSVERSE MAGNETIZATION AND THE MAGNETIC RESONANCE SIGNAL

After the RF pulse, the component of the magnetization in the *transverse plane* (transverse magnetization) induces a current in RF receiver coils (according to Faraday's law). The detected signal actually wobbles or oscillates at the same frequency as the magnetization vector which passes by it. This is analogous to creating an electrical current in a generator by moving a magnet past a coil of wire (Fig 1–9).

In the quantum theory model the RF energy generation is explained as the emission of energy as the *nuclei* move to lower energy states. This is analogous to the emission of characteristic x-rays by *electrons* as they move to lower orbits in x-ray imaging. However, the x-rays contain much more energy. Even a soft x-ray photon contains over 10^{12} times the energy of one RF photon in NMR.

The detected RF output makes up the MR signal. All MR contrast effects, whether due

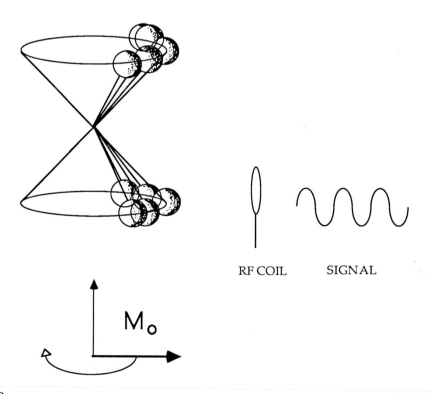

RF COIL   SIGNAL

M_o

FIG 1–9.
The protons precessing in coherence result in a component of the magnetization vector in the transverse plane. The output of the receiver coil or antennae is shown as an oscillating signal.

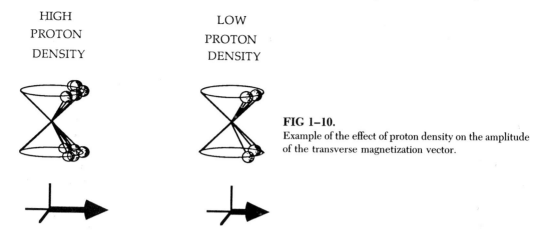

HIGH
PROTON
DENSITY

LOW
PROTON
DENSITY

FIG 1–10.
Example of the effect of proton density on the amplitude of the transverse magnetization vector.

MAGNETIZATION VECTOR

to T1, T2, flow, spin density, chemical shift, magnetic susceptibility, or other factors, manifest themselves as alterations in the transverse magnetization detected by the RF coil.

The initial amplitude of the signal is proportional to number of protons in the sample or the proton density: the more protons present, the greater the intensity of the magnetization. This results in a larger value of the signal detected by the RF coils (Fig 1–10).

STATIONARY VS. ROTATING FRAME OF REFERENCE

When examining the transverse magnetization detected by the receiver coils it is important to consider the perspective or frame of reference. To the outside stationary observer, the magnetization vector will continue to precess and change direction due to RF excitation and relaxation. Each time the vector passes by the RF coil, the signal intensity will be positive. This value will continue to oscillate with the precession of the vector around the transverse plane (Fig 1–11). Precession results in the vector tracing a roughly spherical rotary path as excitation, relaxation, and precession all determine its course (Fig 1–12). This process that combines precession with a change in the angle of the net magnetization vector is referred to as *nutation*.

In order to simplify the observation of this phenomenon, it is possible to observe the magnetization vector from a "rotating frame" which is analogous to climbing on the carousel at a circus to better observe the up and down motion of the horses. By observing from the rotating frame the rotary aspect of motion may be eliminated which allows a closer inspection of the relaxation processes (or the motion of the horses). From now on the effects of excitation and relaxation on the magnetization vector will be discussed from the perspective of this rotating frame.

T2* AND FREE INDUCTION DECAY

The amplitude of the detected MR signal after a 90 degree pulse does not stay constant but actually rapidly decays to zero. This damped oscillation is called a *free induction decay*

(FID). As has been discussed, the amplitude of the FID is proportional to the number of protons present in the sample or proton density. The rate of decay is characterized by the exponential decay term T2* (pronounced "tee-too-star") (Fig 1–13).

The signal decays because all magnetic fields are imperfect and protons in the sample in slightly different areas of the magnet experience slightly different magnetic fields. From the Larmor relationship it is known that the magnetic field experienced by the protons determines the frequency of precession. Thus the different local fields will produce different precessional frequencies. In other words the faster protons speed up and the slower protons slow down resulting in loss of coherence or transverse dephasing (Figs 1–13 and 1–14).

The loss of coherence translates into loss of induced current in the RF receiver coil. Protons that are in phase produce a high amplitude RF signal. If the same number of protons are precessing out of phase, the RF signal detected by the coil will be much less (Fig 1–14). Because this decay depends on the magnetic field imperfections rather than the patient, T2* contains little useful information about the *sample* and must be eliminated (Fig 1–15).

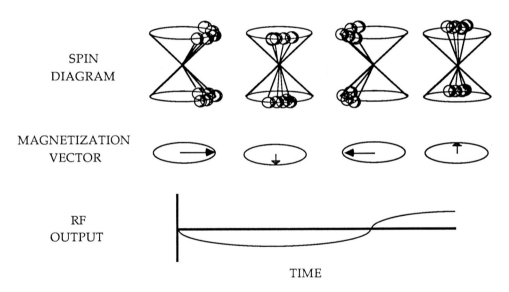

FIG 1–11.
Precession of protons resulting in variation of RF output with time.

FIG 1–12.
Stationary vs. rotating frames of reference.

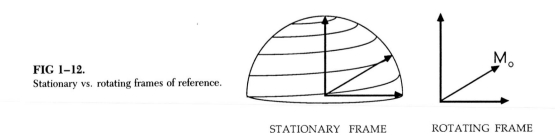

STATIONARY FRAME   ROTATING FRAME

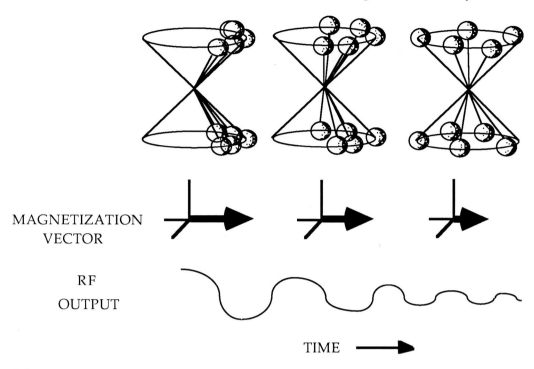

MAGNETIZATION VECTOR

RF OUTPUT

TIME

FIG 1–13.
Dephasing of protons due to magnetic field inhomogeneities (T2* effects). As dephasing occurs the transverse vector decreases resulting in a smaller RF signal.

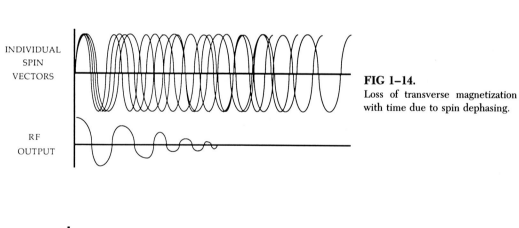

INDIVIDUAL SPIN VECTORS

RF OUTPUT

FIG 1–14.
Loss of transverse magnetization with time due to spin dephasing.

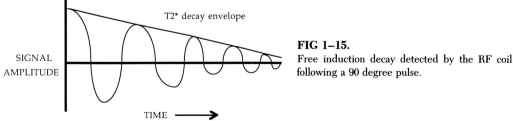

T2* decay envelope

SIGNAL AMPLITUDE

TIME

FIG 1–15.
Free induction decay detected by the RF coil following a 90 degree pulse.

SPIN ECHO, GRADIENT ECHO

It is important to now consider how a signal with any useful information for imaging is obtained. In order to cancel out the spurious T2* information from the signal it is necessary to bring the protons back into coherence. This is accomplished by the application of a 180 degree RF pulse (Fig 1–16).

This second RF pulse reverses the direction of precession and thus refocuses the protons. This causes the protons to regain coherence in the transverse plane and again to produce a signal in the RF receiver coil. A popular analogy for this process is runners on a track. Imagine a quarter-mile track which represents the transverse plane. Three runners of various skills are at the starting line. One is an Olympic sprinter, the second is an average college runner, and the third is an overweight radiologist. When the gun sounds all runners take off from the blocks, initially in phase. But very quickly as they precess around the track, they begin to lose coherence or dephase. The Olympian is far in the lead with the college runner in the middle and the radiologist bringing up the rear.

At this point the starting gun again fires and all runners turn around and run in the opposite direction on the track. Everyone is still out of phase but now the Olympian is bringing up the rear and the radiologist is in the lead. Because of their different rates of running the Olympian and the college runner eventually catch up with the slow radiologist and once again they are in phase (assuming they maintain their individual speeds), which occurs as the runners cross the starting line. They only remain together for a split second (the echo) and then begin dephasing around the track in the other direction. When this refocusing is done with protons instead of runners and with a 180 degree RF pulse instead of the gun, it is known as a *spin echo* (Figs 1–16 and 1–17).

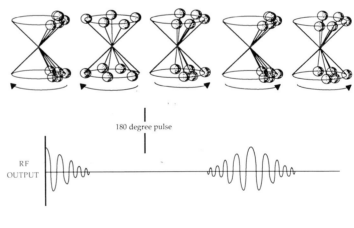

FIG 1–16.
Diagram showing rephasing of the protons with a 180 degree RF pulse to produce a spin echo. As the protons regain coherence, the signal is again generated in the RF coil.

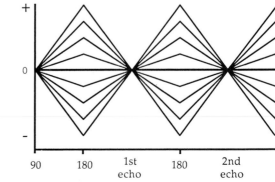

FIG 1–17.
Spin phase graph showing phase relationships during echo generation. Protons rapidly dephase after 90 degree pulse. A 180 degree pulse reverses this process and results in echo formation.

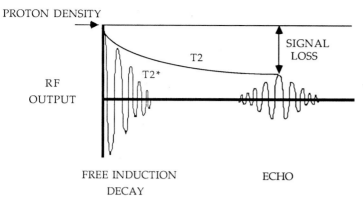

PROTON DENSITY

RF OUTPUT

T2

T2*

SIGNAL LOSS

FREE INDUCTION DECAY

ECHO

FIG 1–18.
Diagram of unexplained loss of signal detected in receiver coils despite reversal of T2* effects through the use of the echo.

Rephasing can also be accomplished by rapidly reversing the magnetic field gradients instead of the 180 degree pulse. The resulting recovered signal using this technique is referred to as a *field* or *gradient echo* and will be covered in more detail later. Either process can be represented diagrammatically as a spin phase graph[22] (see Fig 1–17). After the echo, the protons again lose coherence. Multiple echoes can be obtained by reapplication of refocusing RF pulses or gradients.

Although the echoes cancel out T2* effects due to magnetic field nonuniformities, *the recovered signal at the echo is still less than its original height as determined by the proton density* (Fig 1–18). To understand this loss it is necessary to begin to understand other relaxation processes not corrected by the echo. This important decrease in transverse magnetization is due to irreversible losses in the sample itself due to T1 and T2 relaxation effects, which depend on the local environments of the protons in the sample reflecting chemical structure, and ultimately human anatomy.

T2 RELAXATION

One source of irreversible signal loss is due to T2 relaxation effects, which is measured as the spin-spin or transverse relaxation time. T2 (like T2*) results from magnetic field inhomogeneities. However, unlike the reversible dephasing that occurs due to static field T2* effects, T2 dephasing is due to randomly varying intrinsic magnetic fields created by adjacent nuclei in the patient. For this reason these effects are essentially irreversible and are not corrected by the spin echo or gradient echo. The term *spin-spin* refers to the fact that interactions between protons determine the rate of T2 relaxation. No energy is actually lost but rather energy is exchanged between protons. Called *transverse relaxation*, the T2 dephasing effects occur in the transverse plane (Fig 1–19). The biologic significance of T2 will be considered in greater detail below.

Like exponential radioactive decay, T2 is the time constant for a first-order exponential decay process. T2 (milliseconds) may be thought of as the time necessary to reduce the transverse magnetization to 37% of its original value following the RF pulse (Fig 1–20). The

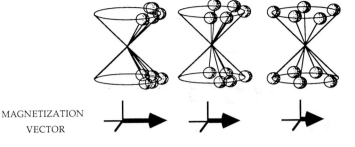

FIG 1–19.
Loss of transverse magnetization due to T2 relaxation effects.

MAGNETIZATION

VECTOR

FIG 1–20.
Time intensity curve for T2 relaxation. One T2 time is the time in milliseconds necessary to lose 63% of the signal.

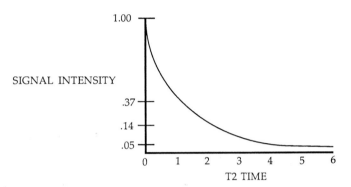

relationship of signal intensity (I) to time for T2 relaxation depends on the time from the 90 degree pulse until the echo (known as the echo time or TE) as well as the T2 of the tissue. The TE or echo time is the time in milliseconds from the 90 degree RF pulse until the echo is received. This relationship may be expressed as

$$I = f(e^{-(TE/T2)})$$

Unlike T2*, T2 is the time constant for irreversible proton dephasing due to *intrinsic sample* properties. Typical values for T2 in biological tissues are in the range of 50 to 500 msec (always ≤T1). T2, unlike T1, is also essentially independent of magnetic field strength.

T1 RELAXATION

The RF stimulation adds energy to the system and causes protons to move to a higher energy state. The process of dissipation of this energy to the chemical lattice and returning of protons to the lower energy state is known as *T1 relaxation* (Fig 1–21). The word *lattice* is a throwback to the days when NMR was used to investigate molecules in a crystalline lattice. Currently the definition has been broadened to mean the surrounding magnetic environment. The lattice fields result from other nuclei and paramagnetic molecules. Just as the rate of oscillation of the RF affects the efficiency of stimulation, the frequency of lattice field fluctuations also affects the efficiency of T1 relaxation.

Because MR imaging techniques require multiple repetitions of RF stimulations, the detected transverse magnetization depends on more than the spin density and T2 relaxation time. The longitudinal magnetization prior to the sampling RF pulse is also reflected in the transverse magnetization detected by the coils. In other words, if another RF pulse is given before full T1 relaxation recovery has occurred the height of the subsequent FIDs will be diminished. Therefore, the rate of longitudinal relaxation characterized by the T1 relaxation time also affects transverse magnetization and image contrast.

T1 in milliseconds is the time required for 63% of the longitudinal magnetization to recover following the RF pulse (Fig 1–22). The relationship of signal intensity (I) to time for T1 relaxation depends on the time between 90 degree RF pulses (repetition time or TR) as well as the T1 of the tissue. The TR or repetition time is the time in milliseconds from the beginning of the first 90 degree RF pulse through the entire spin echo pulse sequence until another 90 degree pulse is given to start the whole process again. The relationship may be expressed as

$$I = f(1 - e^{-[TR/T1]})$$

Like T2, this parameter is dependent on sample and, therefore, provides useful medical information. Typical T1 values for biological materials are 200 to 2,000 msec (>T2). While

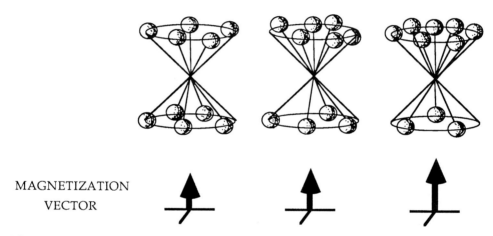

MAGNETIZATION
VECTOR

FIG 1–21.
Recovery of longitudinal magnetization with time.

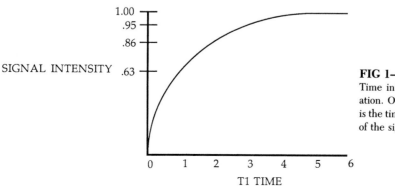

SIGNAL INTENSITY

T1 TIME

FIG 1–22.
Time intensity curve for T1 relaxation. One T1 time in milliseconds is the time required to recover 63% of the signal.

tissue T2 values show very little dependence on field strength, T1 tissue values actually increase slightly with increasing magnetic field strength. This is because the precessional frequencies and thus the efficiency of T1 relaxation are dependent on the strength of the applied external magnetic field (B_0).[23] Although T1 and T2 relaxation both occur simultaneously and affect the image quality, they are essentially independent of one another.

PULSING SEQUENCE

The MR signal intensity (I) due to the transverse magnetization which is represented as pixel brightness on MR images is a reflection of T1 and T2 relaxation times as well as several other factors. Proton density (N), proton flow (f(v)), proton susceptibility, as well as RF pulse characteristics, also affect the signal intensity.

The relative contributions of some of these factors to the transverse magnetization may be manipulated by controlling the timing of the RF pulses (known as a pulsing or pulse sequence) to form the image. The timing values are the repetition time (TR) and echo time (TE). For example, a short TR and TE will result in an image which emphasizes the T1 characteristics of the tissue and is said to be "T1-weighted." A longer TR and TE will result in a more "T2-weighted" image. Some of these relationships are summarized in the following equation for spin echo sequences:

$$I = N \cdot f(v)(e^{-(TE/T2)})(1 - e^{-(TR/T1)})$$

While many equations describe signal intensity in MR, this simplified form will be used in our discussions. This equation is fundamental to understanding MR contrast relationship in imaging and will be examined in detail in subsequent chapters.

SIGNAL-TO-NOISE

The ratio of NMR signal to background noise (SNR) is one of the most important factors in MR imaging. High SNR can be traded off for higher spatial resolution, contrast resolution, or faster scan time. One of the simplest ways to improve SNR is through the use of signal averaging.

Signal averaging is a technique where each echo is repetitively observed and summed. The signal is nonrandom and will therefore increase proportionally to the number of observations (n). Since most noise is random, the noise term only increases as the square root of the number of observations (Fig 1–23). In addition to signal-to-noise improvements, averaging also decreases certain types of motion artifacts by a similar process.

This is actually a relatively inefficient way to improve image signal-to-noise since each summation doubles the total scan time, while the signal to noise only improves as the square root as the number of echoes (for small n). For example, one summation of two echoes will double the scan time with only a 40% improvement in SNR (Figs 1–24 and 1–25).

Because of the variety of names for this technique there is some confusion about nomenclature for signal averaging. Names such as NAV (number of averages), averages, excitations, passes, and autostops all are used by different manufacturers. While one manufacturer may consider summing together ten data sets to be "ten averages," another manufacturer may label their images produced by the same technique as "one average" because the SNR improvement was obtained following a single averaging step of the ten data acquisitions.

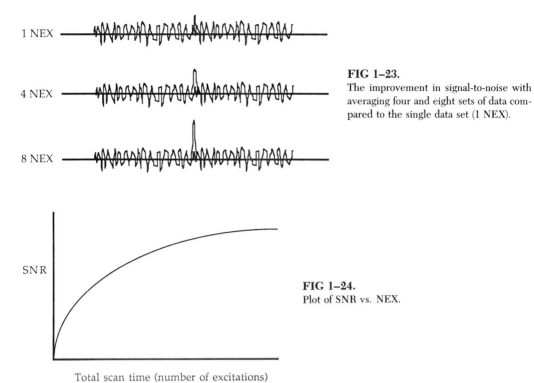

FIG 1–23.

1 NEX

4 NEX

8 NEX

FIG 1–23.
The improvement in signal-to-noise with averaging four and eight sets of data compared to the single data set (1 NEX).

SNR

Total scan time (number of excitations)

FIG 1–24.
Plot of SNR vs. NEX.

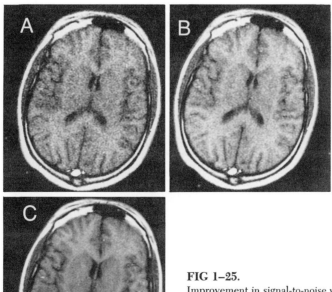

FIG 1–25.
Improvement in signal-to-noise with increasing number of excitations. (**A**) 2 NEX, (**B**) 4 NEX, (**C**) 10 NEX.

Fortunately there is a trend to use the standard term number of excitations (NEX) to indicate the actual number of data sets that are summed.

Signal-to-noise in today's MR systems has improved sufficiently using such techniques as surface coils, quadrature detection coils, bandwidth reductions, and optimized system electronics to the point where signal averaging is less necessary and often images are routinely obtained with one excitation on many scanners.

REFERENCES

1. Andrew ER: *Nuclear Magnetic Resonance.* Boston, Cambridge University Press, 1969.
2. Stark D, Bradley W: *Magnetic Resonance Imaging.* St Louis, CV Mosby, 1987.
3. Bloembergen M: *Nuclear Magnetic Relaxation.* New York, WA Benjamin, 1970.
4. Christianson: Nuclear magnetic resonance, in Curry TS, Dowdey JE, Murry RC (eds): *Introduction to Physics of Radiology,* ed 3. Philadelphia, Lea & Febiger, 1984, pp 461–505.
5. Fullerton G: Basic concepts for nuclear magnetic resonance imaging. *Magnetic Resonance Imaging* 1982; 1:39–55.
6. Oldendorf W, Oldendorf W: *The First Book of MRI.* Boston, Martinus Nijhoff, 1988.
7. Heiken JP, Glazer G, Lee JKT, et al: *Manual of Clinical Magnetic Resonance Imaging.* New York, Raven Press, 1986.
8. Dixon RL, Ekstrand KE: The physics of proton NMR. *Med Phys* 1982; 9:807–818.
9. Gadian DG: *NMR and Its Applications to Living Systems.* Oxford, England, Clarendon Press, 1982.
10. Kaufman L, Crooks LE, Margulis AR: *Nuclear Magnetic Resonance Imaging in Medicine.* New York-Tokyo; Igaku-Shoin, 1981.
11. Roth K: *NMR-Tomography and -Spectroscopy in Medicine.* New York, Springer-Verlag, 1984.
12. Pykett IL, Newhouse JH, Buonanno FS, et al: Principles of nuclear magnetic resonance imaging. *Radiology* 1982; 143:157–168.
13. Bradley WG, Newton TH, Crooks LE: Physical principles of nuclear magnetic resonance, in Newton TH, Potts DG (eds): *Modern Neuroradiology: Advanced Imaging Techniques.* San Anselmo, Calif, Clavadel Press, 1983.
14. Kramer DM: Basic principles of magnetic resonance imaging. *Radiol Clin North Am* 1984; 22:765–778.
15. Wong W, Tsuruda J, Kortman K, et al: *Practical MRI.* Rockville, Md., Aspen, 1987.
16. Morgan CJ, Hendee WR: *Introduction to Magnetic Resonance Imaging.* Denver, Multi-media Publishing, 1984.
17. Jones JP, Partain CL, Mitchell MR, et al: Principles of magnetic resonance, in Kressel HY (ed): *Magnetic Resonance Annual 1985.* New York, Raven Press, 1985.
18. Morris PG: *Nuclear Magnetic Imaging in Medicine and Biology.* Oxford, Clarendon Press, 1986.
19. Stepisnik J, Erzen V, Kos M, et al: *Magnetic Resonance Imaging in the Earth's Magnetic Field.* San Francisco, Society for Magnetic Resonance in Medicine, 1988.
20. Zukav G: *The Dancing Wu Li Masters.* New York, Bantam Books, 1986.
21. Capra F: *The Tao of Physics.* New York, Bantam Books, 1984.
22. Singer JR: NMR diffusing and flow measurements and an introduction to spin phase graphing. *Phy E Sci Instrum* 1978; 11:281–291.
23. Fullerton GD, Cameron IL, Ord VA: Frequency dependence of magnetic resonance spin lattice relaxation of protons in biological materials. *Radiology* 1984; 151:135–138.

Chapter 2

Magnetic Resonance Contrast Mechanisms

Robert B. Lufkin, M.D.

Image contrast is based on the difference in signal intensity between areas of different structure or composition in an image. Superior soft tissue contrast resolution is one of the greatest advantages of magnetic resonance imaging (MRI) over computed tomography (CT). In x-ray imaging, attenuation of the beam by the patient is the major source of image contrast. The amount of attenuation reflects the electron density of the material. Therefore the intensity or the brightness of the pixel on the CT image depends on the electron density modulated to some extent by any infused contrast material.

Magnetic resonance image contrast, on the other hand, arises from a complex relationship of many different factors including proton density, T1, T2, magnetic susceptibility, and flow. Because the transverse magnetization or signal intensity is the only variable that can be directly measured, it may be difficult to segregate the relative contribution to image contrast of all these terms from a single image.[1-5]

The main approach to MR image tissue characterization through contrast effects is to rescan the patient with different combinations of *pulse sequence* parameters [repetition time (TR) and echo time (TE)]. For reasons that will be covered shortly, a short TR, TE sequence produces a T1-weighted image and a long TR, TE sequence produces a T2-weighted image. By observing the change in signal intensity in each sequence, the tissue characteristics (long T1, short T2, low proton density, etc.) can be inferred.[6] In addition, by changing the pulse sequence parameters, image contrast may be manipulated with MR in ways not possible with CT.

Much of the power of MR contrast can be understood by analyzing one form of the spin echo equation

$$I = N*f(v)(e^{-(TE/T2)})1 - e^{-(TR/T1)})$$

where I = signal intensity, N = proton density, and f(v) = proton flow.

Most of the terms of this equation were covered in Chapter 1. Note that the T2 expression $(e^{-(TE/T2)})$ is similar to the T1 expression $(1 - e^{(TR/T1)})$ except that the "1-minus" term is missing. This means that the effects on signal intensity for T1 and T2 prolongation are opposite and thus tend to offset one another. This can be a problem because the majority of pathologic conditions that affect the cell, whether neoplasia, inflammation, or edema, all tend to prolong T1 and T2 due to increased free water.

This means that the effects of T1 and T2 on image intensity tend to cancel out and may even result in an area of abnormality being invisible on an image. The use of various pulse sequences with different amounts of T1 and T2 weighting will help to avoid this situation. To better understand the effects of pulse sequences on image contrast it is necessary to analyze the contribution of each term to the signal intensity, or transverse magnetization (I).

PROTON DENSITY

Proton density has a unique position in the MR spin echo equation. Unlike the complex exponential terms describing T1 and T2 effects, the proton density term (N) is merely multiplied times everything else in the equation. Although there are protons throughout the body, the protons of interest for MR are those that make up the nucleus of the hydrogen atom. In fact the only protons that contribute significantly to the MR signal are the nuclei of hydrogen atoms in water molecules or on some groups in fat molecules. Thus proton density in MR actually reflects only a subset of all protons in fat and water molecules (mobile protons).

In Chapter 1, it was shown that proton density in a sample determines the initial NMR signal amplitude or the height of the free induction decay. If there is a large number of mobile protons there will be a strong signal. This strong signal will then be further affected by the other terms in the equation such as T1 and T2 to produce either a strong or weak signal depending on this host of other factors. Materials with high proton density include fat, cerebrospinal fluid (CSF), blood, and other fluids (Table 2–1).

On the other hand, if there are relatively few mobile protons in the tissue, then there will be a zero or small value for N in the equation. Because this zero term is multiplied by everything else, the effects of T1 and T2 and the other parameters are negated (zero multiplied times anything is still zero). Therefore, regardless of how the pulse sequence is changed, if there are few mobile protons, the image will be black (Fig 2–1).

This low proton density situation is somewhat unique and can be valuable for analyzing pathology. Other causes for low signal on certain images (such as tissues with a short T2 or long T1) may appear black on a single pulse sequence but will often change intensity as other pulse sequences are obtained. Rapid or turbulent flowing blood or CSF may appear black on many pulsing sequences but is often recognizable by other characteristic artifacts. However, materials with low proton density will usually remain at a low signal level. Examples of tissues that can have this appearance are air, calcifications, dense cortical bone, fibrous tissue, and plastics and other implanted materials.

TABLE 2–1.

Proton Density Effects on the Magnetic Resonance Image

Low proton density — dark
  Calcium, air, cortical bone, fibrous tissue
High proton density — variable appearance depending on pulse sequence
  Fat, fluids

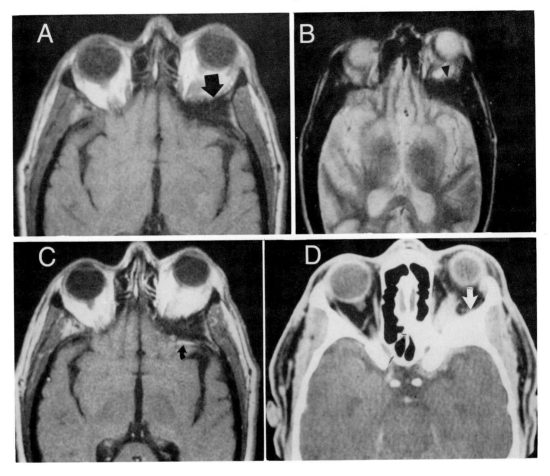

FIG 2–1.
Sphenoid wing meningioma. **A,** T1-weighted image (SE/500/30) shows a large area of low signal in the region of the sphenoid wing representing hyperostosis *(arrow).* **B,** on a T2-weighted image (SE/2000/85) the region remains low signal *(arrowhead).* **C,** following gadolinium-DTPA infusion there is some enhancement by the tumor *(arrow)* but the low-signal region is unchanged. **D,** computed tomographic scan confirms the presence of low-proton-density hyperostosis *(arrowhead).*

Because of the lack of signal from low proton density materials such as calcium it has been said that MR cannot show cortical bone. This is true in the sense that cortical bone does not result in a signal on MR. However, to say one cannot see cortical bone on MR is like saying one cannot see air on CT. Although it is seen as black on CT, air can of course be seen because of the tissue around it. For the same reasons, cortical bone is also visible on MR because of the tissue around it. Although CT detects calcium better than MR, in most cases MR is able to provide adequate information.

Certain pulse sequences on MR are referred to as proton density or spin density images. These are produced using combinations of relatively long TR and short TE. This has the effect of decreasing both T1 and T2 weighting which results in greater contribution to image contrast by the spin or proton density. This also has the effect of greatly increasing the image signal-to-noise.

TABLE 2–2.

Comparison of Representative Proton Density, T1 and T2 Values
for Various Tissue Types at Midfield Strength

Tissue	Proton Density	T1 (msec)	T2 (msec)
CSF	10.8	2000	250
Gray matter	10.5	475	118
White matter	11.0	300	133
Fat	10.9	150	150
Muscle	11.0	450	64
Liver	10.0	250	44

T1 AND T2 CONTRAST MECHANISMS

If proton density were its sole source of contrast, in many ways magnetic resonance (MR) would not be better than CT as far as contrast resolution. MR would still have advantages in other areas but as far as soft tissue contrast resolution, the proton density of tissue on MR and electron density on CT varies only about 10% throughout soft tissues of the body. Fortunately there are other more powerful sources of soft tissue contrast in MR.

T1 and T2 relaxation effects provide this remarkably superior soft tissue contrast resolution in MR compared to CT. This is because many substances with similar proton and electron densities will still result in different signal intensities on MR due to the marked differences in T1 values and T2 values (Table 2–2).

There are several models that may be used to understand how MR relaxation contrast mechanisms work. By considering the two large groups of protons in the body, that is, fat and water, it is possible to make some observations about relaxation times and contrast behavior on MR.

Molecular Motion and Relaxation Efficiency

Water and similar substances such as cerebrospinal fluid (and other pure fluids in the body) have both a long T1 and a long T2 relaxation time while protons in fat tend to have a short T1 and an intermediate-to-short T2 time. Fat is bright on T1-weighted image and intermediate signal on T2-weighted images. From these basic observations conclusions about the behavior of these molecules in terms of MR can be made.

Water is made up of small molecules that have a high rate of molecular motion. These rotational or translational movements occur very rapidly and are due to thermal effects (brownian motion) (Fig 2–2). Cholesterol is an example of a large lipid molecule. The mobile protons on these molecules have much slower rates of molecular motion due to the greater inertia of the larger molecule.

The rate of T1 relaxation depends on how efficiently energy is distributed back to the lattice. In order to optimally add energy to the system the radiofrequency (RF) field should fluctuate at the resonant frequency of the system. By the same token energy can be redistributed most efficiently when the magnetic fields of the lattice are fluctuating at or near this resonant frequency.

If there is a close correlation between the Larmor frequency and the rate of field fluctuation due to molecular motion, a very efficient transfer of energy and thus a short T1 time results. Small molecules like water have a much higher rate of molecular motion than the

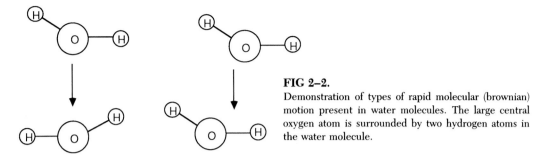

FIG 2–2.
Demonstration of types of rapid molecular (brownian) motion present in water molecules. The large central oxygen atom is surrounded by two hydrogen atoms in the water molecule.

ROTATION   TRANSLATION

Larmor frequency for any of the current MR instruments (high or low field). They are, therefore, inefficient at returning energy to the lattice and have long T1 relaxation times.

Protons in medium-sized molecules, such as cholesterol, with slower molecular motion are closer to this range and thus are most efficient in T1 relaxation. Larger molecules such as long-chain fatty acids tumble at frequencies well below the resonant frequency. However, rotation of terminal fatty acid groups at higher frequencies allow efficient T1 relaxation for these fats also.

In addition to molecular size, other factors (protein binding effects) affect the rate of molecular motion and thus the efficiency of transfer of energy back to the lattice which determines the relaxation time.

Protein Binding and Relaxation

Pure fluids like water tend to have a high rate of molecular motion and thus long T1 relaxation times. In the body, most water is not in the pure state but rather is present in solutions of proteins and other macromolecules. This occurs not only within the cell but in large extracellular fluid collections as well.

Pure water or *bulk water* has a high rate of molecular motion and very long T1 due to inefficient energy transfer to the lattice. However, as protein or large macromolecules with hydrophilic binding sites are added to the solution the rapidly moving free water becomes *structured* (motionally perturbed but not bound) around the macromolecule. Finally, *bound* water is that water that is actually hydrogen bonded to a fixed polar or ion site on the macromolecule. All water molecules that are affected by macromolecules (bound and structured water) are referred to as *hydration layer* water. This process slows down the rate of molecular motion, therefore, bringing it closer to the Larmor frequency of the system and thus increasing the efficiency of relaxation (Fig 2–3).

Therefore, the presence of hydration layer water around macromolecules results in shortening of T1 relaxation times. By this mechanism, solutions of water containing a high protein content or a large amount of cellular debris may have a T1 relaxation time similar to that of cholesterol or other fats. This is an important aspect of MR interpretation: *fluids can have a variety of appearances based on their protein content.*

Factors Affecting T2 Relaxation

In T2 relaxation, energy is not transferred to the lattice but is rather exchanged with the spins in the excited and ground states. This results in a loss of coherence of the precessing nuclei which reduces the detected transverse magnetization. T2 relaxation efficiency is increased by the presence of static or low-frequency intrinsic magnetic fields (large molecules and solids). These fields alter the local magnetic field value and cause the spins to precess at slightly higher or lower frequencies, which results in phase dispersion and loss of coherence.

Solids and large molecules have relatively slowly varying fields which result in large intrinsic fields and relatively rapid T2 relaxation. Smaller molecules like water have high rates of molecular motion. The high frequencies tend to average out the intrinsic fields to zero so that the magnetic field is determined by that of the external field and spin phase is maintained for a longer period of time (long T2).

In the case of solutions of macromolecules, the intrinsic fields increase with the amount of solid in solution. This results in greater dephasing and shorter T2 relaxation times in fluids with macromolecules compared to pure fluids.

EFFECTS OF T1 AND TR ON IMAGE CONTRAST

T1 relaxation times allow certain types of tissue to be distinguished on MR. Substances with a short T1 (high signal) can either be fat, lipid-containing molecules, or proteinaceous fluid. Subacute hemorrhage, melanin, or other paramagnetic substances in low concentration such as gadolinium may also shorten the T1. Substances with long T1 (low signal) include neoplasms (both benign and malignant), inflammation, and any kind of cellular alteration that opens up cell membranes and increases bulk water. The differences in image intensity due to T1 relaxation values (T1 contrast) can be increased by the use of certain pulse sequences to produce a T1-weighted image (Table 2–3).

Throughout this manual new pulse sequences, image tricks, motion artifact suppression, gradient moment nulling, reduced bandwidth, and all sorts of developments to improve the MR scanning process will be discussed. Any time a new improvement is considered, it is necessary to find out what its costs in terms of image quality, signal to noise, scan time, spatial resolution, contrast resolution, etc.

One tradeoff to examine is the relationship between signal amplitude (I) and TR time.

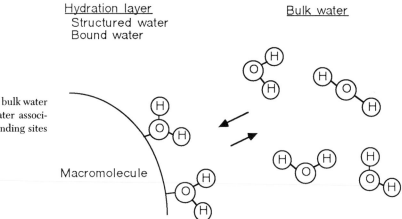

FIG 2–3.
Comparison of unbound bulk water with hydration layer water associated with hydrophilic binding sites on the macromolecule.

TABLE 2–3.

T1 Effects on Image Appearance (T1-Weighted Image)

Short T1 — bright
   Fat, proteinaceous fluid, subacute bleed (methemoglobin),
   Other paramagnetic substance with proton-electron dipole-dipole interaction in low concentration (gadolinium,
      melanin?)
Long T1 — dark
   Neoplasm, edema, inflammation, pure fluid, CSF

In the spin echo equation, this is represented by the exponential expression:

$$I = (1 - e^{-(TR/T1)})$$

An easier way to show this relationship is with a graph. Two substances with different T1 relaxation times are graphically represented in Figure 2–4. The substance in the upper curve has a shorter T1 than the material in the lower curve. Thus, for any value of TR, the shorter T1 substance has a higher signal intensity.

In order to maximize the difference in signal intensity based on tissue T1 times (T1 contrast), the TR time in the pulse sequence is shortened. This results in a T1-weighted image. With longer TR time, the tissues have both fully recovered their longitudinal magnetization and have similar signal intensities and little contrast.

A short TR sequence will therefore maximize T1 contrast but this also affects other aspects of image quality. As the TR is shortened, although the T1 contrast increases, the overall signal-to-noise decreases. Thus in order to optimize signal to noise it is necessary to use a relatively long TR compared to the T1 of the tissues (i.e., TR = 2,000 to 3,000 msec).

This concept will be used again when fast scanning techniques like field echoes are discussed because very short TR times will be used which can result in extremely T1-weighted images at the expense of signal-to-noise.

EFFECTS OF TE AND T2 ON IMAGE CONTRAST

TE and T2 also affect image signal and contrast. T2 relaxation times (like T1 and other tissue parameters) allow certain types of tissue to be distinguished. Substances with a short T2 (low signal) are often iron containing (such as blood breakdown products and nonheme

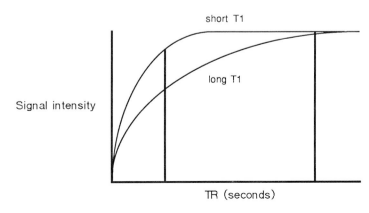

FIG 2–4.
Effects of TR and tissue T1 values on image intensity and contrast. The upper curve material has a short T1 and the lower curve a longer T1. T1 contrast is maximal with a short TR and ratio of NMR signal to background noise (SNR) is highest with a long TR.

TABLE 2–4.

T2 Effects on Image Appearance (T2-Weighted Image)

Short T2 — dark
Iron deposition in the liver, magnetic susceptibility effect (hemosiderin, deoxyhemoglobin, ferritin)
Long T2 — bright
Neoplasm, edema, inflammation, gliosis, pure fluid, CSF

forms of iron such as ferritin). Neoplasms (both benign and malignant), inflammation, and practically any kind of cellular alteration that opens up cell membranes to increase the intracellular water content (and therefore free water) are all substances with long T2 relaxation times (high signal) (Table 2–4).

The differences in image intensity due to T2 relaxation values can be increased by the use of certain pulse sequences to produce a T2-weighted image. The relationship of signal intensity (I) and TE for various T2 tissues is shown by the exponential relationship:

$$I = (e^{-(TE/T2)})$$

Similar to the T1 expression (except that the "1-minus" term is missing), this results in a different appearance to the graph compared to that for T1. Two tissues with different T2 relaxation times are graphically represented in Figure 2–5. The tissue in the upper curve has a longer T2 than the material in the lower curve. Thus, for any value of TE, the longer T2 substance has a higher signal intensity.

In order to maximize the difference in signal intensity based on T2 times, the TE time in the pulse sequence is lengthened. This results in a T2-weighted image. With a shorter TE time, the tissues have similar signal intensities and little contrast. This is because sufficient time has not elapsed for differences in T2 to cause dephasing of the spins.

A long TE sequence will therefore maximize T2 contrast at a cost of image quality. As the TE is lengthened, although the T2 contrast increases, the overall signal-to-noise decreases. In order to optimize signal-to-noise it is necessary to use a short TE relative to the T2 times of the tissue (i.e., 20 to 30 msec).

In order to make a heavily T1-weighted image a short TR is used to maximize T1 contrast and a short TE to minimize T2 contrast. By the same token, to make a heavily T2-weighted image, a long TE to maximize T2 contrast and a long TR to minimize T1 contrast is used.

FIG 2–5.
Effects of TE and tissue T2 values on image intensity and contrast. The substance in the upper curve has a long T2 compared to that in the lower curve. T2 contrast is maximized with a long TE and SNR is highest with a short TE.

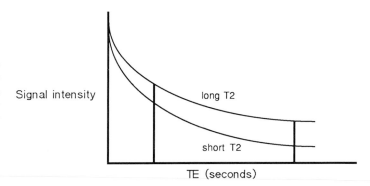

Finally, a short TE and long TR sequence would maximize the signal to noise in the image. This is accomplished at the expense of T1 and T2 contrast. Because of the lack of strong T1 or T2 contrast, these high signal-to-noise images are sometimes referred to as *proton density* or spin density images.

EFFECT OF FLIP ANGLE ON SIGNAL AND T1 AND T2 CONTRAST

In later chapters, fast scanning techniques which employ flip angles less than 90 degrees and magnetic field gradients to refocus the spins will be covered. Although the contrast effects are complex, when the flip angle is changed, the image contrast also varies (Fig 2–6). In general, for a given TR and TE that results in a T1-weighted image with a 90 degree flip angle, decreasing the flip angle will decrease T1 weighting. With TR prolongation, decrease in T1 contrast is accompanied by an increase in signal-to-noise as the image becomes more spin density weighted. Further decreases in flip angle eventually result in decreased signal to noise and an increase in T2 (or T2*) contrast.

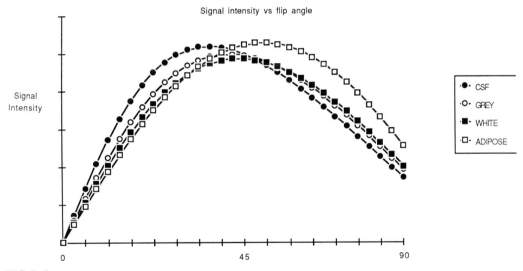

FIG 2–6.
Effects of theta (θ, tip or flip angle) on image intensity and contrast. TR and TE are constant. The CSF *(black circles)* has a long T1 and T2 compared to the other tissues. Maximum T1 contrast is obtained with a 90 degree flip angle for this pulse sequence. Intermediate flip angles (Ernst angles) yield the maximum signal to noise. A low flip angle results in greatest T2 (or T2*) contrast (Courtesy of Jay Butterman, Ph.D.)

CALCULATED T1 AND T2 IMAGES AND VALUES

Since the only thing that can be directly measured in MR is the transverse magnetization, any attempt at T1 and T2 measurements must actually be calculations from manipulations of this signal. This is usually done by solving for T1 or T2 from the pulse sequence equation (one form or another) after repetitive acquisitions.

$$I = N*f(v)(e^{-(TE/T2)})(1 - e^{-(TR/T1)})$$

For example, if everything is kept constant and the TR is varied to produce two values for the image intensity (I), then T1 can be calculated. Similarly, T2 can be calculated from multiple (at least two) determinations of signal intensity with different values of TE and all other terms constant. For a number of reasons these determinations have turned out to have little widespread clinical application.

One problem is that this technique, like all cross-sectional image based measurements, is limited by partial voluming errors. That is, any measurement based on the image signal intensity is actually the average determination for the entire voxel and as such induces errors in the estimate.

An even more serious problem comes from the assumption that all terms (other than the one being solved) are constant in the MR equation. This is a clear oversimplification that ignores flow, magnetic susceptibility, and chemical shift effects, among others. This greatly reduces the accuracy of relaxation measurements in situations where these other terms play a significant role. Most solutions for T1 and T2 also assume a single exponential decay term. This is not actually the case. T1 decay is actually different for the fat and water compartments in the sample. This assumption adds even more error to the measurement.

A final problem is that even if the determination of T1 and T2 could be made accurately, many experts now believe that T1 and T2 measurements in themselves are not that specific. It may be more useful for most cases to have high anatomic image detail rather than an extremely accurate T1 value. A more accurate diagnosis can often be made based on the morphology of the T1 or T2 alterations in the image rather than accurate quantification of the actual relaxation times.

T1 VS. T2-WEIGHTED IMAGES

Pulse sequence information is very important in the accurate analysis of MR images. When looking at a CT scan the first thing most people consider is whether intravenous contrast was given. With MR probably the first thing to determine is what pulse sequence (i.e., T1- or T2-weighted) was used.

Later on it will be apparent that the determination of which is the image phase axis and which is the frequency encoding axis is also important because different artifacts occur in different axes. Finally, it is also necessary to determine if a contrast agent was administered in order to appropriately interpret the MR image findings.

There is actually no absolute T1- or T2-weighted image and it all depends on what the image is being compared to. If the T1 values and T2 values of tissues are specified then it is possible to define an ideal T1 weighted image as one that will reflect the T1 components of the tissue. The same will be true for T2 contrast (Table 2–5). From the relaxation time values, a relatively T1-weighted image will result in black CSF, gray gray matter, and white white matter. A relatively T2-weighted image, on the other hand, will have white CSF, white gray matter, and gray white matter (Fig 2–7).

TABLE 2–5.

Typical Normal Brain Relaxation Times for a Midfield System

Tissue	T1 (msec)	T2 (msec)
CSF	2,700	1,200
Gray matter	450	100
White matter	270	80

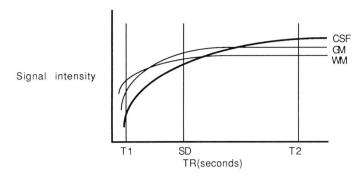

FIG 2–7.
Graph of signal intensity vs. TR for cerebrospinal fluid (CSF), gray matter (GM), and white matter (WM). The intensity values for T1-weighted (T1), spin density (SD), and T2-weighted (T2) images are shown.

A problem occurs in the intermediate range with images results with black CSF, gray white matter, and white gray matter. CSF still has its T1-weighted appearance yet the gray and white matter relationship is clearly T2-weighted (Fig 2–8). It is important to realize that all images are only *weighted* toward T1 or T2 to various degrees and all contain *both* T1 and T2 information.

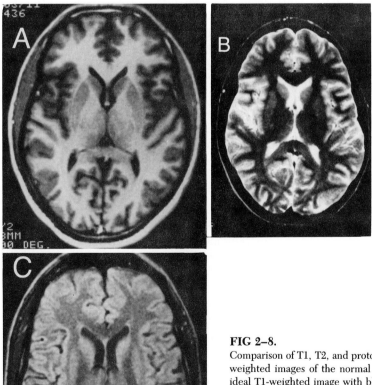

FIG 2–8.
Comparison of T1, T2, and proton density weighted images of the normal brain. **A,** ideal T1-weighted image with black CSF, white white matter, and gray gray matter. **B,** ideal T2-weighted image with white CSF, gray white matter, and white gray matter. **C,** proton density image with black CSF, gray white matter and white gray matter.

TABLE 2–6.

Magnetic Susceptibility Phenomena

Type	Electrons	Susceptibility	Mechanism
Diamagnetic	Paired	-10^{-6}	No permanent spin moment
Paramagnetic	Unpaired	$+10^{-3}$	Noninteracting permanent moment
Superparamagnetic	Unpaired	$+10^{+2}$	Noninteracting domains
Ferromagnetic	Unpaired	$+10^{+2}$	Interacting domains

MAGNETIC SUSCEPTIBILITY

Another important source of contrast in MR is that due to magnetic susceptibility effects. All substances respond when placed in a magnetic field. The degree to which the substance becomes magnetized or the ratio of the applied magnetization to the resultant magnetic field of the substance is the *magnetic susceptibility* (Table 2–6).

This response to an externally applied magnetic field is determined by the electronic rather than the nuclear configuration of the component atoms. This is because the orbital angular momentum of the electron is much greater than the dipole generated by the nucleus. Thus, although the MR resonance phenomenon creating the image is based on the nucleus, the overall magnetic environment that also affects the image is based on the presence of paired or unpaired *electrons.*

The majority of tissues in the body have no unpaired electrons and thus the spin angular momentum is cancelled. However, when placed in a B_0 field (B_0 = vector representing a large external magnetic field), the individual orbital momentum of each electron results in the induction of a weak magnetic field in the opposite direction of the applied field. These tissues have a slightly negative susceptibility and are called *diamagnetic.* That is, when placed in a magnetic field they magnetize slightly in the opposite direction of the applied magnetic field (Fig 2–9).

A smaller group of materials share the characteristic of having unpaired electrons. These unpaired electrons respond to the B_0 field in a similar manner as the weaker unpaired nucleons. Although not all orient with the field, as with the nucleons, a statistically significant portion do. If the unpaired electrons are present in sufficient quantity then this effect dominates the weaker diamagnetic effects and a strong magnetization results parallel to the applied field as a positive susceptibility.

Substances with unpaired electrons may be paramagnetic, superparamagnetic, or ferromagnetic. Materials with positive magnetic susceptibility have interesting effects on image contrast. While they produce no MR signal themselves, the materials significantly change image contrast by producing *relaxation enhancement* of adjacent proton MR signals. This may appear as either T1 or T2 shortening.

PARAMAGNETISM

Paramagnetic materials (like ferromagnetic and superparamagnetic substances) have unpaired electrons that result in a positive magnetic susceptibility. The effect of paramagnetic substances is several orders of magnitude weaker than that of the other substances with

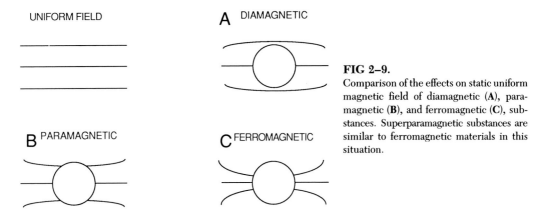

UNIFORM FIELD

A DIAMAGNETIC

B PARAMAGNETIC

C FERROMAGNETIC

FIG 2–9.
Comparison of the effects on static uniform magnetic field of diamagnetic (**A**), paramagnetic (**B**), and ferromagnetic (**C**), substances. Superparamagnetic substances are similar to ferromagnetic materials in this situation.

positive susceptibility. Paramagnetic materials have independent magnetically dilute moments. The induced magnetization returns to zero when the applied magnetic field is turned off (Fig 2–10).

As was covered in Chapter 1, protons in the absence of nearby unpaired electrons realign with the main magnetic field through spin lattice and spin-spin relaxation mechanisms. This occurs as a result of variations in the local magnetic field produced by the motion of other water protons. When unpaired electrons are present an even greater magnetic dipole is produced by the greater spin and angular momentum of the electron resulting in increased efficiency of both T1 and T2 relaxation. This is referred to as a *proton-electron dipole-dipole interaction.*

Paramagnetic substances exert their influence on the MR signal by this mechanism and improve the efficiency of T1 and T2 relaxation. Although both T1 and T2 relaxation efficiency is improved, in most situations, the T1 effect predominates (Fig 2–11). Because the effect of the proton-electron dipole-dipole interaction decreases as the sixth power of the distance between the dipoles, the unpaired electrons have to be accessible to the water protons in order for these dipole-dipole interactions to occur. Therefore, there is a proximity effect (within 3 angstroms or so) and substances containing unpaired electrons must usually be in aqueous solution in order for the water protons to get close enough to them.

There are endogenous as well as exogenous paramagnetic substances that shorten T1 relaxation times. Examples of paramagnetic substances are gadolinium, methemoglobin, and melanin. They appear bright on T1-weighted images. Importantly, paramagnetic materials

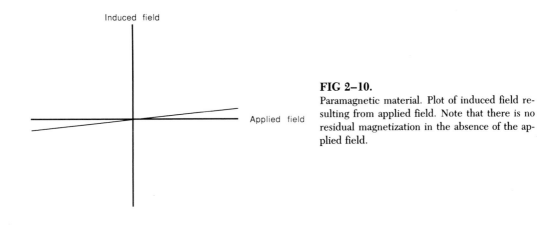

Induced field

Applied field

FIG 2–10.
Paramagnetic material. Plot of induced field resulting from applied field. Note that there is no residual magnetization in the absence of the applied field.

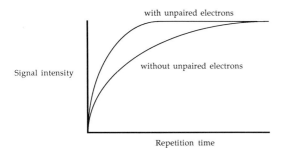

with unpaired electrons

Signal intensity

without unpaired electrons

Repetition time

FIG 2–11.
Plot of intensity vs. repetition time for a diamagnetic substance (without unpaired electrons) and a paramagnetic substance (with unpaired electrons). There is relaxation enhancement with a paramagnetic material.

have no signal of their own. These substances instead alter the signal from the existing protons in aqueous solution. There is also no significant field strength dependence of proton-electron dipole-dipole interactions. The effect occurs to essentially the same extent on both high- and low-field MR instruments.

Gadolinium is a lanthanide metal with unpaired electrons which is paramagnetic.[7] Although the free metal is toxic, when bound to diethylene triamine pentaacetic acid (DTPA) or other chelates it is safe for human use. It is the first major paramagnetic intravenous (IV) contrast agent to be approved for MR use. Gadolinium has similar pharmacokinetics as iodinated contrast in CT; it also has a similar volume of distribution and is cleared by the kidneys. It appears to be much safer. Lower doses are used and as yet there have been no idiopathic anaphylactoid reactions to gadolinium-DTPA.

The advantages of MR contrast agents are obvious for the evaluation of the blood–brain barrier. On T2-weighted images gliosis or edema is visible but it is often important to detect the actual blood–brain barrier disruption. Contrast-enhanced MRI is also valuable in the evaluation of leptomeningeal disease and the postoperative patient. Also, because the changes with gadolinium are T1 effects, higher signal-to-noise T1-weighted images may be used to optimally show enhancement (Fig 2–12).

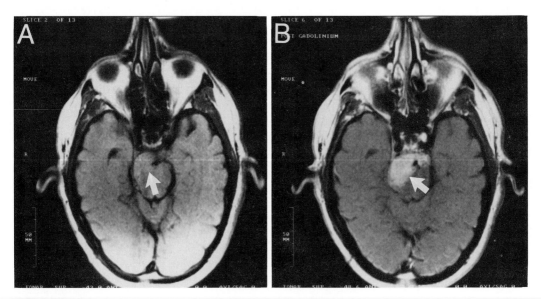

FIG 2–12.
Meningioma. Pre- and postgadolinium administration. **A,** on the noncontrast study (SE/800/30) there is an isointense mass distorting the brain stem *(arrow).* Contrast between the tumor and midbrain is low. **B,** following gadolinium, the meningioma *(arrow)* shows dense staining on the same pulse sequence.

While gadolinium DTPA and other new MR contrast agents are not seeing the ubiquitous application that is present with iodinated contrast agents in CT, they are playing an increasing role for a variety of both central nervous system (CNS) and body applications. Newer, low osmolality gadolinium complexes are also currently under investigation for human uses. Other chelates as well as ferromagnetic and superparamagnetic materials are also being investigated and may soon be available for general MR use. Researchers are also trying to tag monoclonal antibodies with paramagnetic substances or ferromagnetic substances for more specific contrast enhancement.

Melanin is another endogenous substance that is paramagnetic. Some of the earliest work in MR showed T1 prolongation of all malignant human tumors tested except for melanoma which showed T1 shortening. It was recognized early on that melanin is a stable free radical that is paramagnetic.[8] Later literature suggests that T1 shortening in the appropriate clinical situation may strongly suggest the presence of melanin.[9]

The problem with relying on T1 shortening as a reliable indicator for a melanoma on MR is that other things such as fat, subacute blood, and melanoma may bleed, show gadolinium uptake, or contain small amounts of lipid thus lowering the specificity of the finding of T1 shortening for melanoma. Also, amelanotic melanomas have no significant melanin or T1 shortening which limits the sensitivity of T1 shortening as a sign for melanoma.

A second form of relaxation enhancement occurs when the substance with unpaired electrons cannot approach close enough to the protons for proton-electron dipole-dipole interactions to occur (perhaps due to molecular geometry) yet is heterogeneously distributed in the tissue (such as inside a RBC). The higher magnetic susceptibility of the heterogeneously distributed material results in local magnetic field heterogeneity. When water protons diffuse through the field inhomogeneities, variations in Larmor frequency and thus phase will result which are not corrected with spin echo or gradient echo refocusing strategies. This loss of phase and thus decreased transverse magnetization is manifested as a short T2 relaxation time. Interestingly, T1 relaxation is unchanged by this process (Fig 2–13). In another words, T2 relaxation is enhanced, which results in a low signal. Because the enhancement preferentially affects the transverse relaxation, the signal gets lower and lower with heavier T2 weighting.

Unlike proton-electron dipole-dipole interactions, this T2 relaxation enhancement has a field strength dependence. With spin echo imaging it is a very strong dependence (1/T2 is proportional to field strength *squared*). High field units have a significant advantage in detecting these effects when spin echo imaging is used.

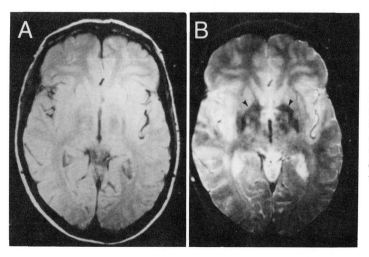

FIG 2–13.
Brain iron deposition **A,** on the proton density image (SE/1000/30), the ferritin is poorly seen. **B,** the preferential T2 shortening of the ferritin results in decreasing signal *(arrowhead)* with heavier T2-weighting (SE/2000/90).

When pulse sequences that use magnetic field gradients to refocus the protons are employed, this effect (1/T2) is only proportional to field strength. Using this technique it is possible to examine iron and other ferromagnetic materials with low-strength machines as well as high-field strength machines. The important thing is that the shortening preferentially affects T2 relaxation times. There is no parallel T1 effect.

In addition to the work with contrast agents and other exogenous substances, there are situations where endogenous materials alter MR contrast due to preferential T2 shortening. This occurs in nonheme iron deposition states in the liver, brain, and other areas[11]. The characteristic lowering of signal as the images have greater and greater T2 weighting strongly suggests a magnetic susceptibility effect due to iron.

SUPERPARAMAGNETISM

The dipoles of unpaired electrons may act even more strongly in closely packed crystalline structures. Groups of electron dipoles may act together as a unit called a *domain* within these structures. When the crystal is similar in size to the domain, the electron groups act as independent domains.

These substances are termed *superparamagnetic*. Although the magnetic susceptibility is 100 to 1,000 times stronger than with paramagnetic substances, superparamagnetic materials also return to zero magnetization after removal of the applied magnetic field (Fig 2–14). Superparamagnetic materials are typically solid particulates (rather than aqueous solutions) that act as independent domains. These materials have pronounced effects on image contrast *(T2 shortening)* and are being investigated as potential MR particulate contrast agents.

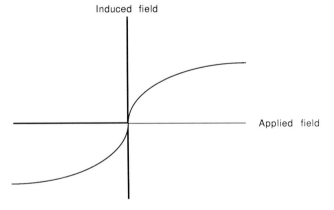

FIG 2–14.
Superparamagnetic material. Plot of induced field resulting from applied field. Although susceptibility is greater than with paramagnetic materials, no residual magnetization is present after the field is turned off.

FERROMAGNETISM

In materials with interacting domains the orientation of the magnetic dipoles reaches a magnetic equilibrium based on the crystal structure. These materials also have a high magnetic susceptibility, however, unlike para- and superparamagnetics, they have a permanent residual magnetization even when the applied field is removed (Fig 2–15). Materials with interacting domains are termed *ferromagnetic*. A common example of such materials is an ordinary bar magnet. Ferromagnetic materials are made up of solid phase microscopic interacting domains.

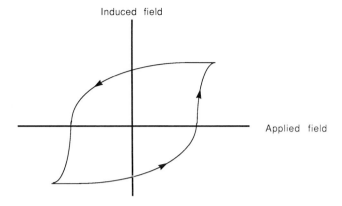

Induced field

Applied field

FIG 2–15.
Ferromagnetic material. Plot of induced field vs. applied field. Note residual magnetization after the applied field is removed.

HEMORRHAGE

One of the most common types of relaxation enhancement encountered in MR images is that due to hemorrhage. The appearance of hemorrhage on MR is complex and involves both mechanisms of relaxation enhancement. Thus in order to understand the appearance of hemorrhage it is necessary to use both the model of proton-electron dipole-dipole interactions in aqueous solutions as well as magnetic susceptibility effects of iron molecules containing unpaired electrons resulting in a T2 shortening effect.[12]

The characteristic signal changes of MR of hemorrhage are due to the iron in the blood. In CT the characteristic signal changes of hemorrhage are due to electron-dense protein. Thus, CT is very good for the examination of acute hemorrhage when large amounts of protein are present but in a matter of hours to days when the protein breaks down the CT examination becomes equivocal or negative. Because the MR signal depends on the more persistent iron the effects last weeks, months, or even years later. Although MR is unquestionably more sensitive than CT for subacute or chronic hemorrhage, its final role in acute hemorrhage is still being worked out. Computed tomography is valuable for acute hemorrhage, but MR is beginning to play a greater role with T2*-sensitive imaging techniques such as gradient echo imaging.[13]

Iron occurs in the body in several forms, not only as an oxygen transport system but also as a storage protein and in enzyme systems. In all cases it is tightly bound because free iron is toxic. In the case of evolving hematomas, iron undergoes changes in chelation and electron spin states as well as in molecular geometry and compartmentalization which manifest themselves as characteristic changes on the MR image. In fact, the orderly evolution of the iron states of the hematoma on MR (affected to some extent by local considerations of pH and oxygen partial pressure or tension [PO_2]) allows hematomas to be staged on MR as acute, subacute, or chronic with far greater accuracy than with CT or other imaging techniques (Fig 2–16) (Table 2–7).

The normal carrier state for oxygen in the red blood cells (RBCs) is oxyhemoglobin. This reversibly converts to deoxyhemoglobin depending on the PO_2 and pH in the lungs and capillary beds. The iron in oxyhemoglobin is in the ferrous (Fe^{2+}) state but has one unpaired electron in the outer shell and is diamagnetic. In a simple acute intraparenchymal hemorrhage the RBCs contain oxyhemoglobin. The bleed is essentially isointense with brain parenchyma because neither of the two relaxation enhancement effects take place. Although the actual bleed may be isointense at this point, early edema may be high signal on the T2-weighted images.

TABLE 2–7.

Iron in Magnetic Resonance Imaging*

	Oxidation State	Unpaired Electrons	Proton-Electron Dipole-Dipole Interaction	Preferential T_2 Shortening
Oxyhemoglobin (HbO$_2$)	Fe^{2+}	1	−	−
Deoxyhemoglobin (Hb)	Fe^{2+}	4	−	IRBC + LRBC −
Methemoglobin (MHb)	Fe^{3+}	5	+	IRBC + LRBC −
Hemosiderin (lysosomes)	Fe^{3+}	>10,000	−	+ +
Ferritin (intracellular)	Fe^{3+}	>10,000	−	+ +

*IRBC = intact red blood cell membrane; LRBC = lysed red blood cells.

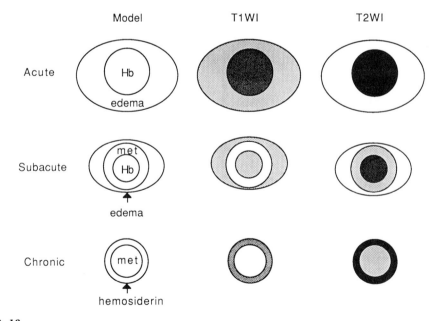

FIG 2–16.
Hemorrhage diagram. The model shows the location of edema, deoxyhemoglobin (Hb), methemoglobin (met), and hemosiderin. The effects on signal intensity are shown in simplified form for T1-weighted (T1WI) and T2-weighted (T2WI) images for acute (<72 hours), subacute (72 hours-1 week), and chronic hemorrhage.

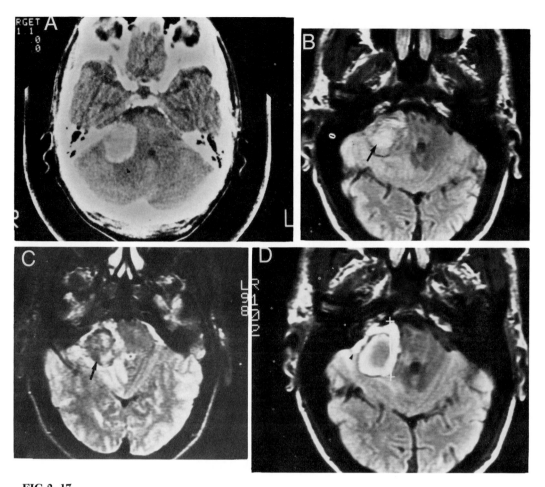

FIG 2–17.
Acute hemorrhage into an acoustic neuroma. **A,** contrast-enhanced CT shows a large acoustic neuroma on the right (*arrowhead*). **B,** proton density (SE/2000/20) MR performed at the same time shows intermediate signal within the mass (*arrowhead*). **C,** T2-weighted image (SE/2000/70) at the same time shows low signal within the mass (*arrow*) consistent with preferential T2 shortening due to deoxyhemoglobin in the acute hemorrhage. **D,** proton density image (SE/2000/20) obtained 6 days later shows characteristic increased signal of methemoglobin in both the mass as well as the adjacent subarachnoid space (*arrow*).

After a few minutes to hours the oxyhemoglobin is desaturated to deoxyhemoglobin (Fig 2–17). Although deoxyhemoglobin is still Fe^{2+}, it has four unpaired electrons. Because of the molecular geometry, the unpaired electrons cannot get close enough to the water protons for proton-electron dipole-dipole interactions to occur. However, because of the positive magnetic susceptibility of this material and the fact that it is heterogeneously distributed in the intact RBCs, dephasing causes irreversible loss of signal or T2 shortening.

This preferential T2 shortening results in low signal on T2 images and a less significant effect on T1-weighted images. This often occurs in the most central portion of the hematoma first which is often the most hypoxic. Surrounding high signal due to edema is often present on T2-weighted images in the brain with acute hemorrhage. Because of the lack of field strength dependence of the signal changes of acute hemorrhage that this model predicts, the role of clot retraction is also under investigation.

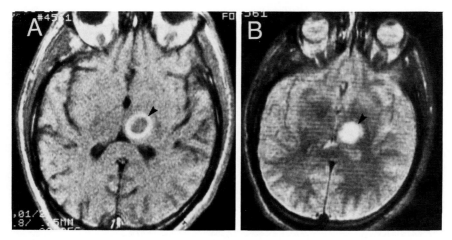

FIG 2–18.
Subacute hemorrhage at cryothalomotomy site. Image obtained 4 weeks following freezing procedure of the left thalamus shows characteristic blood breakdown products. **A,** T1-weighted image (SE/500/30) shows high signal rim of methemoglobin *(arrowhead).* **B,** T2-weighted image shows fluid-containing necrotic center *(arrowhead).*

With continued hypoxia, irreversible oxidation of deoxyhemoglobin to methemoglobin occurs in the RBCs. Methemoglobin has five unpaired electrons and because of its geometry allows water protons to move close enough for proton-electron dipole-dipole interactions to occur.[14] In intact cells it is also heterogeneously distributed so some T2 shortening may occur although the T1 effects usually predominate (Fig 2–18). Typically the increased signal of methemoglobin is at the periphery of the hematoma and with continued oxidation gradually fills in with time (Fig 2–16). Methemoglobin formation usually begins to occur at 72 to 90 hours. This appears as high signal on T1-weighted images and may also be seen as high signal on T2-weighted images. It is important not to mistake contrast enhancement by gadolinium-DTPA for methemoglobin in subacute hemorrhage. In order to avoid confusion with subacute hemorrhage, a noncontrast MR should be performed.

The last stage occurs when methemoglobin is converted to hemosiderin. Hemosiderin is a large molecule with 10,000 or more unpaired electrons. When heterogeneously distributed in macrophages, a profound T2 shortening effect results such as is present with deoxyhemoglobin and ferritin. Its appears as a black rim on T2-weighted images. It may also be visible on T1-weighted images, although often it is not as dark as the T2-weighted chronic hemorrhage.

At this point in the chronic hemorrhage the edema usually resolves leaving a high signal methemoglobin center gradually replaced by a growing rim of low signal hemosiderin in macrophages. The amount of hemosiderin present may reflect the presence of blood-brain barrier disruption. The more rapidly the blood-brain barrier recovers, the more hemosiderin will remain, presumably because the macrophages have limited access to the bloodstream. The value of this in differentiating simple hemorrhage with an intact blood-brain barrier vs. hemorrhage into a tumor with chronic blood-brain barrier disruption is under investigation.[15]

REFERENCES

1. Wehrli FW, MacFall JR, Newton TH: Parameters determining the appearance of NMR images, in Newton TH, Potts DG (eds): *Modern Neuroradiology: Advanced Imaging Techniques.* San Anselmo, Calif, Clavadel Press, 1983.

2. Edelstein WA, Bottomley PA, Hart HR, Smith LS. Signal noise, and contrast in nuclear magnetic resonance (NMR) imaging. *J Comput Assist Tomogr* 1983; 7:391–401.

3. Wehrli F, Macfall JR, Shutts D, et al: Mechanisms of contrast in NMR imaging. *J Comput Assist Tomogr* 1984; 8:369–380.

4. Hendrick RE, Nelson TR, Hendee WR: Optimizing tissue contrast in magnetic resonance imaging. *Magn Reson Imaging* 1984; 2:193–204.

5. Hendrick RE, Newman FD, Hendee WR. MR imaging technology: Maximizing the signal to noise from a single tissue. *Radiology* 1985; 156:749–752.

6. Lufkin R, Keen R, Rhodes M, et al: Simulator for instruction in pulse sequence selection in MRI. *AJR* 1986; 147:199–202.

7. Carr DH, Brown J, Leung AWL, et al: Iron and gadolinium chelates as contrast agents in NMR. *J Comput Assist Tomogr* 1984; 8:385–389.

8. Damadian R, Zaner K, Hor D, et al: Human tumors detected by nuclear magnetic resonance. *Proc Natl Acad Sci USA* 1974; 71:1471–1473.

9. Gomori JM, Grossman RI, Shields JA, et al: Choroidal melanomas: Correlation of NMR spectroscopy and MR imaging. *Radiology* 1986; 158:443–445.

10. Spencer G, Lufkin R, Simons K, et al: MR of a melanoma simulating ocular neoplasm. *AJNR* 1987; 8:921–922.

11. Drayer B, Burger P, Darwin R, et al: MRI of brain iron. *AJR* 1986; 147:103–110.

12. Gomori JM, Grossman RI, Goldberg HI, et al: Intracranial hematomas: Imaging by high field MR. *Radiology* 1985; 157:87–93.

13. Edelman RR, Johnson K, Buxton R, et al: MR of hemorrhage: A new approach. *AJNR* 1986; 7:751–756.

14. Bradley WG, Schmidt PC: Effect of methemoglobin formation on the MR appearance of subarachnoid hemorrhage. *Radiology* 1985; 156:99–103.

15. Grossman RI, Gomori J, et al: MR of hemorrhagic conditions. *Acta Radiol Suppl* 1986; 361:53–55.

Chapter 3 _____

Magnetic Resonance Image Formation

Robert B. Lufkin, M.D.

To create medical images with magnetic resonance (MR) it is essential to be able to accurately localize the nuclear magnetic resonance (NMR) signal. For useful medical applications it is a further requirement that the measurement be done nondestructively, noninvasively of various points in a human being. The techniques of MR image formation are most interesting because most are different from anything done with computed tomographic (CT) scanning or other imaging modalities.[1, 2]

In the past many approaches to NMR imaging have been tried. Only a few are in use today but the others are of interest in order to understand the development of NMR imaging. The earliest method was with a *sequential point measurement* (Fig 3–1,A). The point method was accomplished by distorting the magnetic field so the NMR process only occurs in small part in the body which is in resonance with the RF pulse. After the 90 to 180 echo sequence is performed, the patient or the magnetic field is moved so that a different sensitive volume may be sampled. The whole process is then repeated as many times as there are pixels to produce the entire scan. The problem with this approach is that MRI is slow and a single-point method could take several hours for even a moderate resolution image.

A better technique is the *sequential line technique* (Fig 3–1,B). In this case an entire line of data is sampled at the same time. This approach is a little faster than the sequential point method but still not appropriate for clinical use. Today most operators using magnetic resonance imaging (MRI) for clinical purposes use even faster image formation by *sequential plane [two-dimensional (2-D)] imaging*, which finally allows clinically practical scan times (e.g., 2 to 10 minutes per image set acquisition) (Fig 3–1,C). *Volume imaging [three-dimensional (3-D)]* techniques are also presently under investigation that are extremely promising for certain clinical applications (Fig 3–1,D).

The display strategy for the MRI signal using the concepts of voxels and pixels is probably familiar to everyone from the days of CT scanning. The sample volume is a specific volume of tissue, which is known as a volume element or *voxel* (Fig 3–2). An array of voxels form the image slice. The slice thickness is defined by the voxel thickness. One surface of the voxel is called the picture element or *pixel*. The entire voxel determines the NMR signal and appears on the image as an intensity value for that pixel.

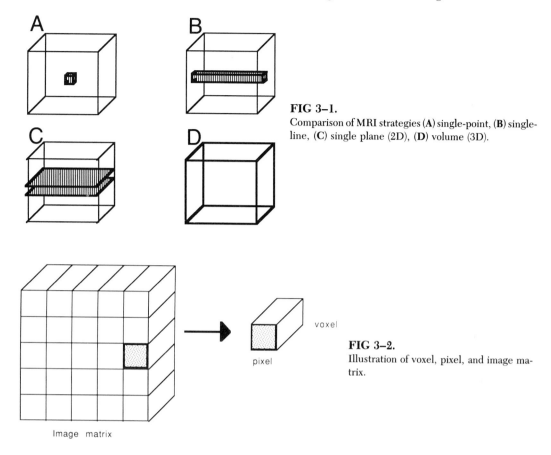

FIG 3–1.
Comparison of MRI strategies (**A**) single-point, (**B**) single-line, (**C**) single plane (2D), (**D**) volume (3D).

FIG 3–2.
Illustration of voxel, pixel, and image matrix.

MAGNETIC FIELD GRADIENTS

Magnetic field gradients are the key tools that permit MR imaging to be possible by allowing the MR signal to be localized in space. A *gradient* is a variation in magnetic field with distance or specifically a linear variation in magnetic field from weaker to stronger along one dimension of the patient (Fig 3–3). The amount of variation is actually very small, typically two to three *orders of magnitude* less than the static magnetic field of the system (e.g., gradients of 10 mT/m for a 0.5-T system).

When a magnetic field gradient is superimposed on the existing static magnetic field, the resonant frequency of the protons varies along the gradient according to the local magnetic field. Thus, the frequency of the protons varies with spatial location along the axis of the applied gradient.

Slice Select Gradient

MRI employs magnetic field gradients to spatially encode the signal in three fundamental ways. First, in order to select a slice, a linear magnetic field gradient is applied during

FIG 3–3.
Linear magnetic field gradient. The heighth of the arrows is proportional to field strength. The magnetic field varies linearly with distance along the gradient.

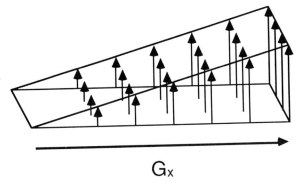

$$G_x$$

application of the 90 degree radiofrequency (RF) pulse in order to stimulate a plane of finite thickness.

In other words, for a patient on the table, an axial slice may be selected by turning on the gradient that runs from head to toe. This has the effect of speeding up the resonant frequency from the top of the head and slowing down the protons near the feet. Concomitant with this gradient, the 90 degree pulse is applied. Because this gradient allows the selection of the image slice it is referred to as the *slice-select gradient* (Gss) (Fig 3–4).

The *location of the slice* along the gradient is determined by the center frequency of the 90 degree RF pulse. In other words, the distance of the excited plane from the magnet center is completely determined by the strength of the Gss and by the difference between the frequency of the excitation pulse and the resonant frequency of the background field. A higher frequency pulse will tend to select image planes nearer the head and lower frequency pulses will select slices nearer the feet.

The *slice thickness* can be determined by controlling the range of frequencies used in the 90 degree pulse (Fig 3–5,A). This range of frequencies is called the *bandwidth*. A larger bandwidth will result in a thicker slice.

Alternatively, the frequency may be held constant and the slice select gradient amplitude varied (Fig 3–5,B). The field gradient controls the mapping of frequency onto space. Therefore a shallow gradient will map a given bandwidth of frequencies onto a thicker slice than a steep gradient. Slice thickness can therefore be varied by either changing the bandwidth or the gradient amplitude. The drawback is that as thinner slices are produced, there are fewer mobile protons in the sample so that the signal amplitude (and thus signal-to-noise) decreases.

FIG 3–4.
Slice select gradient. The slice select gradient is turned on during the application of the 90 degree RF pulse to allow selective stimulation of a plane of protons.

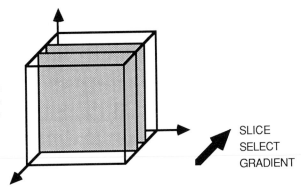

SLICE
SELECT
GRADIENT

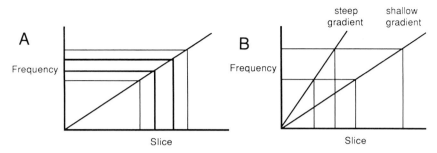

FIG 3–5.
Variation in slice thickness is possible by either changing bandwidth (**A**) or gradient amplitude (**B**).

Scan Plane Selection

The slice select gradient also determines the *scan plane orientation*. Three physical gradients in the MR instrument are referred to as Gx, Gy, and Gz which are orthogonally oriented in space. Any of these physical gradients can be assigned to the task of slice selection. The gradient from head to toe used as the Gss produces axial images. When slice selection is performed with the gradient from right to left, sagittal images will result. Unlike CT where the scan plane is determined a priori by the detector-tube axis, scan planes in MR are determined by the selection of the gradients. The slice selection step is only the beginning. Image formation with MR requires a veritable symphony of gradient switching, all with precision timing.

Back Projection Reconstruction

One of the orthogonal magnetic field gradients has been used to select the scan plane. Two more spatial dimensions remain to be encoded and two remaining gradients are available to accomplish this. One method is similar to that found in CT-back projection reconstruction.

As an example, consider two vials of water as the image phantom. After delivery of a 90 degree RF pulse to the system, a free induction decay (FID) will be detected by the RF receiver. For the purposes of this discussion assume that T2* effects are negated and refocusing is unnecessary.

The FID signal contains the single resonant frequency of the water and although it decays as its amplitude decreases, the entire process occurs at one frequency. At this point it is necessary to review the technique of *Fourier transformation*.[3] Jean-Baptiste Joseph Fourier narrowly escaped being beheaded in the French Revolution and went on in later years, while accompanying Napoleon to Egypt, to develop the mathematical tool that bears his name.[4]

This device allows the transformation from one representation of frequencies to another. There are at least two ways to display frequencies. One is plotting amplitude vs. time graphically (Fig 3–6). The signal frequency is represented as a sine wave. Because signal amplitude is plotted vs. time, this is referred to as the *time domain*.

Sometimes it is useful to display the signal in another way that is not amplitude vs. time but amplitude vs. frequency. This is sort of a "radio dial" representation with each peak corresponding to a different frequency. So instead of actually displaying the sine wave, a single spike on the radio dial corresponds to the frequency. Because amplitude is plotted vs. frequency, this is referred to as the *frequency domain*.

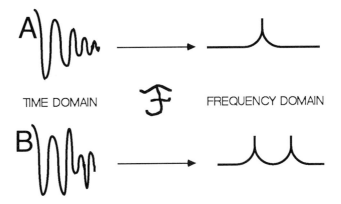

FIG 3–6.
The use of the Fourier transformation (F) to transform the RF output signal from the time vs. amplitude domain to the frequency vs. amplitude domain for a signal of a single frequency (first line) and two frequencies (line two).

TIME DOMAIN   FREQUENCY DOMAIN

The Fourier transformation is thus a tool to go back and forth from these two representations-from time domain to frequency domain (i.e., from the sine wave representation to the radio dial representation and back and forth). This approach is fundamental to all computed tomographic scanning techniques including MRI, x-ray CT, positron-emission tomography (PET), and single-photon emission tomography (SPECT).

The Fourier transformation is also used in MR spectroscopy. In order to perform NMR spectroscopy the FID is collected. However, instead of looking at something like water in the sample, the system is often tuned to a more chemically heterogeneous sample such as phosphorus-31 instead of protons. In this case the frequencies of the individual chemical components such as adenosine diphosphate (ADP) or adenosine triphosphate (ATP) vary.

Following Fourier transformation, instead of producing one peak (as in the case of water) several peaks for all the components containing phosphorus-31 are produced (Fig 3–7). Separation of the peaks on the frequency domain mapping reflects different chemical environments of the components, or chemical shift information. High-field systems maximize chemical shift information that is valuable for spectroscopy. Unfortunately, this increased chemical shift also results in increased artifacts in MR high-field images.

Unlike spectroscopy where frequency shifts encode chemical environment information, for imaging it is assumed that the proton-containing compounds are chemically homogeneous and frequency is instead used to encode spatial information. In order to do this a gradient must be turned on during signal collection.

With the gradient turned on during the FID a simple signal with one frequency is not obtained. Instead, turning on this gradient during the FID produces a much more complex signal (Fig 3–8).

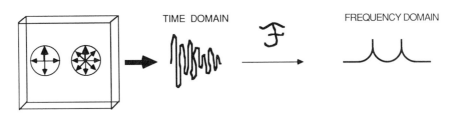

TIME DOMAIN   FREQUENCY DOMAIN

FIG 3–7.
NMR spectroscopy is performed without magnetic field gradients and uses the Fourier transformation to display different frequencies reflecting differing chemical species in the sample rather than the physical location of the sample.

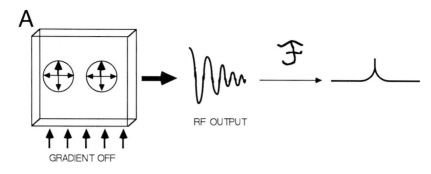

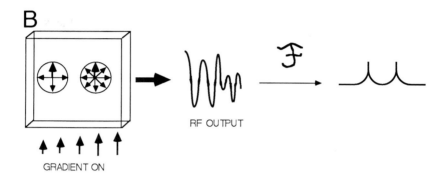

FIG 3–8.
Effect of gradient on RF output signal. With the gradient off, the Fourier transformation of the outputted signal is a single peak reflecting the resonant frequency of water (**A**). No spatial information is present. When the gradient is applied, the resonant frequency of the water protons changes according to the location along the gradient. This is reflected in the Fourier transformation of the outputted data (**B**).

To better understand this complex signal, the Fourier transformation is used to switch to the radio dial or frequency domain representation. When this is done the signal obtained with the gradients on is actually two frequency peaks. The two frequencies correspond to two water-resonant frequencies. The gradient changes the frequency of the two water vials because each vial now experiences a slightly different magnetic field depending on its location along the gradient.

The gradients spread the proton resonances out in a spatial distribution. In the case of the two vials, the frequency domain representation is two peaks. This representation is actually a one-dimensional spatial projection of this phantom. It is like a shadow projected on the wall.

Once this projection is obtained it is a straightforward matter to go back and obtain more and more projections in different directions by electronically rotating the gradients around the patient. As is known from CT scanning, it is possible to create a 2D image by filtered back projection reconstruction if enough of these projections are obtained (Fig 3–9).[5]

While most CT scanners still use this approach, it was also used in the early MR scanners. There are, however, several major drawbacks to this approach (Table 3–1). Therefore, most modern MR scanners use a better method called 2D Fourier transformation (2D-FT) reconstruction.[6] Unfortunately 2D-FT doesn't work with CT and these machines must still use backprojection techniques.

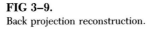

FIG 3–9.
Back projection reconstruction.

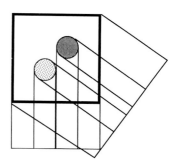

There are several differences between these methods. First, the artifacts in projection reconstruction are star-shaped due to the radial form of reconstruction that is done. With the 2D-FT technique most artifacts are rectilinear (cross-shaped) in form, which is often less disruptive to the image.

The point spread function is a measure of the way spatial information is encoded in the image. With projection reconstruction this function is gaussian. With 2D-FT imaging this is a *sinc function* (sin x/x) which is much sharper. Next and importantly for MR imaging, projection reconstruction is very sensitive to magnetic field uniformity, whereas 2D-FT is much more forgiving. Finally, 2D-FT methods allow the acquisition of nonquadratic data matrices, which is not possible with projection reconstruction. This allows spatial resolution to be traded off against improvements in image acquisition time along one axis while spatial resolution is preserved in the other axis.

TABLE 3–1.

Reconstruction Techniques

	Projection Reconstruction	2D-FT
System	CT or MR	MR only
Artifact form	Star pattern	Rectilinear
Point spread function	Gaussian	Sinc (sharper)
Sensitivity to magnetic field uniformity	High	Lower
Nonquadratic acquisition	No	Yes

2D-FT IMAGE FORMATION

2D-FT imaging is accomplished using three distinct steps which each encode a different spatial axis of the 2D slice: slice selection, phase encoding, and frequency encoding.

Slice Selection

Slice selection in 2D-FT imaging is, fortunately, like that for projection reconstruction (see Figs 3–4 and 3–5). One gradient is activated during the 90 degree pulse and this gradient becomes by definition the slice select gradient. The RF pulse excites a certain bandwidth of frequencies, a certain center frequency, and thus selects a volume of protons. If thinner slices are desired, steeper gradients or narrower bandwidths are used as long as acceptable signal to noise is present.

Phase Encoding

The next step uses a concept called *phase encoding* that is not entirely familiar from CT experience. To simplify things, consider a slab of tissue with only nine protons that will be localized in space (Fig 3–10). The frequency of the spins is indicated by the number of arrows present and the phase is indicated by the direction of the large arrow. One gradient has already been used to select the slab. Two gradients are left with which to encode the remaining two spatial dimensions and to make the image.

As shown in Figure 3–10,A, all the protons have the same phase angles following the 90 degree RF pulse (T2* effects are ignored for now because they are handled by the echo). The frequency is also the same for all nine protons because all are experiencing the same magnetic field as determined by the main magnet.

Activating one of the two remaining gradients has the effect of changing the magnetic field strength slightly along its axis. This in turn changes the Larmor frequencies of the protons according to their position along the gradient (Fig 3–10,B). The locations of the protons along this axis are thus mapped with their frequencies. When the gradient is first activated, the protons are still in phase.

After a few milliseconds an interesting thing occurs along this gradient. Because the protons have different frequencies according to their location along the gradient, they no longer stay in phase (Fig 3–10,C). The dephasing that occurs, however, takes place in a very specific manner according to the location along the gradient. For example, after a period of time the protons at the lower field end have a lower frequency and a phase angle of 3 o'clock. The intermediate protons have higher frequency and a phase angle of 6 o'clock. The protons at the high field end then have the highest frequency and a phase angle of 9 o'clock.

Figure 3–10,D depicts the last step in the process. At this point the gradient is turned off and all the protons return to a constant frequency as determined by the main magnetic field strength. Briefly, the spatial location of the spins along the gradient was encoded by their frequency. When the gradient was turned off, all the protons returned to uniform frequency and the spatial information was lost. Or was it?

Actually the "memory" of that gradient was preserved by the spins in the form of their phase angles. Although the frequencies all return to a constant, the phase angles remain different according to the location along that axis. In our example if it is determined that a proton has a phase angle of 3 o'clock, then it is known that the proton is somewhere in the left column. For a phase angle of 9 o'clock, then that proton is somewhere in the right column.

Thus, location has been encoded with phase. For this reason, this gradient is called the *phase encoding gradient* and the image axis along the gradient is called the *phase encoding axis.* Note that unlike the Gss, which must be activated during the 90 degree RF pulse, the phase encoding gradient is turned on and off in the absence of any RF stimulation.

Frequency Encoding

One last spatial dimension remains to be encoded and one last gradient is available to use. Before this last gradient is turned on, the spins are all at the same frequency as shown by Figure 3–11,A. The phase angles are different depending on the location of the spins along the other axis from the prior application of the phase encoding step.

When the third gradient is activated, the magnetic field changes along the gradient and the frequencies of the protons change according to their spatial location (Fig 3–11,B). The only thing different in this instance is that this gradient is turned on *during the echo collection.*

Therefore, this frequency encoded spatial information is detected in the RF output of the echo. For this reason, the last gradient is referred to as the *frequency encoding gradient*

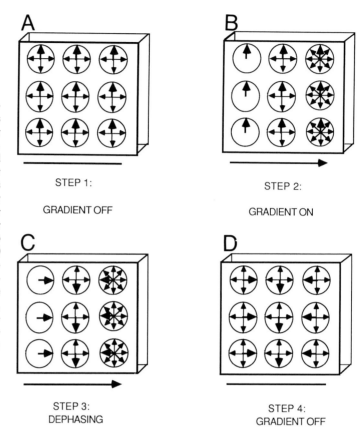

FIG 3–10.
Phase encoding. Frequency is indicated by the number of arrows present and phase is indicated by the direction of the large arrow. With the gradient turned off (**A**) all protons are at the same frequency and phase. When the gradient is turned on, the protons immediately change frequency according to their position along the gradient (**B**). After a few milliseconds the protons also dephase along the gradient (**C**). (**D**) Finally, the phase encoding gradient is turned off and all the protons return to precesssing at the same frequency. The phase angles, however, remain changed according to the position along the gradient that was turned on moments before.

FIG 3–11.
Frequency encoding. **A,** with the gradient turned off, all protons are precessing at the same frequency. The phase angles are different due to the effects of the prior phase encoding step. **B,** when the gradient is turned on, the spin frequencies change according to the location along the gradient.

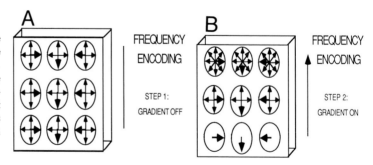

and the image axis along the gradient is the frequency encoded or readout axis. The frequency encoding gradient thus creates a one-to-one correspondence between the frequency of the returned signal and the source's position along the readout direction. Again, the location of the proton along the frequency encoded axis can be determined completely from the strength of readout gradient and the difference between the return signal frequency and resonant frequency of the background field.

When the echo signal is read, detectors that are sensitive to signal amplitude (pixel brightness) as well as phase and frequency (proton location) are used. Thus any protons that produce a signal must ideally fulfill the following conditions:

1. They must be within the selected slice (from the slice selection step).
2. Their locations along the phase axis will be proportional to their phase angle (from the phase encoding step).
3. Their location along the frequency axis will be proportional to their frequency (from the frequency encoding step).

The slice selection gradient determines the scan plane. It is important which is the phase-encoded and frequency-encoded axis because certain artifacts occur only in the phase encoding axis and other artifacts only occur in the readout axis. Therefore, depending on the artifact and the anatomy, it may be necessary to project one artifact in one direction or another by changing these axes.

Pulse Sequence Timing Diagram

As the 2D-FT imaging techniques are better understood it is apparent that split second timing is required for turning on and off the slice select, phase encoding, and frequency encoding gradients and coordinating them with the 90 degree RF pulse and the echo. Just as the symphonic score allows the conductor to follow and understand complex actions that the orchestra will perform, the *pulse sequence timing diagram* allows a better understanding of the actions of MR image formation (Fig 3–12). This graphic display includes not only the 90 and 180 degree RF pulses, the FID, and the echo, but also one timing line for each of the three gradients.

The slice select gradient (G slice) is turned on during the 90 degree RF pulse and the readout gradient (G read) is turned on later when the echo occurs. The phase encoding gradient (G phase) is turned on by itself when no RF activity is occurring.

In practice the pulse sequence waveforms are slightly more complex (Fig 3–12,B). The protons respond the same whether they are experiencing a phase encoding, slice selection, or a frequency encoding gradient. Every time a gradient is turned both the frequency and the phase change.

When the slice selection gradient is on, not only do the frequencies change, but dephasing of the protons also occurs. Thus phase encoding also occurs along this axis when the gradient is activated. In order to negate the phase encoding effects of the slice select and frequency encoding gradients, these gradients are turned on in the opposite direction, resulting in new gradient shapes called *compensatory gradients* (Figs 3–12 and 3–13).

In the pulse sequence timing diagram, these gradients are in the same direction for the readout axis, however, because the action occurs on either side of the 180 degree RF pulse the effects are opposite. No compensatory gradients cancel out phase shifts of the phase encoding gradients for obvious reasons.

The concept of compensatory gradients to zero phase shifts is important. While the present example illustrates the use of such gradients to zero phase shifts for stationary protons, this approach may be applied to correct for higher-order motion terms such as constant velocity, or even acceleration of protons during the duty cycle. These advanced concepts will be covered in Chapter 4.

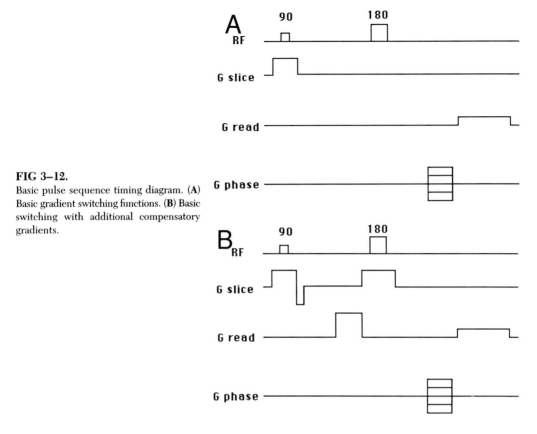

FIG 3–12.
Basic pulse sequence timing diagram. **(A)** Basic gradient switching functions. **(B)** Basic switching with additional compensatory gradients.

Image Formation Matrix

Despite the complexity of gradient actions necessary to spatially encode the signal that is detected in the echo, that single signal is not enough to make an entire image. Instead this process must be repeated many times. Each repetition is referred to as a view, level, or phase encoding step. Modern MR instruments typically acquire from 128 to 384 of these steps to form an image.

Unlike back projection reconstruction where one-dimensional radial projections are sequentially sampled, with 2D-FT the slice select and readout gradients are kept constant while the phase encoding gradient is stepped through many different levels. The slice select

FIG 3–13.
Phase compensation gradient (for stationary spins). The application of the slice select gradient not only changes the proton-resonant frequencies but also causes dephasing. In order to eliminate this unnecessary phase change the gradient is pulsed in the opposite direction (this works well as long as the protons are stationary).

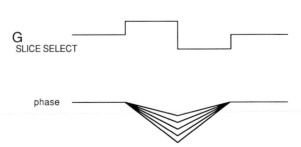

gradient must be turned on the same amount with each view in order to repetitively select the same slice. The readout gradient also remains the same with each of these steps. The only thing that changes between views is the phase encoding gradient which varies through many different steps from very shallow to very steep. The shallow gradient acquisitions sample low spatial frequency information in the image and steeper portions sample its high spatial frequency aspects.

Each time the phase encoding gradient is turned on an echo is collected. The echoes are then digitized and loaded into a 2D data acquisition matrix (Fig 3–14). This display nomenclature is referred to as *k* space. The data are then Fourier transformed in two dimensions (thus 2D-FT) and the phase-frequency information is mapped onto the image by location and the signal amplitude for each pixel is displayed as brightness (Fig 3–15).

NORMAL SPIN ECHO K SPACE DATA ACQUISITION

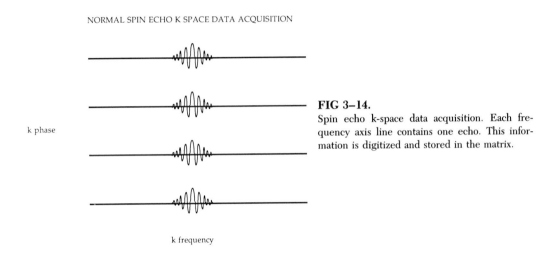

FIG 3–14.
Spin echo k-space data acquisition. Each frequency axis line contains one echo. This information is digitized and stored in the matrix.

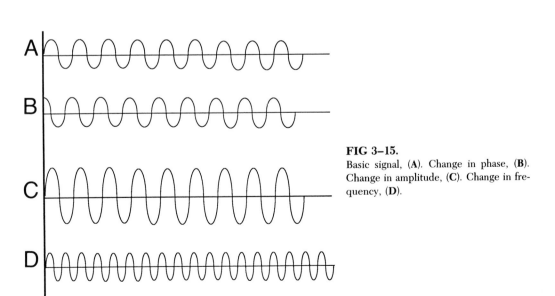

FIG 3–15.
Basic signal, (**A**). Change in phase, (**B**). Change in amplitude, (**C**). Change in frequency, (**D**).

This representation of the untransformed data in the matrix is very interesting because it is essentially holographic information. The raw MR data is like a hologram in that each portion of the data storage plane contains the entire image. The raw data is in holographic form and is converted to an image by the 2D-FT. If the image data is cut into four pieces, four separate sections of the original image will be obtained with spatial resolution of the original image. If the holographic data are divided into four sections, each subset after 2D-FT will contain the entire image but at lower signal-to-noise than the original. This aspect of image information is exploited with fast MR imaging techniques that only acquire a subset of the MR data, thus shortening scan time at the expense of signal-to-noise.

An interesting thing occurs in MR images produced using 2D-FT techniques as a result of the way these data are loaded into the matrix. There is an asymmetry in the two image axes. Not only in the way they are encoded, but also in the way spatial resolution is represented in the image.

The spatial resolution along the frequency axis is determined by how finely the echo is digitized into matrix pixels. If spatial resolution in the frequency axis is to be increased, the signal is subdivided into a larger number of bins. Although there is a decrease in signal-to-noise there is relatively little penalty in image acquisition time because each echo is acquired in just a few milliseconds (Fig 3–16).

To increase the spatial resolution in the phase encoding axis, however, requires more phase encoding steps. The problem here is that each phase encoding step takes one TR time. Therefore spatial resolution is very expensive along this axis. Unlike the frequency encoded axis, spatial resolution along the phase axis costs image acquisition time.

Because of this MR images routinely have higher spatial resolution in the frequency than in the phase encoding axis. Often images are acquired on a 256 × 128 matrix. The axis with the 128 resolution is almost always going to be the phase encoding axis with the higher resolution along the readout axis.

Spatial Resolution

Because extensions of disease are often recognized by subtle alterations in normal anatomy or slight blurring of fascial planes, spatial resolution in MR imaging is very important. A complete discussion of the issues of spatial resolving power for MRI depends on signal-to-noise ratio (SNR), image contrast, motion, and other factors and is beyond the scope of this text.

The limits of spatial resolution are determined in classical optics theory by the wavelength of the electromagnetic radiation forming the image. When a higher spatial resolution is needed

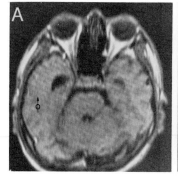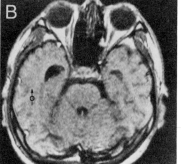

FIG 3–16.
Spatial resolution improvement by increasing the number of phase encoding steps. (**A**) 128 × 256 image. (**B**) 512 × 256 image. The improvement in spatial resolution along the phase axis (θ) is obvious.

it is necessary to use higher and higher frequency radiation to achieve shorter wavelengths.

Since the wavelengths used for MR imaging are on the order of 40 m, according to this theory it should not be possible to resolve an elephant much less human anatomy with MR. These rules are obviously not applicable in this situation. Magnetic resonance image formation works on a completely different principle than conventional optics. In fact the limits of MRI spatial resolution are determined by diffusion rates of protons within the voxel; MR images with pixels as small as 40 μm have been obtained from biologic specimens.[7]

Spatial resolution in MR images is set by how finely the image is divided into pixels (i.e., image matrix size). The other factor that affects the size of each pixel (and thus spatial resolution) is the size of the image or field of view (FOV). The FOV is determined by the gradient amplitude and bandwidth in a similar manner to the control of slice thickness. Both factors must be considered in determining pixel size.

$$\text{Pixel size} = \frac{\text{Field of view}}{\text{Matrix size}}$$

For example, a 10 × 10 image matrix acquired using a 10-cm field of view will result in 1-cm pixels. Spatial resolution can be increased in two ways. The data matrix can be increased to 20 × 20 with a constant FOV and the pixel size will decrease to 0.5 cm (Fig 3–17). The penalty with this approach is primarily time because of the increased acquisition time due to the greater number of phase encoding steps with the larger matrix size.

Alternatively, the matrix size can be kept constant and the field of view decreased to 5 cm. This also results in a 0.5-cm pixel. The major drawback here is that signal to noise is lower and certain types of artifacts (aliasing or wraparound) are more common.

Reduced Bandwidth Technique

Image signal-to-noise can be increased by using reduced bandwidth image acquisition.

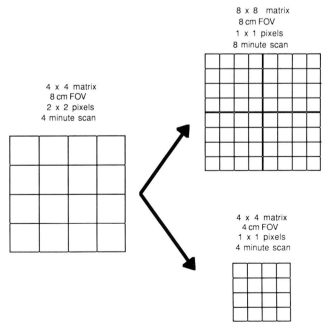

8 x 8 matrix
8 cm FOV
1 x 1 pixels
8 minute scan

4 x 4 matrix
8 cm FOV
2 x 2 pixels
4 minute scan

4 x 4 matrix
4 cm FOV
1 x 1 pixels
4 minute scan

FIG 3–17.
Field of view demonstration showing spatial resolution/time tradeoffs. Spatial resolution can be increased by using a larger matrix at the expense of increased acquisition time. Spatial resolution may be increased while preserving acquisition time by using a smaller field of view at the expense of increased aliasing artifacts and decreased SNR.

The smaller the image bandwidth the narrower the FOV so that in order to maintain the same image size, the gradient amplitude must be lowered. The advantage of this approach is that SNR is increased without any increase in imaging time.[8]

There are several disadvantages to reduced bandwidth technique. The lower gradient amplitude increases certain types of image artifacts such as chemical shift misregistration errors. This is less of a problem on low- to midfield instruments where chemical shift misregistration errors are less pronounced than on high field machines.

Image bandwidth is inversely proportional to sampling time (the time that the signal is sampled around the echo). As sampling time is increased, the minimum echo time that can be used in a given pulse sequence is increased (Fig 3–18,A and B). Therefore this approach is most effective with longer TE sequences (which generally have lower SNR than short TE sequences). Some manufacturers automatically narrow the bandwidth with increasing TE in order to increase the sampling time (Fig 3–18,B and C). Another approach to allow longer sampling times and reduced bandwidth with shorter TE times is to sample asymmetrically around the echo (Fig 3–18,D).

Multiecho Pulse Sequence

The time between 90 degree pulses (repetition time or TR) is also sometimes referred to as the *duty cycle* because it represents the total amount of time required for each view or phase encoding step in image formation. The amount of time in each duty cycle from the

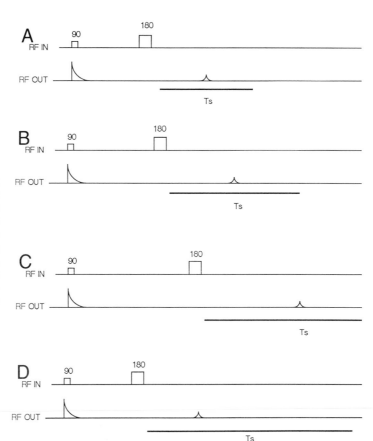

FIG 3–18.
Matched bandwidth illustration. **A** and **B**, increasing the sampling time (Ts) in a given sequence narrows the bandwidth and increases the SNR. As the TE is increased from **A–C**, the Ts may be increased thus allowing a narrower bandwidth. **D**, asymmetric sampling around the echo can further reduce the bandwidth (and increase Ts and SNR) for a given TE.

90 degree pulse until the echo is collected is referred to as the echo time or TE. This time is typically ten or even a hundred times shorter than the TR for many pulse sequences. Therefore, most of the time in the duty cycle is not spent on data collection but rather just waiting. This may seem like a considerable inefficiency because the long TR is what ultimately determines scan time.

The long TR costs scan time and patient throughput. Making the duty cycle shorter by decreasing the TR will result in faster image formation times, but will also affect image quality by lowering the signal to noise and increasing T1 weighting of the image. Although active data collection is not being done during most of the cycle, the long dead time is necessary in order for T1 recovery to occur. This is especially necessary for T2-weighted images.

One thing that can be done to exploit this dead time is referred to as *multiecho technique*. After the first echo is collected it is a simple matter to wait a short amount of time [e.g., 1/2 echo time (TE)] and then give another 180 degree pulse and collect a second echo a short time later (e.g., TE) (Fig 3–19). The second echo data are then collected onto a separate matrix and transformed into a second image. This can be done again and again to produce third, fourth, and fifth echoes. In general, the longer the TR relative to the TE (i.e., greater dead time) the more echoes that can be collected. For practical reasons only a first and second echo are obtained in most situations. Importantly, both the first and second echo images are obtained in the same amount of image acquisition time as the first echo.

Rules for Multiecho Sequences

1. All images must have same repetition time (TR).
2. Echoes are of same slice.
3. Echo times may be nonmultiples—assymetric echo.
4. More echoes are possible with long TR and short TE.

Both first and second echo images will necessarily have the same TR time and be of the same slice (they both have the same 90 degree pulse and slice select gradient). The second image will, of course, be more T2-weighted (because of the longer TE). Originally it was easiest to use TEs that were multiples of each other for multiecho sequences such as TR 2000 with a TE of 28 to 56 or 56 to 112. These are called *symmetrical multiecho* acquisition because of the symmetric TEs.

The problem with multiecho sequences in general is that although they are very efficient timewise (two image sets are obtained in the amount of time it takes to acquire only one), the contrast separation between the two sequences is relatively little. This is because both

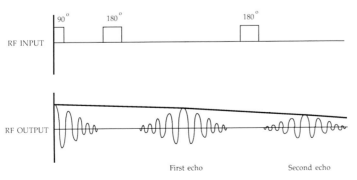

FIG 3–19.
Multiecho pulse sequence. After the first echo is collected following the 180 degree RF pulse a second 180 degree pulse is given to refocus the protons and form a second echo.

sequences have the same TR. Thus the short TE sequence may not be particularly T1-weighted and the long TE sequence may not be particularly T2-weighted.

In an effort to improve this situation, *asymmetric multiecho* acquisition sequences were developed. These allow greater separation of the TE for improved contrast distinction (Fig 3–20). So instead of doing a TR 2000 and TE 28-56 double echo, one can do a 2000/20-90 double echo. Though in many cases this will provide great enough contrast separation of the images, occasionally when heavy T1 and T2 weighting are required it is necessary to acquire two separate pulse sequences (at a greater cost of time).

Multiecho, Multirepetition Rate Pulse Sequence

An alternative approach to obtaining improved contrast separation in two pulse sequences while still saving time compared to individual separate T1- and T2-weighted acquisition is the multiecho, multirepetition rate sequence (MEMR). Although this method takes longer than the double echo, it is still faster than acquiring each sequence separately. Also an equal number of slices for both T1 and T2 sequences is obtained with MEMR. This is faster than the individual acquisition rates but slower than a double echo of SE/2000/90 and SE/2000/20. The greater contrast difference with MEMR than with standard double echo is accomplished by interleaving the duty cycles of each sequence (Figs 3–20 and 3–21).

Multislice Pulse Sequence

The dead time in the duty cycle may also be used to obtain multiple slices. Instead of stimulating a single slice and then waiting, another 90 to 180 degree pulse train may be delivered after the echo to select another slice and obtain multiple slices in the same amount of time it takes to obtain a single slice (Fig 3–22). For this to work, a change in the slice select gradient or the 90 degree RF pulse frequency is needed for each new slice. Thus a new slice is selected in a different location from the first slice so that the relaxation processes don't interfere with one another (Fig 3–23).

In multislice acquisitions, like multiecho, all the slices have the same TR. With a longer TR and a shorter TE, there is more dead time and more slices can be acquired. The slices must be in different locations (they can't overlap) because they are all being acquired simultaneously, otherwise their separate relaxation processes will interfere with each other.

Rules for Multislice Sequences

1. All images must have same TR.
2. More slices are possible with long TR and short TE.
3. Slices cannot overlap.

These rules bring up a problem in the acquisition of contiguous slices with a multislice sequence. The shape of the RF energy delivered during the 90 degree pulse determines the shape of the MR slice profile. Originally most RF slice profiles were gaussian because it was the most simple approach. The convention for determining the thickness of such gaussian profiles is called the "full-width half-maximum" thickness. This nominal slice thickness is determined by measuring the width at the point of the half the maximum of the amplitude (Fig 3–24).

The foregoing condition creates a problem in that although the slice thickness is defined by the full-width half-maximum measurement, a much thicker region of tissue is being

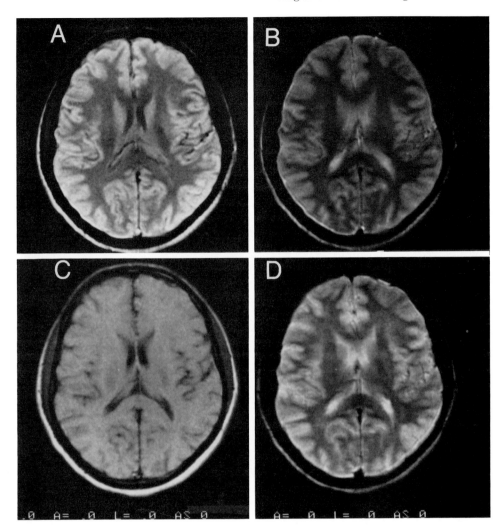

FIG 3–20.
Comparison of multiecho techniques. **A** and **B,** asymmetric double echo (SE/2000/30-85) sequence produces a proton density image (**A**) (SE/2000/30) and a more T2-weighted scan (**B**) (SE/2000/85). **C** and **D,** The MEMR sequence has greater contrast separation. The short sequence (**C**) (SE/366/30) is more T1-weighted than (**A**). The T2-weighted image (**D**) (SE/2381/85) is similar to (**B**).

stimulated because the RF pulse profile is gaussian. Thus if slices are pushed any closer together the tails of the gaussian profiles will overlap and image artifacts will result due to interslice crosstalk (Fig 3–25).

In multislice MRI, the slices are often thinner than the center-to-center offsets, for example, 3-mm slices obtained every 5 mm or 9-mm-thick slices every 12 mm. It is not possible to obtain contiguous slices using gaussian RF profiles because the full-width half-maximum thicknesses result in crosstalk.

There are three ways to obtain contiguous MR slices. The first way is to use gaussian slice profiles and first scan the patient with a single multislice sequence with the required gaps. Then the patient is rescanned with another multislice sequence with gaps shifted one-

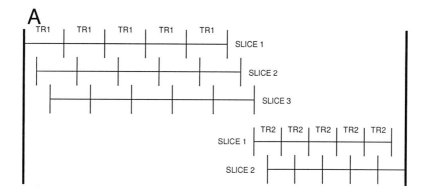

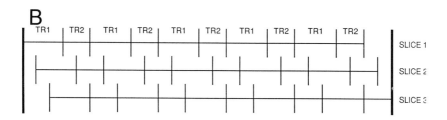

FIG 3–21.
Comparison of standard double acquisition with MEMR acquisition. **A,** In the standard acquisition, the long TR sequence (TR1) produces three slices and the short TR sequence (TR2) produces two slices. **B,** The MEMR sequence allows three slices to be obtained with both TR sequences in less time than for the five slices produced in **A.**

half slice thickness so the acquisitions are interleaved (Fig 3–26). This works well for producing overlapping slices except that the study of course requires twice the scan time of a single multislice acquisition.

Approaches to Contiguous Section MR Imaging

1. Interleaved double acquisition
2. Sinc RF waveform (long TE)
3. 3D-FT acquisition (short TR)

A more elegant and time-effective way to get contiguous slices is to redesign the RF pulse profile. If it were possible to generate square RF profiles instead of the gaussian profiles, slices could be contiguous without having overlapping tails.

The Fourier transform of a gaussian RF slice profile is a gaussian RF slice profile (Fig 3–27). However, it is possible to obtain more of a square-shaped profile in the frequency domain if the shape of the time domain signal is changed to a *"sinc" function.* A sinc function is similar to a gaussian profile with additional curves at its extremes. Mathematically, it is the (sin x/x) function. When this sinc shaped RF pulse profile is Fourier transformed, the resulting slice profile is square in shape. These square profiles permit nearly contiguous slices (i.e., 3-mm-thick slices with a 0.2 mm gap).[9]

The problem is that the additional side lobes of the sinc RF pulse take additional time to deliver. Thus sinc RF pulses limit how short a TE that can be used. If very short TEs are

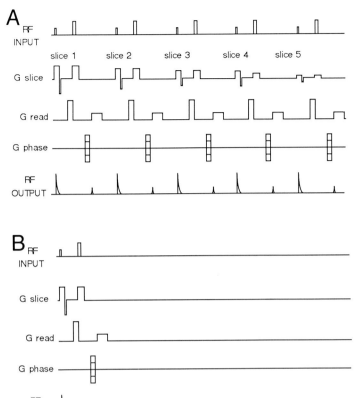

FIG 3–22.
A, multislice pulse sequence timing diagram for a five-slice acquisition. The slice select gradient (G slice) changes for each 90 degree pulse in order to specify a new slice. **B,** standard single slice pulse sequence timing diagram for comparison.

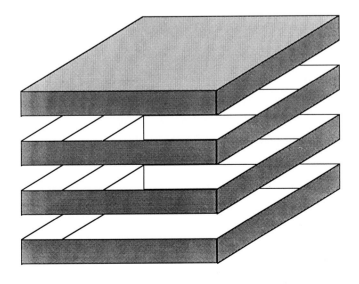

FIG 3–23.
Multislice 2D-FT acquisition.

FIG 3–24.
Gaussian RF slice profile.

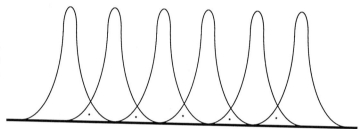

FULL WIDTH
HALF MAXIMUM

millimeter

FIG 3–25.
Interslice crosstalk *(asterisk)* results from attempts at contiguous multislice sequences using gaussian RF slice profiles.

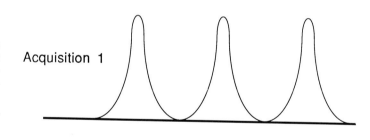

FIG 3–26.
Multislice interleaved acquisition. Acquisition 2 is shifted one-half slice thickness from acquisition 1 and the resulting set of images are interleaved and overlapping. The only problem is that the study takes twice as long as a single-acquisition multislice sequence.

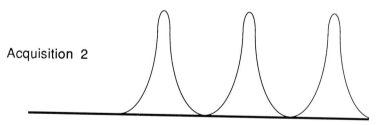

Acquisition 1

Acquisition 2

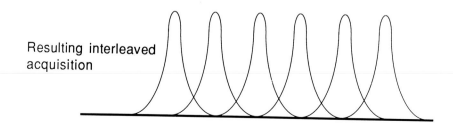

Resulting interleaved acquisition

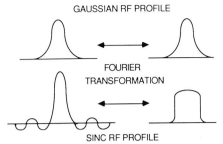

FIG 3–27.
Radiofrequency pulse profile options. The Fourier transformation of a gaussian profile is a gaussian profile. The frequency domain representation of the sinc function, however, is closer to a square wave, which permits closer slices in a multislice acquisition.

used with sinc RF pulses, there is insufficient time to deliver the complex RF pulse (Fig 3–28). Sinc RF pulses are therefore best implemented on pulse sequences with longer TEs. If the number of side lobes is reduced in order to allow short TEs, eventually there will become a simple gaussian RF pulse profile which then requires gaps between slices. To obtain contiguous multislices for short TE, T1-weighted images (without interleaving), a third strategy called three-dimensional Fourier transformation imaging (3D-FT) is necessary, the details of which will be covered below.

Either multislice or multiecho may be used in MR imaging to take advantage of the dead time in the duty cycle. In fact, often both multislice and multi-echo are performed in the same sequence in many cases. The only constraint is the finite time from the TE until the

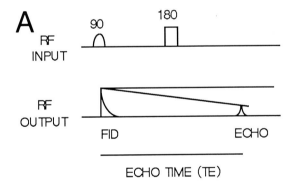

FIG 3–28.
Comparison of gaussian (**A**) and sinc (**B**) RF pulse profiles. The additional RF stimulation time required by the use of sinc RF pulse profiles places lower limits on the TE time in a given pulse sequence.

next 90 degree pulse (i.e., TR-TE). So in a given situation it may be possible to obtain either one slice with ten echoes or ten slices with one echo, or most often combinations such as five slices with two echoes.

Orthogonal Scan Plane Selection

MRI systems have three separate physical magnetic field gradient coils, each capable of creating a gradient field along one of three orthogonal directions. These are usually chosen to coincide with the principal axes of the patient: superior to inferior (Z axis), anterior to posterior (Y axis), and left to right (X axis) (Fig 3–29). If each of the three physical coils is assigned a separate gradient function (slice selection, phase encoding, or frequency encoding), images in the three principal planes may be obtained. For each of these three planes, there are two choices for the phase encoding direction. When an axial scan is set up, Gz is assigned as slice select and there is some default for which is phase encoding and which is readout. The act of selecting the scan plane is the assignment of function to these physical gradients (Fig 3–30).

A given gradient becomes the slice select gradient by virtue of the fact that it turns on during the 90 degree slice select pulse. Another gradient becomes the readout gradient because it is turned on during the readout. Timing is everything and that is why the representation of these choices is called a pulse sequence timing diagram.

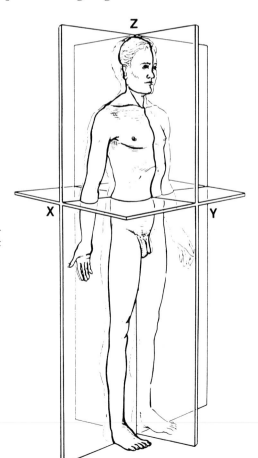

FIG 3–29.
Conventions for scan plane axes relative to the patient. Superior to inferior (Z axis), anterior to posterior (Y axis), left to right (X axis).

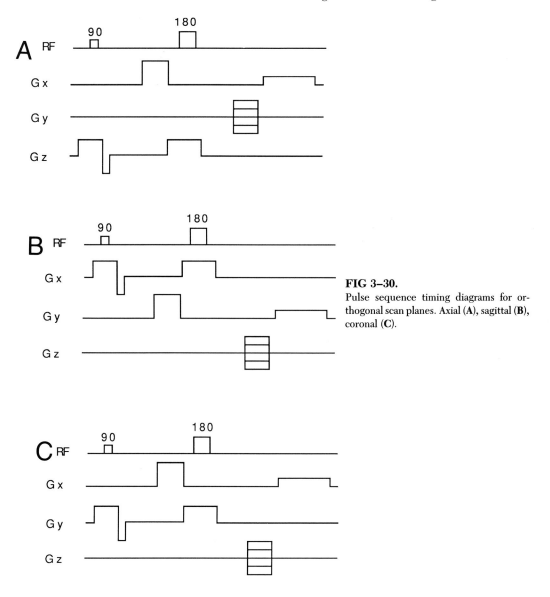

FIG 3–30.
Pulse sequence timing diagrams for orthogonal scan planes. Axial (**A**), sagittal (**B**), coronal (**C**).

Oblique Image Formation

The capability to obtain images in a variety of planes has been heralded as a fundamental advantage of MR. Oblique imaging has been applied to numerous areas, including the spine, knee, heart, and orbits.

Nobody ever said that the principal axes of the image volume, as defined by the slice selection (Gss), frequency encoding (Gf), and phase encoding gradients (Gpe), respectively, must coincide directly with the three principal axes of the gradient coils (Gx, Gy, Gz). In fact, it is possible to define a new coordinate system obtainable through a general rotation.[10]

The magnetic gradient field is a vector whose direction and magnitude changes in a carefully prescribed fashion during the course of a scan. The gradient contributions required in each of the principle axes are easily obtained by multiplying this vector by a rotational matrix to produce a eulerian rotation. As a practical matter, it is easiest to perform the first rotation about the phase encoding axis, due to the similarity between the slice select and readout gradient waveforms (Figs 3–31 and 3–32).

The combination of principal gradients (Gx, Gy, Gz) necessary to define new gradients (Gss, Gf, Gpe) for an oblique imaging plane rotated about the Y axis with a eulerian angle θ, would be

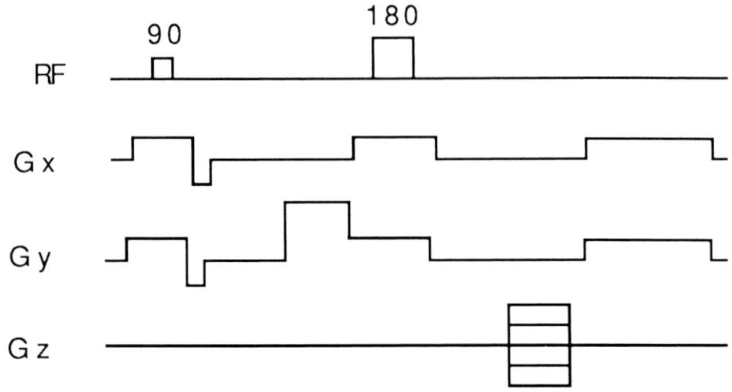

FIG 3–31.
Pulse sequence timing diagram for an oblique image. Slice selection and readout are accomplished by simultaneous application of Gx and Gy to create new functional gradients.

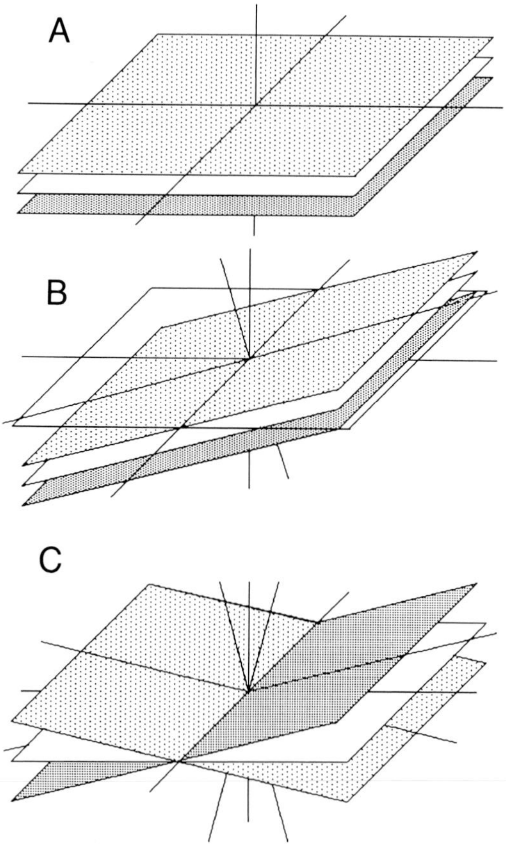

FIG 3–32.
Multislice options. **A,** orthogonal sequence. **B,** oblique sequence. **C,** MAVIN.

$$Gss = Gx \cos \theta - Gz \sin \theta$$

$$Gf = Gx \sin \theta + Gz \cos \theta$$

$$Gpe = Gy$$

Since the phase encoding axis could be chosen to be along the X, Y, or Z axis, oblique images can be obtained ranging between sagittal to coronal, axial to sagittal, or coronal to axial by using a single axis of rotation.

For a more general rotation, the second eulerian angle could be chosen to be a rotation about the frequency encoding gradient. By using two rotation angles, images for any possible slice angles could be obtained. Although oblique images with rotations about a single axis are useful in most situations where obliques are required, generalized obliques using two Euler angles are sometimes valuable in certain areas such as cardiac imaging.

Multiangle Obliques

So far, all images produced by a multislice oblique pulse sequence have been parallel to each other and positioned at a fixed interval. This limitation required that for each separate oblique plane in which images were obtained a separate pulse sequence had to be performed, which resulted in lengthy examination times. In fact there is no absolute requirement that all slices in a multislice oblique section have to have the same angle of obliquity and interslice interval.

Instead what can be done is to independently select each slice angle of obliquity and interslice interval in a single multislice sequence. This new technique is referred to as *multiple-angle, variable-interval, nonorthogonal* imaging technique (MAVIN) (Fig 3–32,C).[11]

MAVIN and other similar techniques allow the independent choice of slice angle and position for each image in a multislice sequence obtained in the same time necessary to perform a parallel slice, fixed interval, multislice sequence with the same number of images (Fig 3–33). Image interpretation is generally easiest (less confusing) if only the first angle of rotation is used, creating imaging planes that vary from axial to sagittal, sagittal to coronal, or coronal to axial.

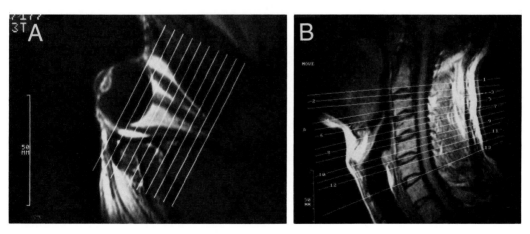

FIG 3–33.
Oblique image options. **A,** all slices parallel, **B,** MAVIN.

Restricting the choices of oblique imaging planes in this way also allows images previously performed in one of the principle axes to be used as a scout or reference scan. The principal gradient combinations (Gss, Gpe, Gf) necessary to define new gradients for a three slice MAVIN sequence with single eulerian rotations of θ_1, θ_2, and θ_3 about the X axis would be as follows

$$Gss1 = Gy \cos \theta_1 - Gz \sin \theta_1$$

$$Gf1 = Gy \sin \theta_1 + Gz \cos \theta_1$$

$$Gpe1 = Gx$$

$$Gss2 = Gy \cos \theta_2 - Gz \sin \theta_2$$

$$Gf2 = Gy \sin \theta_2 + Gz \cos \theta_2$$

$$Gpe2 = Gx$$

$$Gss3 = Gy \cos \theta_3 - Gz \sin \theta_3$$

$$Gf3 = Gy \sin \theta_3 + Gz \cos \theta_3$$

$$Gpe3 = Gx$$

Although the algebra required to perform MAVIN may be simple, the acquisition of quality images in oblique planes requires precise control of individual gradient coils. Any nonlinearity of the gradient response to changes in current invalidates the algebra, necessitating corrections which may be impossible to make. At the point of intersection of multiple planes, local changes in repetition time (interslice crosstalk) result in local loss of signal along the line of intersection. For this reason, scan planes are chosen so that the intersection is away from the region of interest.

Strategies for Fast MR Scanning

There are a number of reasons to develop strategies for fast MR scanning. The speed of scanning determines patient throughput and ultimately cost-effectiveness of MR imaging in any given clinical situation. Patient acceptance also improves with decreasing scan times.

Shorter imaging times often result in improved image quality by the reduction of motion and flow artifacts. With a moderate reduction in scan time, breath holding studies of the abdomen are possible. With even greater improvements in scanning time some researchers are already producing nongated cardiac examinations.

The total time required for a given 2D-FT MR image acquisition is described by the following equation:

$$\text{2D-FT scan time} = \text{TR} \times n \times \text{NEX}$$

where TR equals the repetition time, n equals the number of phase encoding steps (or views) obtained, and NEX equal the number of excitations (or repetitions) used. All techniques for fast scanning in MR are based on the reduction of the time required for one or more of these parameters in the imaging process.

For the purposes of this discussion various fast MR scanning strategies will be examined according to which aspect of total scan time they primarily optimize. For each fast MR scanning technique the time savings will be weighed against the cost in image signal to noise, contrast resolution, and spatial resolution. Any additional artifacts or degradation in image quality associated with a given fast scanning technique will also be covered.

Reduced Number of Excitations

Signal averaging (increasing NEX) was discussed earlier as a technique to improve SNR and MR images. In addition to signal to noise improvements, averaging was also useful in early systems to eliminate certain types of artifacts. A straightforward approach to fast MR scanning is to decrease the number of excitations. Since SNR improves with increasing NEX as the square root of NEX, fewer excitations will result in lower signal to noise.

Fortunately, signal-to-noise in modern MR systems has improved sufficiently using such techniques as surface coils, bandwidth reduction, and optimized system electronics to the point where signal averaging is less necessary and images are routinely obtained with one excitation on many instruments. In order to improve image acquisition speed beyond this point other strategies must be employed.

Reduced Number of Phase Encoding Steps

The next group of strategies for fast MR scanning is based on reducing the number of views (or phase encoding steps) to produce the image. For all techniques listed, the reduction in image time is paid for with reductions in image SNR and other factors.

Conjugate Data Synthesis.—Consider the k-space representation of data required in conventional 2D-FT MR imaging (see Fig 3–14). In this representation, each data line along the X axis is produced from a spin or gradient echo acquired at the TE. These data lines encode spatial information along the X axis and also contribute spatial information to a column along the Y axis. The acquired echo signal plotted along the X axis is called the *time domain signal.*

All the points in a column along a constant value of X after the X axis Fourier transformation will also have the shape of an echo along the column of the Y axis. This Y axis information is called the *pseudo–time domain echo* because it is mathematically equivalent to the signal shape along the X axis (time domain echo) (Fig 3–34).

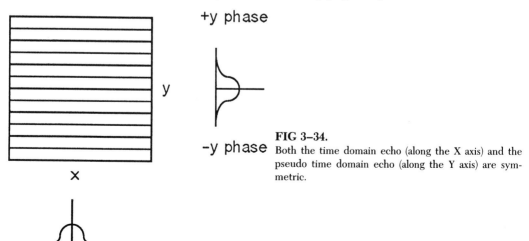

FIG 3–34.
Both the time domain echo (along the X axis) and the pseudo time domain echo (along the Y axis) are symmetric.

The pseudo–time domain echo is symmetric about the Y axis if the T2 of the tissues is much longer than the echo width. This is a reasonable assumption in human imaging. Because of the symmetry about the Y axis it is possible to acquire only one-half of the phase encoding steps to form the echo and then synthesize the other half through a technique known as conjugate data synthesis (Fig 3–35).[12]

While this technique requires additional postprocessing computation, no additional scan time is required. The reduction in scan time is possible with reduction in image signal-to-noise, although contrast and spatial resolution are largely preserved (Fig 3–36).

Zero Filling.—Another approach to fast scanning using a reduced number of phase encoding steps is the technique of zero filling. The computer implementation of the Fourier transformation used in MRI is known as the fast Fourier transformation (FFT). Unfortunately, because the FFT algorithm requires a power of 2 data points in order to run, the data matrix must be 64, 128, 256, or 512 points in size. This limitation places constraints on imaging because while one may want to accept longer scan times than are necessary to fill a 256 matrix with 256 phase encoding steps, the next largest size of 512 may result in an unacceptably long scan time.

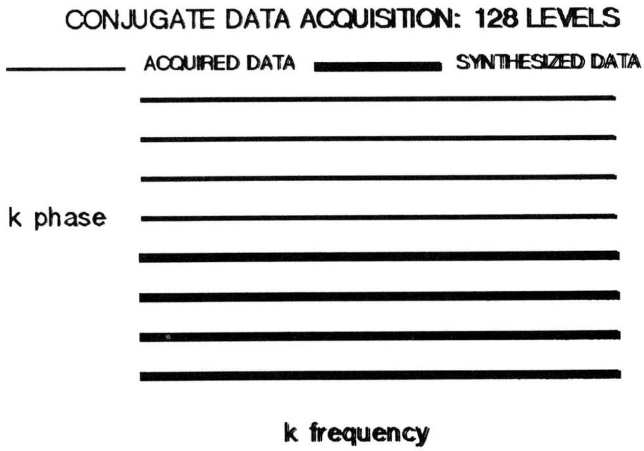

FIG 3–35.
K-space representation of conjugate data synthesis acquisition. Only half the levels are directly acquired (thin lines) and the remaining half are synthesized (bold lines).

CONJUGATE DATA ACQUISITION: 128 LEVELS

_____ ACQUIRED DATA ▬▬▬▬ SYNTHESIZED DATA

k phase

k frequency

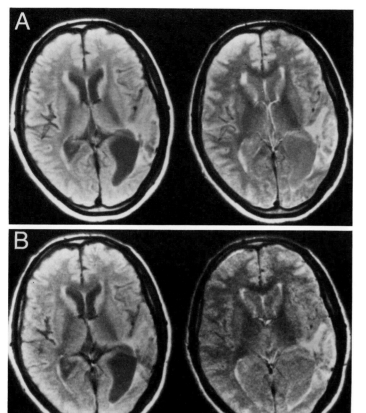

FIG 3–36.
Comparison of conjugate data synthesis with standard techniques in a patient with cortical infarction. **A,** spin echo images (SE/2000/28 and SE/2000/56) with standard data acquisition requiring 8 minutes to obtain. **B,** spin echo images (SE/2000/28 and SE/2000/56) with conjugate data synthesis of the same patient which required 4.2 minutes to obtain. Note minimal loss of signal to noise. (Courtesy of Allan Stein, M.D.)

An alternative to acquiring a full power of 2 data set is possible by acquiring less than a power of 2 dataset and filling the rest of the matrix with zeros. This allows the FFT to run yet makes possible much shorter scan times.[13]

Unlike data conjugation, the technique of zero filling only acquires the central portion of the k-space data set and fills the outer sections with zeros in order to produce a full power of two data set (Fig 3–37). In the case of 50% zero filling, a savings of 50% scan time would be traded off against decreased spatial resolution in the phase encoding axis only as well as a slight increase in artifacts in the same axis known as truncation errors. These will be discussed in Chapter 4. Interestingly, signal-to-noise is largely preserved and spatial resolution in the frequency encoding access is also unchanged. Like conjugate data synthesis, zero filling also produces reductions in scan time with no significant change in contrast resolution. Zero filling techniques are widely used throughout the industry by virtually every manufacturer although in many cases the applications are transparent to the user.

Echo Planar Imaging.—The most dramatic reductions in MR imaging time to date are those obtained using the technique of *echo planar imaging.*[14] In *echo planar* imaging, successive spin echoes in a given acquisition line are used to encode position information. That means that complete image encoding can be acquired from a train of successive spin echoes within one TR interval rather than phase encoding a separate line of data with every TR interval.

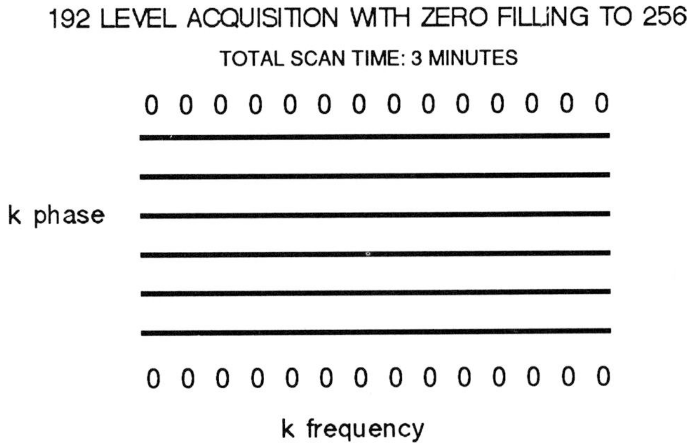

192 LEVEL ACQUISITION WITH ZERO FILLING TO 256

TOTAL SCAN TIME: 3 MINUTES

0 0 0 0 0 0 0 0 0 0 0 0 0 0

k phase

0 0 0 0 0 0 0 0 0 0 0 0 0 0

k frequency

FIG 3–37.
Zero filling. K space representation of a 256 × 256 matrix zero filled to allow a 192 × 256 acquisition. By acquiring fewer levels, the scan time is 25% less than that required for the full 256 matrix.

The limiting step is the time of T2 decay. For human soft tissues this is approximately 50 msec. Therefore, in order to encode an entire image of a 128 data points the entire process must be accomplished within 50 msec. This is obviously an incredibly demanding process for the imaging gradients which in this situation require an echo interval of 25 msec. Echo planar imaging therefore usually requires specialized hardware as well as software for implementation. Because of these limitations pure echo planar imaging is difficult to implement on an image matrix sizes larger than 64 or 128 data points.

Despite these limitations, in some clinical situations the compromises in signal to noise, spatial resolution, in contrast resolution of echo planar imaging are acceptable in order to have total imaging scan times in the order of 50 msec.

Hybrid Imaging.—Because of the technical difficulties of implementing echo planar imaging, a hybrid form combining echo planar with 2D-FT MRI has been developed.[15] Rather than sampling all of k-space with oscillating phase encoding gradients during a single repetition time, hybrid techniques sample additional levels with generally two or four echoes during each excitation (Fig 3–38).

In addition to making less demands on the imaging gradients, hybrid techniques are a significant time savings over 2D-FT techniques although they are much slower than pure echo planar imaging. Compromises in signal-to-noise and spatial resolution are also made compared to conventional 2D-FT imaging (Fig 3–39). The fact that multiple data points are acquired during subsequent echoes for a given image results in alterations in contrast resolution compared to standard 2D-FT techniques.

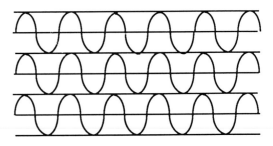

k phase

FIG 3–38.
Hybrid k-space acquisition. Each excitation samples three lines of k space.

k frequency

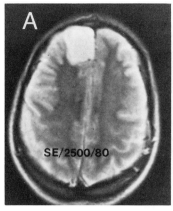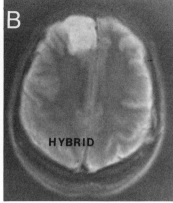

FIG 3–39.
Comparison of standard 2D-FT technique with hybrid scanning in a patient with a frontal glioma. **A,** axial (SE/2500/80) image (NEX = 1) which required 10.6 minutes to obtain. **B,** axial (SE/2500/80) hybrid image which required 2.6 minutes for acquisition. There is some loss of signal-to-noise (Courtesy of Lee Chui, M.D.)

Reduced Repetition Time

The last group of techniques for fast MR scanning reduce acquisition time by reducing the TR. In standard 2D-FT spin echo imaging, a long TR time is necessary to allow longitudinal magnetization recovery in order to obtain T2-weighted images. Therefore, shortening of the TR time also results in increased T1 weighting as well as significant decreases in image signal-to-noise.

Driven Equilibrium.—Driven equilibrium or driven equilibrium Fourier transform (DEFT) techniques decrease the amount of time required for T2-weighted images by allowing shorter TR times to be used in imaging.[16] The DEFT technique depends on the fact that after data collection a second 180 degree RF pulse may be applied to refocus the transverse nuclear magnetization so that it can be easily reoriented with a driven equilibrium RF pulse.

A conventional 90 to 180 degree pulse train is used and the first echo collected. A second 180 degree refocusing pulse is delivered and a second echo is generated. Gradients are also applied in such a way that at the point of the echo dephasing effects due to previously applied gradients cancel out. The key to the pulse sequence is that at this point a 90 degree RF pulse is applied which rotates a transverse magnetization back into the equilibrium position with the static magnetic field. The affect of this second 90 degree pulse is to drive the transverse magnetization back to the equilibrium position thus simulating an infinite TR time (Fig 3–40).

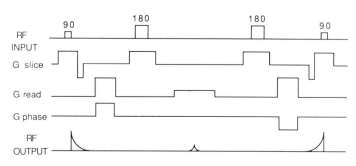

FIG 3–40.
Driven equilibrium (DEFT) pulse sequence timing diagram.

With driven equilibrium it is possible to obtain T2-weighted images without having to wait the amount of time for long TR periods necessary with standard 2D-FT techniques. A driven equilibrium T2-weighted image may be obtained in the same or less time as a heavily T1-weighted image. While driven equilibrium has been implemented in the laboratory it is exceedingly difficult to perform in clinical practice and has so far seen little widespread clinical application.

Magnetic Field Gradient Echo Technique.—This technique allows extremely fast MR scanning through the marked reduction of repetition time. Because of the time required to deliver a 180 degree RF pulse, the production of a spin echo is not feasible when the TR is extremely short. Instead, refocusing is accomplished using magnetic field gradients to refocus the spins in the transverse plane. The elimination of the 180 degree pulse also lowers the RF energy deposition which can be a concern with high-field imaging. This use of magnetic field gradients allows for a TR as short as 30 msec.[17]

With a short TR, however, SNR drops because little time is left for longitudinal magnetization recovery before the next 90 degree pulse. An improvement in SNR can be achieved for short TR sequences by using flip angles less than 90 degrees (Figs 3–41 and 3–42). This leaves a residual vector of magnetization in the longitudinal plane at the beginning of the duty cycle. In addition to improving signal-to-noise, the narrow flip angles also affect contrast and T2-weighted contrast relationships are possible with very narrow flip angles and short scan times.

Because of the decreased efficiency of refocusing the spins the technique is extremely sensitive to magnetic field homogeneity (T2* effects). Fortunately, most static magnetic fields in MRI have acceptable uniformity for the implementation of this technique. However, in clinical images there is a dramatic increased sensitivity to magnetic field inhomogeneity within the patient due to magnetic susceptibility effects of iron or implanted ferromagnetic surgical clips (Fig 3–43).

This phenomenon has both good and bad effects. It improves the detection of small areas of deoxyhemoglobin in acute hemorrhage or areas of hemosiderin. It also increases artifacts

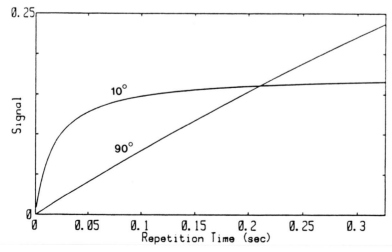

FIG 3–41.
Plot of signal vs. repetition time for 10 degree and 90 degree flip angles. For shorter TRs (<200 msec) the narrower flip angle gives an improved signal.

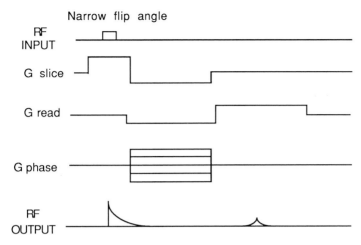

FIG 3–42.
Simplified gradient echo pulse sequence timing diagram.

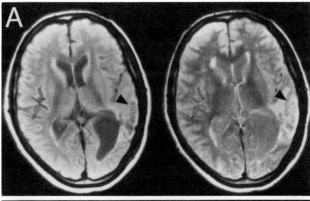

FIG 3–43.
Comparison of field echo with standard spin echo technique in a patient with hemorrhagic cortical infarction (also seen in Figure 3–36). These images were obtained at 0.35 T. **A,** spin echo images (SE/2000/28 and SE/2000/56) with standard data acquisition show an area of high signal consistent with cortical infarction (*arrowhead*). **B,** field echo images with narrow flip angle to emphasize T2* weighting show focal areas of decreased signal (*arrowhead*) due to deoxyhemoglobin in the acute hemorrhage (Courtesy of Allan Stein, M.D.)

from ferromagnetic implanted materials and areas of differing susceptibility. While the effect increases in proportion to field strength with gradient echo sequences, the dependence on field strength is less than with spin echo where it is proportional to field strength squared.

The technique also is extremely sensitive to flow because selective 180° pulses are not used for refocusing. Flow void effects (which will be covered below) primarily occur at extremely high velocities or with turbulence, and most structures appear as increased signal proportional to velocity.

This technique, known by the generic name of *field echo* or *gradient echo,* has been implemented on virtually every MR system today and has a variety of acronyms developed by the manufacturers such as FLASH (fast low-angle shot) and GRASS (gradient recalled acquisition in a steady state) scanning.

Fast MR scanning may be accomplished through a number of strategies as discussed above. Each technique trades off improvements in scan time for compromises in signal to noise, spatial resolution, contrast resolution, and/or other imaging artifacts. Fortunately, most imaging systems now have significant signal-to-noise improvements accomplished through electronics or coil technology to such an extent that this is often an acceptable compromise for improvement in scanning time.

The scanning strategies discussed are in a variety of stages of clinical implementation although several are already in widespread use. The techniques were discussed separately for convenience, however, most strategies can be combined in order to have a further improvement in imaging time.

THREE-DIMENSIONAL FOURIER TRANSFORMATION IMAGING

Instead of acquiring multiple single-slice sequences (2D-FT), another technique of MRI acquires an entire volume of information by an approach known as three-dimensional Fourier transform imaging (3D-FT). The volume acquisition is made up of multiple contiguous voxels which may be cubic (isotropic) or oblong (anisotropic) (Fig 3–44). By acquiring anisotropic voxels a larger volume may be covered in the same scan time while still permitting contiguous slices. Isotropic acquisition is particularly valuable (although it takes longer to acquire than anisotropic) because it allows reformation of image data in any plane without significant loss of resolution.

The advantages of 3D-FT is that since the entire volume of the image has been acquired, images in any plane can be generated after the patient has left the clinic (recall that to obtain a new plane in high resolution with 2D-FT the patient must be rescanned). In addition, the

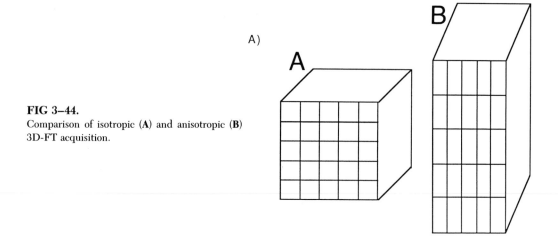

FIG 3–44.
Comparison of isotropic (**A**) and anisotropic (**B**) 3D-FT acquisition.

interslice interval is generally very small since it is determined by the space between the voxels. 3D-FT is thus a way to obtain contiguous slices without having to use sinc RF pulses or interleaved acquisitions.

In general terms, 3D-FT imaging is accomplished by exciting the whole volume without turning on any gradients during the slice selection step, that is, by stimulating the whole head. Then phase encoding is done in two axes. Finally, readout occurs in just one direction (Fig 3–45).

This additional axis of phase encoding results in a much longer scan time compared to 2D-FT imaging. While 2D-FT scan time is determined by the following equation:

$$2\text{D-FT scan time} = \text{TR} \times n \times \text{NEX}$$

the time for a 3D-FT imaging sequence is determined by a different equation:

$$3\text{D-FT scan time} = \text{TR} \times n1 \times n2 \times \text{NEX}$$

Therefore 3-D imaging is very time-intensive. Because of this, T1-weighted images are the most practical to obtain. Short TR sequences using gradient echo technique are particularly useful.

3D-FT is primarily valuable in areas of the body where anatomy is a priority and tissue signal information is less important. This is because with 3D-FT the patient is placed in the scanner and for 20 minutes data from the whole head are acquired, so retrospectively images are generated in different planes and directions. There is still only one pulse sequence, that is, a T1-weighted image. Depending on the clinical problem, rather than angling 5 degrees and looking at anatomy in different projections, in many cases it is more helpful to have a T2-weighted image. Areas where 3-D imaging is particularly useful are regions of complex anatomy like the pituitary, lumbar spine, etc. where T1-weighted images are often sufficient.

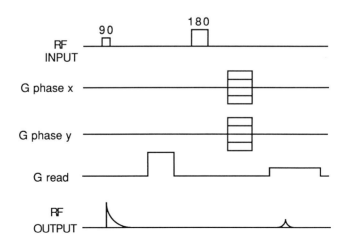

FIG 3–45.
Simplified 3D-FT pulse sequence timing diagram. The gradients are off during the slice selection step so that the whole image volume is stimulated by the 90 degree pulse. Instead of a slice select gradient, two-phase encoding gradients are used for data encoding.

EFFECTS OF VARYING ECHO TIME AND REPETITION TIME

Varying TR and TE has many effects on MR image quality in addition to mere changes in contrast. Slice thickness, degree of slice contiguity, imaging time, signal-to-noise, and number of echoes or slices in a simultaneous acquisition all also depend on TR and TE.

For example, as TE increases a number of things occur. In addition to increasing the T2 weighting of the image, the overall signal-to-noise is lowered. The SNR effect is somewhat offset because with a longer TE greater bandwidth reduction is possible for SNR improvement.

Since the dead time decreases as TE increases with a constant TR, the number of slices or echoes possible in multimode decreases. Longer TE times mean that we have more time so that sinc RF pulses may be used for contiguous slices, or steeper gradients may be used for thinner slices or higher-resolution images.

A longer TE can also mean greater sensitivity to motion and flow artifacts. On the other hand, a longer TE allows higher-order correction of these artifacts using gradient moment nulling strategies. Interestingly, lengthening TE has no effect on overall scan time.

The effects of decreasing TR are increased T1 weighting and overall reduction in signal-to-noise. This SNR loss is somewhat offset by the decreased overall scan time with a shorter TR. This allows some improvement in SNR through signal averaging in the same scan time. Finally, as the dead time decreases (as TR decreases with a constant TE) the number of slices or echoes possible in multimode decreases.

REFERENCES

1. Kumar A, Welti D, Ernst R: NMR zeugmatography. *J Magn Reson* 1985; 18:69–85.
2. Bottomley PA: NMR imaging techniques and applications: A review. *Rev Sci Instrum* 1982; 53:1319–1337.
3. Farrar TC, Becker ED: *Pulse and Fourier Transform NMR.* Orlando, Fla, Academic Press, 1971.
4. Roth K: *NMR-Tomography and -Spectroscopy in Medicine.* New York, Springer-Verlag, 1984.
5. Lauterbur PC, Lai CM: Zeugmatography reconstruction from projections. *IEEE Trans Nucl Sci* 1980; 27:1227–1231.
6. Edelstein WA, Hutchinson JMS, Johnson G, et al: Spin warp NMR imaging and applications to human whole-body imaging. *Phys Med Biol* 1980; 25:751–756.
7. Johnson GA, Thompson MB, Gewalt SL, et al: Nuclear magnetic resonance imaging at microscopic resolution. *J Magn Reson* 1986; 68:129–137.
8. Hendrick RE: Sampling time effects on SNR and CNR in spin echo MRI. *Magn Reson Imaging* 1987; 5:31–37.
9. Feinberg DA, Crooks LE, Hoenninger JC, et al: Contiguous thin section MR imaging by two dimensional fourier transform techniques. *Radiology* 1986; 158:811–817.
10. Murphy WA, Gutierrez FR, Levitt RG, et al: Oblique views of the heart by magnetic resonance imaging. *Radiology* 1985; 154:225–226.
11. Reicher MA, Lufkin RB, Smith S, et al: Multiple-angle, variable-interval, nonorthogonal MRI. *AJR* 1986; 147:363–366.
12. Feinberg DA, Hale JD, Watts JC, et al: Halving MR imaging time by congugation: Demonstration at 3.5 kg. *Radiology* 1986; 161:527–531.
13. Yoon HC, Lufkin RB, Smith SD, et al: The effects of zero-filling in magnetic resonance imaging. *J Med Imag* 1988; 2:184–190.
14. Mansfield P, Mosley AA, Baines T: Fast scan proton density imaging by NMR. *J Phys E* 1976; 9:271–278.
15. Haacke EM, Bearden FH, Clayton JR, et al: Reduction of MR imaging time by the hybrid fast scan technique. *Radiology* 1986; 158:521–529.

16. Van Uijan CMJ, Den Boef JH: Driven equilibrium radio frequency pulses in NMR imaging. *Magn Res Med* 1984; 1:502–507.

17. Meulen P, Groen J, Cuppen J: Very fast MR imaging by field echoes, in *Small Angle Excitation, Magnetic Resonance Imaging,* vol 3, 1985, pp 297–299.

Chapter 4

Flow, Motion, and Artifacts

Robert B. Lufkin, M.D.

Although the basic effects of proton density, T1 and T2 relaxation times on the image are modeled by the spin echo pulse sequence equation, a number of important factors that alter the appearance of the image are not included in the equation. This chapter will examine several of these effects including flow, motion, edge phenomenon, and other system artifacts that must be recognized and understood in order to accurately interpret magnetic resonance (MR) findings.

FLOW MECHANISMS

Our model for MR imaging (MRI) assumes that protons are stationary during the entire duty cycle. If protons do not remain in one position, the MR signal will change. Flow can cause regions to be higher or lower signal than that predicted by the proton density, T1 and T2 relaxation times, and susceptibility effects. Unfortunately there is not one cohesive model for flow in MR. Instead a group of smaller models or empirical observations exist that are useful in understanding the MR appearance of flow.[1-4]

Flow effects can be analyzed in two general ways. First, flow can be considered in terms of its mechanism and grouped into two categories. The first group consists of effects that alter T1 or longitudinal magnetization. These are called *time of flight effects* or *velocity effects* and include such things as entry phenomena and high-flow void. These effects depend on the radiofrequency (RF) history of the spins and vary depending on whether spin echo or gradient echo acquisitions are used.

A second group is due to the interaction of flowing protons with magnetic field gradients. Because the spins accumulate phase as they move along a gradient, flow alters phase.[5] This second group of phase effects thus alter the transverse magnetization. Flow effects such as even echo rephasing, odd echo dephasing, image harmonics, and ghost images are all examples of phase effects due to flow. Motion artifacts and flow artifacts are often similar because they both involve moving protons whether in a blood vessel or the wall of a beating heart.

The phase shift (ϕ) depends on factors other than flow velocity and may be described as follows:

$$\phi \approx \Delta V \cdot G \cdot TE \cdot \gamma$$

where ΔV is the velocity of the protons, γ is the gyromagnetic ratio, G is the gradient amplitude, and TE is the echo time. In order to minimize phase changes due to flow, low values of TE and G may be selected.

Rather than analyzing flow by its mechanism it is preferable to use a more practical approach that will be more valuable when actually interpreting images. Thus, instead of considering flow by grouping the phenomena by mechanisms, flow effects will be grouped according to appearances on the image.

INCREASED FLOW SIGNAL INTENSITY

If a region of the image is higher signal than is predicted from T1 or T2 mechanisms, the list of flow effects can be considered to try to see if any of the conditions are met. The first group causes increased signal intensity due to flow.

Entry Phenomenon

The first effect is *entry phenomena* or, as it is sometimes called, paradoxical or slow flow enhancement. This is an example of a time of flight flow effect or longitudinal magnetization effect. It depends on the RF history of the spins, that is, what RF pulses the flowing protons have experienced in the past.[6]

In a stationary situation all the spins stay in the plane of section during the RF stimulation and the echo collection. They experience repeated 90 degree pulses and are partially saturated (they are still recovering longitudinal magnetization). Just outside the plane of section, the spins that have not experienced a prior 90 degree pulse are unsaturated (fully magnetized). The unsaturated spins have a large longitudinal magnetization, because they have not been beaten down by repeated 90 degree pulses.

In the stationary situation there are no effects on the image of these outside spins, but as soon as slow laminar flow occurs through the plane of section, these unsaturated spins begin moving into the slab. When a 90 degree pulse is applied to this unsaturated magnetization vector, a large transverse magnetization and high signal result (Fig 4–1). This artificially

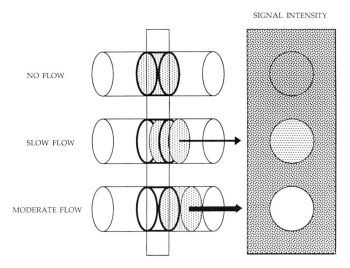

SIGNAL INTENSITY

NO FLOW

SLOW FLOW

MODERATE FLOW

FIG 4–1.
Variation in vessel lumen signal intensity with velocity in a single-entry slice with laminar flow. In the no-flow situation, protons in both the vessel and surrounding tissue are saturated and produce moderate signal. With increasing flow velocity, a greater percentage of unsaturated protons enter the image volume and return a higher signal in the vessel lumen.

high signal is called *entry phenomenon*. The magnitude of the effect depends on many factors. Since it reflects relative magnetizations, the effect is more pronounced on high-field systems. On all systems it is proportional to slice thickness and inversely proportional to repetition time (TR).

For example, in a stack of axial multislice images through the abdomen, flow-related enhancement is often seen in the vena cava in the caudal slices and in the aorta in the cephalad slices. Actually it occurs in not just the first slice but throughout several slices in a stack of multislice images.

Entry phenomena in multislice imaging is complex and beyond the scope of this discussion. If a stack of slices with flow through the stack are imaged (and assume consecutive slice excitation and ignore countercurrent and cocurrent effects) the amount of entry phenomens that occurs in progressive slices decreases depending on the flow characteristics in the blood (Fig 4–2). Entry phenomena occurs not only with flowing blood but also with flowing cerebrospinal fluid (CSF) and other fluids.[7]

Entry phenomena can be useful. The entry slice in a multislice sequence will show maximum enhancement, thus giving clues as to the direction of flow. Entry phenomena can also be confusing. The increased signal as well as associated phase errors can degrade image quality (Fig 4–3).

Presaturation Pulses

Because of these problems with entry phenomena a technique was developed to get rid of it called *presaturation*.[8] It decreases phase errors as well as largely eliminating artifacts due to unsaturated spins entering the plane of section. The technique works in a multislice sequence by delivering RF pulses on either end of the stack to saturate the spins (Figs 4–4 and 4–5). Now there are effectively no unsaturated spins moving into the plane of section. It is possible to use more involved approaches and saturate two, four, six, or all eight surfaces of the image cube.

Presaturation adds 3 to 6 ms to each view acquisition time because of the time necessary to deliver the extra RF pulse at the end. The additional RF pulse also increases energy deposition. Presaturation techniques correct intensity variations, unlike gradient moment nulling (GMN) approaches (MAST) and other techniques which will be discussed which mainly correct phase modulations.

Even Echo Rephasing

A second cause of increased signal intensity is *even echo rephasing*.[9] It is also an example of the second mechanism of flow effect which affects the transverse magnetization due to alteration in phase relationships. Recall that if there is no flow when the gradients are applied, the phase angles disperse and can be effectively refocused.

However, when there is flow along the gradient, the moving spins acquire different amounts of phase depending on their velocity. Since in laminar flow the velocity profile varies across the lumen of the vessel, significant phase dispersion occurs (Fig 4–6).

After the 180 degree pulse the moving spins are not in phase at the time of the echo and the signal intensity will be decreased from the level of the stationary protons. This may be shown on a spin phase graph (Fig 4–7).[10]

Assuming that the laminar flow velocity is constant, because of the symmetry of this phase dispersion, if a second, symmetric echo is collected, after the second 180 degree pulse the spins will come into phase and there will be second echo rephasing. In fact this occurs with not only the second echo but also every even echo thereafter. The second echo will

SIGNAL INTENSITY

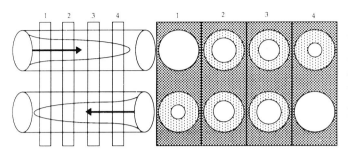

FIG 4–2.
Entry phenomenon in a four-slice multislice sequence (assuming consecutive excitation and ignoring cocurrent and countercurrent effects). The signal intensity is maximal at the entry slice and (with laminar flow) decreases in successive slices.

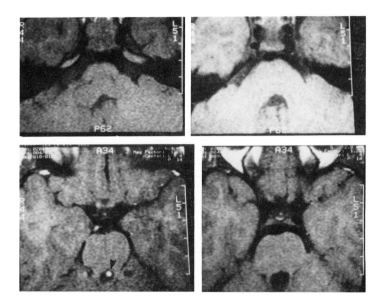

FIG 4–3
Entry phenomenon due to CSF motion. An area of high signal intensity *(arrowhead)* is present in the superior aspect of the fourth ventricle on this T1-weighted (SE/700/25) sequence. This is due to unsaturated protons in CSF entering the image stack during normal CSF pulsations.

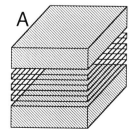
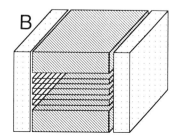

FIG 4–4.
Presaturation pulses added in various positions (**A**) at either end of the image stack or (**B**) on four sides.

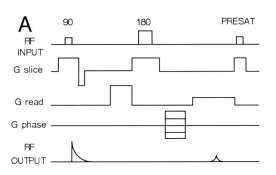

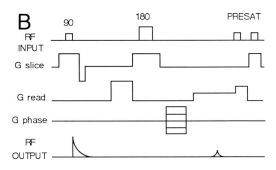

FIG 4–5.
Pulse sequence timing diagram for presaturation pulses.
A, presaturation pulse necessary to produce correction
shown in Figure 4–4, A. **B,** additional pulse in order to
produce correction shown in Figure 4–4, B.

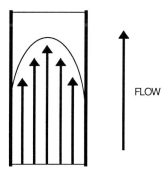

FIG 4–6.
Velocity and phase relationships of moving protons. With laminar flow, velocity (proportional to arrow length) varies across the vessel lumen.

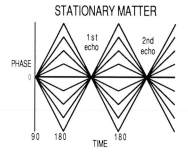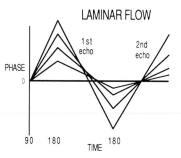

FIG 4–7.
Spin phase graph: comparison of phase relationships of stationary matter and laminar flow. With laminar flow, there is incomplete rephasing at the first echo.

appear to be higher signal than the first echo of the same vessel. On the image it appears as an absolute increase in signal intensity on the even echoes and negative calculated values for T2. This rephasing occurs for the constant velocity component of motion with linear gradients only. Higher-order terms (acceleration or pulsatility) for flow or the gradients are not corrected by the even echoes.

Even echo rephasing occurs with slow laminar flow *multiecho* sequences only, but importantly it only occurs in *symmetric* echoes. That is the TEs have to be multiples, that is, 28, 56, 84, or 112. If asymmetric echoes such as a 2000/20, 2000/90 sequence are employed the symmetry required to refocus the spins on the second echo is destroyed and even echo rephasing does not occur.

Diastolic Pseudogating

Another cause of increased signal intensity related to flow is *diastolic pseudogating*.[1] The concept of gating should be familiar to readers from nuclear medicine and other cardiac studies. Images can be acquired synchronized to a periodic movement in order to effectively stop the motion.

In the case of MR, image acquisition can be coordinated with the R wave. If the 90 degree pulse is given at the beginning of the R wave or some fixed point relative to it all the slices in a multislice sequence will be fixed relative to heart motion. The images will be acquired over several heart beats. When blood flow is stopped image intensity in vessels will vary depending on the point in the cardiac cycle. In images obtained during rapid flow (systole) the signal will be low, during slow or absent flow (diastole) the signal will be higher (Fig 4–8). When a cardiac gated study is performed this effect is anticipated and it is not a problem. It can be a problem in the interpretation of images if it unintentionally occurs.

It is possible to cardiac gate in a patient without hooking up any electrodes or peripheral pulse oximeters. If a patient has a heart rate of 60 beats per minute and the TR is set to 1,000 (assuming a constant heart rate) then cardiac gating will effectively take place. In other words, the pulse sequence image acquisition will be synchronized with the patient's heart rate and images obtained throughout the cardiac cycle. Flow at one point will be high signal in the vessel and another point it will be low signal due to the fact that blood flow is imaged at different times during systole and diastole (see Fig 4–8). A direct one-to-one correspondence between TR and R-wave to R-wave (R-R) interval is not necessary. Multiples of one or the other can also produce interference effects. A TR of 2,000 with a heart rate of 60 beats per minute will result in two regions of systole and diastole in the slice train.

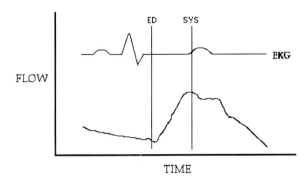

FLOW

TIME

FIG 4–8.
Variation in flow rates during different phases of the cardiac cycle. Considerable variation in velocity is present between end-diastole (ED) and systole (SYS).

When imaging the abdominal aorta, blood may be low signal at one level and high signal on another. The location of the high-signal slices will depend on the phase relationship of the pulse sequence and the cardiac cycle. If a high signal in a vessel is not in the entry slice, then entry phenomena do not explain it, and if it is not the second echo, even echo rephasing is not the cause. Diastolic pseudogating is another possibility. Like all flow effects, this can occur not only in blood vessels but also in cerebrospinal fluid.

DECREASED FLOW SIGNAL INTENSITY

High-Flow Void

Decreased signal intensity may result from rapidly flowing blood and is called *high-flow void*. This occurs because in order to get a transverse magnetization (and thus any signal back) in RF coils it is necessary for the spins to remain in the plane of section long enough to be acted on by both the 90 and 180 degree pulses.

With stationary protons, flow void does not occur because the spins experience both pulses. Flowing protons that are in the plane of section during the 90 degree pulse will have moved out of the section by the time the 180 degree pulse is delivered. Similarly, flow within the section when the 180 degree pulse is given will not have received a 90 degree pulse and thus will also not return a signal (Fig 4–9).

Selective 180 degree pulses (limited to a small region) are used in multislice sequences because nonselective pulses result in interslice crosstalk. Spins in sequences with selective 180 pulses will move out of the plane, miss the 180 pulse, and thus will not return a signal (Figs 4–9 through 4–11).

For spin echo imaging, high-flow blood moving out of the plane of section returns no signal. The amplitude of the returned signal is thus a linear function of velocity and depends on the proportion of spins that leave the slice before experiencing the 180 degree pulse (see Fig 4–10). With spin echo imaging as the velocity is increased the intensity of the signal from the vessel decreases. The lumen gets darker and darker until at high velocity there is no signal.

This effect is not necessarily true for gradient echo images. The signal is returned to a greater extent with gradient echoes because protons are refocused by the gradients even after they have left the section. They still return the signal, because the gradients are

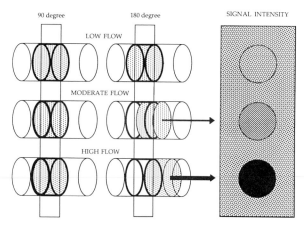

FIG 4–9.
Variation in vessel lumen signal intensity with high-velocity flow in a spin echo acquisition with selective 180 degree pulses. In the low-flow situation, protons in the vessel remain in the slice during both the 90 and 180 degree RF pulse and thus return some signal. With increasing flow velocity, a greater percentage of protons leave the image volume before they can be refocused by the selective 180 degree pulse and thus fail to return a signal in the vessel lumen resulting in "high-flow void."

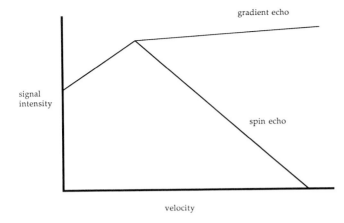

FIG 4–10.
Graph of signal intensity vs. velocity for spin echo and gradient echo sequences. With increasing velocity, a greater percentage of protons escape the selective 180 degree pulse of spin echo imaging and remain dephased (and low signal intensity). This does not occur with gradient focusing techniques. The effects of turbulence are ignored in this example.

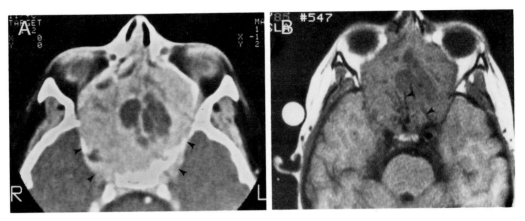

FIG 4–11.
Flow void in a large juvenile angiofibroma. **A,** computed tomography scan with contrast shows a staining mass *(arrowhead)* arising from the nasal cavity and extending into the middle cranial fossa. **B,** magnetic resonance scan (SE/500/30) also shows the mass but in addition tubular areas of low signal which represent parasellar feeding vessels *(arrowhead).*

nonselective and will refocus the spins even if they are three slices downstream. This is because the refocusing gradients by their nature occur over the whole image volume. It is very hard for even rapidly moving spins to escape the refocusing effects of the gradients.

The spins receive the 90 degree pulse in the first slice and then refocus with gradients downstream. If this is attempted with a 90 to 180 degree pulse train the spins leave the slice and no longer refocus, because the 180 degree pulse selectively acts on that slice. High-flow void is sometimes called exit phenomena or washout effect because it is due to washing out or exiting of the spins from the sections.

Turbulence

Turbulence produces irreversible loss of coherence due to random fluctuations in velocity of the spins. This appears as loss of signal intensity. Although turbulence increases with higher velocity, other factors also play a role. The onset of turbulence can be predicted by the Reynold's number (Re) in the following relationship:

$$Re = \frac{d \times V \times \text{tube diameter}}{\text{Viscosity}}$$

where d is density and V is velocity of the blood. Laminar flow is usually present in situations with a Re < 2100 and turbulent flow occurs with Re > 2100. Turbulent flow is thus increased in regions of vessel bifurcation, pulsatile flow, and atheromatous changes in the vessel wall (Fig 4–12).

Turbulence is an important cause for loss of signal because it occurs in both gradient and spin echo pulse sequences. In gradient echo imaging, because of the decreased effects of high flow void most of the flow is high signal, but low signal may be present due to turbulent flow.

FIG 4–12.
Dephasing and signal loss due to turbulence in spin echo imaging of flow. As tubes of larger and larger diameter are used, increasing turbulence causes loss of signal (compared to Figure 4–10). Laminar flow is maintained at higher velocities with smaller tube diameters. (Adapted from Bradley WG, Waluch V: *Radiology* 154:443–450, 1985.)

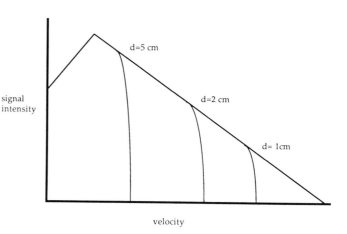

MAGNETIC RESONANCE ANGIOGRAPHY

The ability to produce an image of even moderate spatial resolution of the three-dimensional (3D) course of blood vessels with MR could have significant advantages over conventional invasive angiography which requires ionizing radiation and contrast material injection. Several researchers are already producing relatively high-resolution MR angiograms using a variety of techniques.

By definition, MR angiography does not require the addition of any intravascular contrast agents and the signals are produced entirely by the effect of the RF pulses and magnetic field gradients on the spinning protons. Essentially all techniques of MR angiography use variations of the following three steps to produce the image:

1. A projection image
2. Suppression of background static material
3. Production of a flow-sensitive image

Projection Image

A projection image is necessary for the adequate display of tortuously flowing blood vessels as they course through the body. In most cases, vessels are not adequately represented with a thin-section tomographic image.

Projection imaging may be accomplished during the acquisition of the data by using thick-slab two-dimensional (2D) Fourier transform sections.[11] This is accomplished by making slice select RF bandwidth or magnetic field gradient changes which result in the direct acquisition of a projection image without the necessity for postprocessing (Fig 4–13). This technique has been particularly effective with gating and phase shift imaging strategies.

A projection image may be obtained from a stack of tomographic 2D sections as a postprocessing procedure or directly from a three-dimensional Fourier transformation (3D-FT) acquisition.[12, 13] The advantages of this approach are that the projection can be varied to produce a variety of views from the original data set after the patient has left the clinic. This is not possible with thick-slab techniques.

Suppression of Background Static Material

While projection imaging improves the visualization of flow in tortuous blood vessels it also decreases the overall conspicuity of these same structures. This is due to an increase in

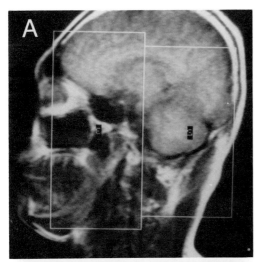

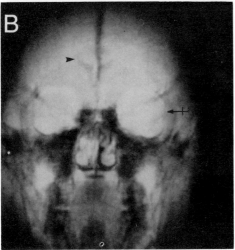

FIG 4–13.
Image projection using thick direct 2D-FT image acquisition. **A,** scout (SE/1200/40) image in the sagittal plane is used to select thick-slice coronal projection images in this normal patient. **B,** resulting thick-slice coronal projection image includes both the lateral ventricles *(arrowhead)* and orbital fat *(arrow)* in the same slice. (Courtesy of Lee Chui, M.D.)

the dynamic range of the image due to the superimposition of large areas of static material. Therefore, in order to regain the contrast in the flowing blood compared to the surrounding static material it is necessary to implement a technique to suppress the signal from this material.

A technique borrowed from conventional and digital angiography for static background material suppression is that of subtraction (Fig 4–14). One technique uses simple magnitude subtraction of a flow-sensitized or velocity-compensated image from a flow-desensitized background image.[14] A second subtraction strategy uses phase differences for subtracting phase-positive or phase-negative flow images from phase-neutral background images. Flow subtraction strategies have the advantage of relatively simple postprocessing requirements. A major drawback to subtraction strategies is that any patient motion between the two images severely degrades image resolution. These misregistration errors may be minimized by interleaving the data acquisition of the two scans.

Postprocessing techniques of image projection using vessel extraction by image analysis also effectively remove static material. The most powerful form of this technique is to acquire a single 3D-FT gradient echo sequence and then suppress background signal by using a ray tracing algorithm combined with thresholding.[15]

Production of a Flow-Sensitive Image

The last requirement for MR angiography is a production of a flow-sensitized image. Three techniques are currently employed

1. Gating of pulsatile flow
2. Time of flight effects
3. Phase shift effects

The most straightforward strategy is to stop or slow pulsatile flow by cardiac gating. This is accomplished by judicious selection of the imaging delay after the R wave so that image formation occurs during diastole (Fig 4–15).

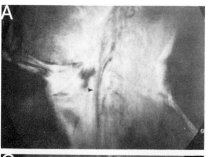
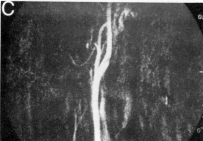
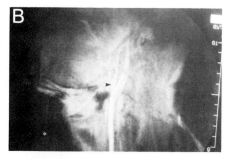

FIG 4–14.
Background suppression using image subtraction. **A,** sagittal scout view of the neck (SE/1200/40) showing flow void in the region of the carotid artery (*arrowhead*). **B,** same plane and imaging technique except now acquired with the use of flow compensation gradients. Note increased signal in the carotid artery (*arrowhead*). **C,** subtraction of image (**A**) from image (**B**) yields flow image of carotid bifurcation. (Courtesy of J. Phillips, M.D.)

One problem with cardiac gating as a method of flow sensitization is that only pulsatile flow is effectively tagged. Therefore venous flow as well as slow flow in some arteries may be difficult to image. In addition, considerable experimentation is often necessary in individual patients to determine the proper delay for diastole in different regions of the body. Also, since subtraction is necessary, misregistration errors degrade image quality.

A second method of flow sensitization is through the use of phase shift effects. All standard spin echo and gradient echo refocusing techniques return spins in stationary material to coherence in the transverse plane during the echo collection. This is not true for nonstationary protons because moving spins dephase along magnetic field gradients. Therefore transverse magnetization at the time of echo is decreased because of variations in phase angles from the motion of the spins along the gradients prior to the echo.

Just as time of flight effects depend on the excitation history of the spins due to RF pulses, phase shift effects depend on the magnetic field history of the spins due to the magnetic field gradients. In the case of phase shift effects, both the amplitude as well as the phase of the signal depend on the flow history of the spins. Examples of phase shift effects on standard MR images are even echo rephasing and odd echo dephasing.

By using bipolar gradients, flow sensitization may be accomplished using a phase difference technique.[16, 17] To obtain maximal signal in the transverse plane (complete rephasing) the phase angle at the echo should be set to zero. By manipulating the magnetic field gradients in the pulse sequence it is possible to accomplish this and sensitize to higher-order flow terms (such as acceleration and change in acceleration or pulsatility) in the MR imaging sequence. The problem is that even high-order flow compensation may not refocus the spins at areas of vessel stenosis or bifurcation. Vortices at these points lead to stochastic velocity distributions known as turbulence.

The third general strategy for flow sensitization is the use of time of flight flow effects. This class of effects depends on the excitation history of the spins due to RF pulses. In this strategy the flow affects the longitudinal magnetization and can be thought of as a T1 clock. Although the signal amplitude depends on flow, the phase is undefined. Gradient echo pulse sequences are particularly sensitive to time-of-flight flow effects for the reasons mentioned previously.

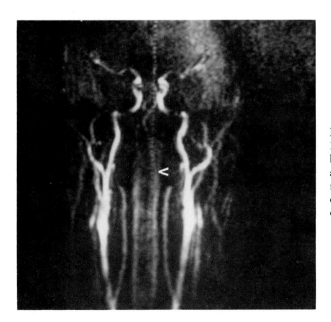

FIG 4–15.
Magnetic resonance angiogram obtained by subtraction of systolic and diastolic images. Coronal projection image of the normal head and neck shows some detection of transmitted CSF *(arrowhead)* and venous pulsations in addition to arterial flow.

There is a bewildering variety of techniques for MR angiography currently under investigation. Researchers use practically all combinations of image projection, static material suppression and flow sensitization to produce MR images of flowing blood and CSF. Some of the most popular techniques currently employ 2D-FT thick-slab imaging for projection, phase difference or magnitude subtraction to suppress static material, and some type of flow sensitization using phase shift effects. One of the most powerful new approaches to MR angiography uses 3D-FT gradient echo acquisition with thresholding and ray tracing to define blood vessels. The choice of the MR angiography strategy depends on the region of anatomy under study and the flow characteristics present. No one technique is ideal for all indications.

For most techniques of MR angiography there are several obvious advantages over dye injection conventional angiography or digital angiography. The MR techniques are fast, non-invasive, and may be done at a cost comparable to or less than conventional angiography. While the physics and instrumentation are technically difficult the actual procedure requires no additional technical personnel as all the manipulations are done under computer software control. Finally, because of the physics of MR angiography it is possible to obtain a projection image in virtually any plane rather than being limited by the standard x-ray angiographic projections. Similarly, by doing selective excitation it is possible to do selective flow studies in a relatively small area of anatomy and effectively eliminate overlying vascular images through limited projection.

The disadvantages of MR angiography at this early stage of development are significant and in many ways limit clinical applications of the technique in its present form. Spatial resolution is limited and is currently less with MR angiography than either digital or cut film angiography. Due to techniques of excitation it is generally not possible to image selective areas by vessel (such as a left internal carotid injection) but rather areas must be imaged by volume. Similarly, it is not possible to do dynamic studies where the arterial, capillary, and venous phases are examined sequentially. In many situations this is a significant problem in detecting slow flow and analyzing vascular runoff.

Some techniques are limited in that they tag only pulsatile flow. Other techniques may tag flow in only one direction and are relatively insensitive to flow in orthogonal directions. Many techniques are insensitive to higher-order flow terms and turbulence in particular.

Despite the significant limitations of MR angiography the strong potential for a clinical application is present. Like most aspects of MRI technology, MR angiography is far from mature and continued development in this area is occurring which will hopefully overcome many of the present limitations of the technique.

ARTIFACTS IN MRI

In addition to the effects of proton density, T1 and T2 relaxation times, flow, and magnetic susceptibility, a number of other artifacts can alter the MR image.[18, 19] The 2D-FT technique used for image reconstruction on most MR instruments is associated with a variety of artifacts that must be recognized and differentiated from normal anatomy and pathology. Artifacts may be classified in a number of ways but for the purposes of this discussion they will be discussed in terms of their appearance.

EDGE ARTIFACTS

Several artifacts occurring at edges due to motion, truncation errors, and chemical shifts may be present in MRI.

Chemical Shift Misregistration Errors

Chemical shift misregistration errors cause accentuation of any fat-water interfaces along the frequency axis of MR images and may be mistaken for pathology. This phenomenon has been described for various materials and tissue types by several investigators.[20-24] The anatomy of most regions of the body outside the CNS is largely made up of fat-muscle and fat-soft tissue interfaces. The deep spaces of the neck, abdomen, and extremities all contain loose areolar tissue which practically defines the anatomy of the region. Unlike the CNS where virtually no MR signal from fat is present, the abundance of fat-water interfaces make chemical shift misregistration artifacts important in studying these regions.

The slightly different Larmor frequency of differing chemical species, such as fat and water (in proton imaging) results in spatial errors in image reconstruction. The artifact appears as dark and light bands along the fat-water interfaces offset along the frequency axis. The bands degrade the image by creating pseudocapsule formation around lymph nodes and other masses. Because chemical shift differences are the result of differing Larmor frequencies of fat- and water-resonant protons, the phenomenon is extremely sensitive to the main magnetic field strength of MR instruments.

The term *chemical shift* refers to the difference in resonant frequency of protons due to local differences in chemical environment. This shift is due to the different electron environments of the protons. Hydrogen atoms associated with different kinds of chemical bonds have different resonant frequencies. The shell electrons act to weaken the effects of the applied magnetic field which results in frequency changes. Chemical shift misregistration artifacts occur because the local field of the protons can vary based on the chemical environment. Protons in water experience a slightly different magnetic field than protons in a fat group, independent of the external applied magnetic field. The external field is uniform, but the internal fields vary based on the local environment. Therefore, water will resonate at a slightly higher frequency than fat. This shift in frequency due to the chemical environment is called *chemical shift*.

Protons in fat and water molecules are separated by a chemical shift of about 3.5 parts per million (ppm) (Fig 4–16). The actual shift in hertz depends on the magnetic field strength of the magnet being used (Figs 4–17 and 4–18). For a 0.3-T system operating at 12.8 MHz, the shift will be 44.8 Hz compared to a 223.6-Hz shift for a 1.5-T system operating at 63.9 MHz. Although the difference at 0.3 T is only 44.8 Hz of 12.7 million, it is a significant enough shift to move the fat and water images apart 1 or 2 pixels on the image. Large chemical shift values are an asset in spectroscopy because of improved separation of chemical isotope peaks with increasing chemical shift. For imaging, however, large shifts in frequency due to chemical shift create artifacts which increase as the field strength of the system increases (see Figs 4–18 through 4–21).

In spectroscopy, frequencies are used to encode chemistry, while in proton imaging frequency is used to encode space. Thus, when fat and water appear in MR scans they will be shifted apart from each other along the frequency encoding axis because they have slightly different resonant frequencies.

Although the main magnetic field strength of the MR system determines the separation in frequency of fat and water nuclei, the mapping of this shift (in terms of pixels and millimeters) is determined by the magnetic field gradients, image bandwidth, and image matrix size. The actual image error in millimeters is determined by a combination of the shift in hertz as well as the amplitude of the magnetic field gradients applied to form the image. Steeper gradients map a given shift in hertz onto a smaller-millimeter displacement (Fig 4–19).

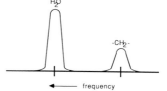

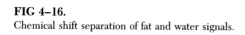

FIG 4–16.
Chemical shift separation of fat and water signals.

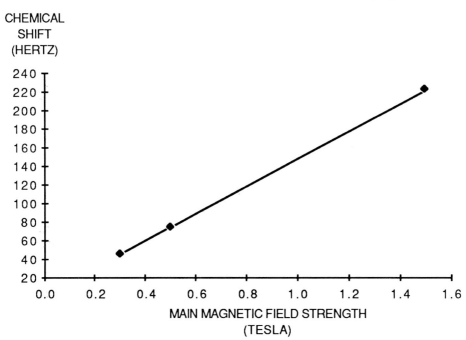

CHEMICAL
SHIFT
(HERTZ)

MAIN MAGNETIC FIELD STRENGTH
(TESLA)

FIG 4–17.
Plot of magnetic field strength vs. chemical shift.

Chemical shift artifacts, even when anticipated and recognized, can obscure normal anatomy and simulate pathology. This is most pronounced in areas of anatomy where fat-water interfaces are common such as the orbit, soft tissues of the neck, retroperitoneum, spine, and pelvis.

Although the option of going from high-field to low-field systems in order to minimize chemical shift is usually not available, several other strategies are available to reduce chemical shift errors. First, since the misregistration offset is present in the frequency or readout axis, the patient may be rescanned with this axis parallel to the fat-water interface (Figs 4–20 and 4–21).

Second, steeper gradients may also be employed to reduce the chemical shift offset in millimeters. The drawbacks to such an approach include the requirement of more powerful gradient power supplies and generally poorer signal-to-noise. The resultant smaller field of view may also lead to aliasing artifacts in the phase axis if the body part being imaged extends beyond the image field of view. Surface coils or other techniques may also be used to reduce aliasing.

A third strategy is to employ specialized pulse sequences. One technique allows the complete separation of fat and water images. These may be analyzed separately or electronically superimposed to eliminate the chemical shift offset. Short T1 inversion recovery sequences (STIR technique) may also be used.[25] By setting the inversion time (TI) of the

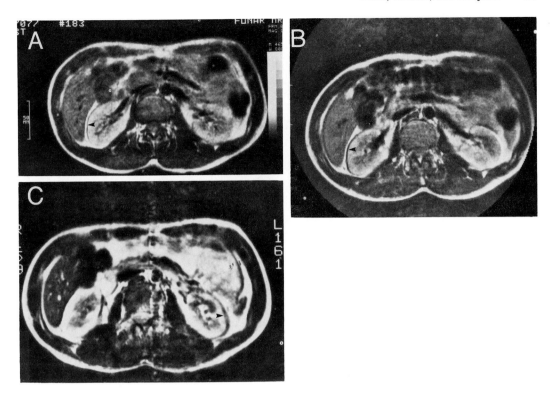

FIG 4–18.
Body coil images of the mid-abdomen of a normal volunteer. All three studies were SE/1000/60 with a 32-cm field of view of the same individual. The frequency encoding axis is along the horizontal dimension of all three scans. The chemical shift artifact *(arrowhead)* at the kidney–fat interface increases with field strength. **A,** 0.3 T, 1 mm offset. **B,** 0.5 T, 1.9 mm offset. **C,** 1.5 T, 2.2 mm offset. Reversed gradient polarity causes the artifact to be on the opposite side.

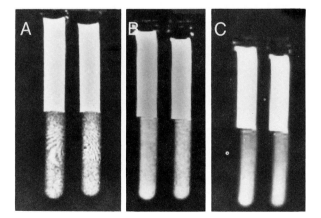

FIG 4–19.
Phantom images (oil and water in a test tube) obtained with varying gradient amplitude. All were obtained using a 256 matrix. Gradients were adjusted to produce effective fields of view of 16, 21, and 35 cm, respectively (decreasing gradient amplitude). The frequency encoding axis is positioned parallel to the oil-water interface. The chemical shift artifact was measured in millimeters and increases with decreasing gradient amplitude. **A,** 16 cm field of view (FOV). **B,** 21 cm FOV. **C,** 35 cm FOV.

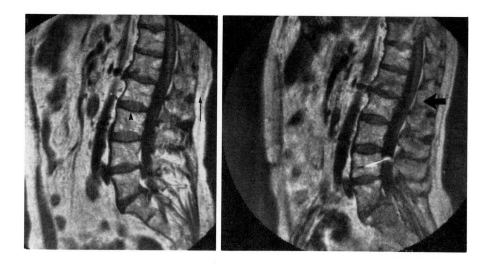

FIG 4–20.
A, effect of changing phase and frequency *(arrow)* axes to diminish chemical shift artifacts. The chemical shift artifact across the vertebral endplates *(arrowhead)* is minimized when the frequency axis is rotated 90 degrees **(B)**. (Courtesy of Michael Anselmo, M.D)

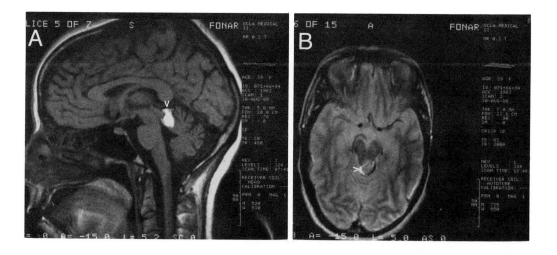

FIG 4–21.
Presumed lipoma of the quadrigeminal plate with chemical shift misregistration artifacts. **A,** on the sagittal scan (SE/480/30) the dark and white bands *(arrowhead)* at the interface between the high signal mass and surrounding brain along the frequency encoding axis confirm its fatty content. **B,** coronal T2-weighted image (SE/2000/85) shows similar findings *(arrow)*.

sequence at 0.69 times the T1 of fat, the signal from fat is suppressed. Implementation of both these approaches requires additional software and, in some cases, additional hardware.

Chemical shift misregistration errors may be distinguished from the other types of edge artifacts by appearance (Table 4–1). Chemical shift misregistration involves the frequency axis primarily. The periodicity is a single offset and it appears as single band on one side or the other. The amplitude is also a single offset which occurs at fat-water interfaces and depends on the different Larmor frequencies of fat and water.

Chemical Shift Phase Cancellation Errors

The differing resonances of fat and water result in another type of chemical shift artifact that occurs primarily with gradient (field) echo imaging. When *180 degree RF pulses* are used to refocus the spins, the differing Larmor frequencies of fat and water have no effect on refocusing because the spins are brought back into phase regardless of their individual frequency. However, when *gradients* are used to refocus the spins this is not the case.[26] From the Larmor relationship, it is known that the fat and water spins will respond differently to the same applied refocusing gradient. The resulting different Larmor frequencies means that phase differences will accumulate between the two different spectral components in the signal (fat and water). Depending on the TE chosen these phase differences will add constructively (in phase) or destructively (out of phase) (Fig 4–22). The frequency of the phase changes with TE also varies with the main magnetic field strength of the MR instrument.

The appearance of signal from voxels that are out of phase and demonstrate phase cancellation will be one of low signal intensity. This occurs in voxels that contain both fat and water components. Cellular bone marrow as well as adipose tissue interfaces with muscle contain components from both groups and thus show dramatic phase cancellation on gradient echo sequences at certain TEs.

Unlike chemical shift misregistration errors which are most pronounced in the frequency encoded axis, chemical shift phase cancellation errors occur on both phase and frequency axes. In addition, although misregistration errors occur in both SE and FE sequences, phase cancellation errors occur only with gradient refocusing techniques (see Table 4–1).

Motion Artifacts

A third type of edge artifact occurs with motion. Motion in various forms is present

TABLE 4–1.

Edge Artifacts in MRI*

	Truncation	Motion	Chemical Shift Misregistration	Chemical Shift Phase Cancellation
Axes involved	Phase and frequency	Phase only	Frequency only	Phase and frequency
Periodicity	Constant for axis	Variable	Single offset	Single offset
Amplitude	Uniform decay	Variable	Single offset	Single offset
Dependent on	Sampling rates	TR, TE, velocity, signal averaging, periodicity	Fat-water interfaces, Larmor frequency	Echo time, field strength
Mechanism	Fourier series truncation	Interference phenomenon	Spatial encoding error due to frequency, Variations	Fat-water phase cancellation
Pulse sequence	SE and FE	SE and FE	SE and FE	FE only

*FE = field echo; SE = spin echo.

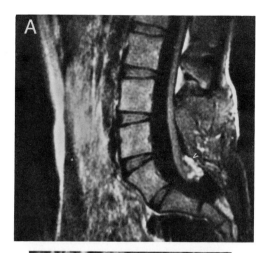

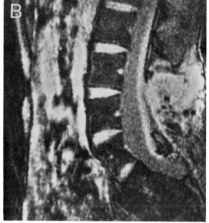

FIG 4–22.
Chemical shift phase cancellation errors in a patient with lipomeningomyelocele. **A,** sagittal T1-weighted spin echo image (SE/500/30) demonstrates the low-lying spinal cord, dilated thecal sac, and dysraphism. The lipoma is easily recognized by its high signal *(arrow)*. **B,** sagittal T1-weighted field echo (SE/200/10/60) image in the same plane shows similar anatomy. Note prominent low-signal chemical shift phase cancellation effects at the lipoma-CSF interface *(arrowhead)* as well as in the vertebral marrow.

throughout the body and may be random from swallowing, or periodic due to respiration, vascular, and CSF flow phenomena. Because of the 2D-FT reconstruction used in MRI, motion has unusual effects on the image which may not be obvious from past experience with CT.[27]

First, there is a slight blurring in the direction of motion. Change in position during the phase encoding levels of image acquisition results in inconsistent image reconstruction along the phase axis regardless of whether the motion is in the phase or frequency direction. These errors in phase location result in "ghost images," or interference phenomena at periodic intervals along the phase axis (Fig 4–23). These image harmonics also tend to be most pronounced at edges or tissue discontinuities. Because phase errors due to flow and motion are proportional to magnetic field gradient amplitude, many experts feel that they tend to be more pronounced with higher field strength systems which must use steeper imaging gradients.

At any given field strength the artifacts may be reduced by using shallower gradient amplitudes or shorter echo times. Changing the phase encoding axis is sometimes also valuable to shift the artifacts away from structures of interest. Because motion is such a common problem in MR images, a number of specific motion artifact reduction strategies have been developed.

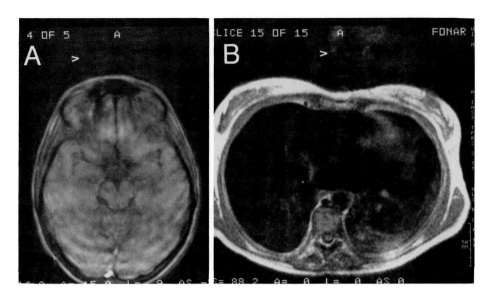

FIG 4–23.
Motion artifacts. **A,** slight head motion produces ghosting along the phase encoding axis. **B,** cardiac movement produces similar artifact in the chest *(arrow).*

Strategies for Motion Artifact Correction

Strategies for motion artifact reduction may be grouped according to the period of motion sensitivity in the pulse sequence timing diagram that they attempt to reduce. Some approaches attempt to reduce motion artifacts by a correction for noise in the image. Other strategies deal specifically with view-to-view motion, that is, that motion that occurs between the 90 degree pulses (duty cycle) (Fig 4–24). Within-view motion, that is, motion occurring between the application of the 90 degree pulse and data collection, is addressed by a third group of artifact reduction strategies.

Signal Averaging.—The first approach considers motion artifacts as noise and decreases them by signal averaging.[28] The random phases of the motion are averaged together and diminished while the nonrandom aspects of the image are preserved. This approach works without regard to view-to-view or within-view aspects of motion. Like other averaging techniques, it does require a doubling of scan time for each signal average. Therefore it is most practical for T1-weighted spin echo images or fast gradient echo imaging.

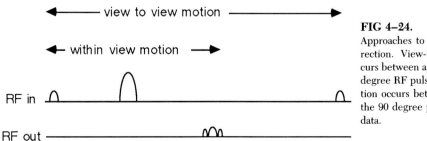

FIG 4–24.
Approaches to motion artifact correction. View-to-view motion occurs between applications of the 90 degree RF pulse. Within-view motion occurs between application of the 90 degree pulse and collection data.

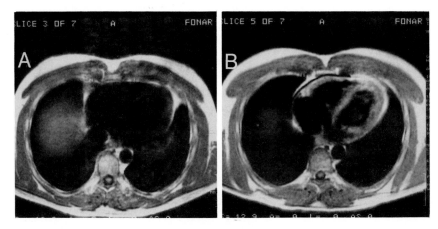

FIG 4–25.
Effect of cardiac gating on image quality. **A,** the ungated study shows considerable motion artifact and poor visualization of internal cardiac anatomy. **B,** with gating, the ghosting decreases and the myocardium is much better seen. (Courtesy of Bobby Keen.)

Improve View to View Consistency.—In this second group of motion reduction techniques, an attempt is made to minimize any displacement of the body part being scanned between each view in order to improve view to view consistency.

Cardiac Gating.—Motion artifacts from periodic motion such as the beating heart may be reduced if the duty cycle is synchronized to the motion in order to minimize view to view inconsistency in the image[29] (Fig 4–25). This is easily accomplished with appropriate hardware. Although the technique works well in specifically imaging the heart, it is less effective in minimizing motion artifacts due to transmitted cardiac motion throughout the body due to dampening effects of the soft tissues.

The hardware used in gating requires additional setup time in addition to the longer scan time required by gating. Although peripheral pulse oximeter gating may be used for some CNS applications, most users still use formal electrocardiogram (ECG) gating for heart MR studies. The fact that the duty cycle is tied to the R-R interval also means that the choice of TR is very limited and the number of slices in either systole or diastole is also constrained in a multislice acquisition.

Respiratory Gating.—The image acquisition may also be gated to the respiratory cycle in order to improve view to view consistency for this type of motion.[30, 31] Here the data are collected at end expiration during minimum motion for each duty cycle. This approach also requires additional hardware and setup time. Actual image acquisition time may be as long as 60% more with respiratory gating. For a number of reasons this approach is not widely used.

Ordered-Phase Encoding.—The order in which the phase encode steps are acquired may be rearranged in order to reduce motion artifacts.[32] This is the basis for centrally ordered-phase encoding (COPE), respiratory ordered-phase encoding (ROPE), and EXORCIST. Ordered phase encoding techniques scan the outer views during maximum motion and the central views during minimum motion. Although scan time is not appreciably lengthened and artifacts are reduced, neither ordered-phase encoding nor gating take into account random phase errors due to within-view motion.

Improve Within-View Consistency: Gradient Moment Nulling.—Even if view-to-view consistency in an image is achieved, random motion occurring between the 90 degree RF pulse and data collection can cause significant artifacts. These result from incomplete re-phasing of the transverse magnetization at the time of slice selection and of data collection (Fig 4–26).

Patanny and co-workers developed a general strategy for nulling these phase errors with magnetic field gradients which is known as gradient moment nulling (GMN).[33] The process is accomplished by solving a set of simultaneous equations which specify gradient profile modifications to the pulse sequence timing diagram. Additional gradient lobes may be added to correct for motion with constant velocity, changing velocity (acceleration), changing acceleration (pulsatility), and even higher-order terms (Figs 4–27 and 4–28). These compensatory gradients may be added to slice select, readout, and phase encoding if necessary to compensate for a flow in all three axes. As a practical matter (the phase encoding gradient is only on for a brief period), it is only necessary to add the compensatory gradients to slice select and the readout axes.

While the compensatory gradients in these techniques do not add to the overall scan time the disadvantage is that they do make considerable demands on the gradient electronics and place practical limitations on the lower limit of echo time, depending on whether higher-order motion corrections are made.

Truncation Artifacts

A fourth type of edge artifact is similar in appearance to motion artifact but is unrelated to movement and is found in both the phase and frequency axes. 2D-FT techniques transform the MR signal to spatial intensity image data with frequency and phase information encoding each axis in the plane of the scan. Complex shapes are specified by a series of sine and cosine waves of various frequencies, phase, and amplitude. Some shapes are more difficult to encode than others. The most difficult shapes to represent with a Fourier series of terms are waveforms with instantaneous transitions, tissue discontinuities, or edges.

To most accurately represent an instantaneous transition with a series of terms for Fourier analysis, a number of frequency-phase terms are necessary. Since the full amount of data is sometimes not practical, the ideal full Fourier series must be *truncated* to a more manageable number of components for patient studies. The truncation of the Fourier series in MR imaging results in errors or approximations in the reconstruction of the appearance of the original object (Figs 4–29 through 4–31). As fewer data terms are used, these errors become more pronounced due to the decreased frequency of ringing and diminished decay rate of ringing amplitude. In images or spatial frequency domain, the oscillations, or ringing, appear as parallel bands of high and low signal adjacent to tissue discontinuities, or edges.[34]

The truncation of the full data series results in a ringing artifact, because of the inability to accurately approximate this tissue discontinuity with a shorter truncated data set. Therefore, the ringing that occurs at all tissue boundaries on MR is called *truncation artifact*. It is sometimes erroneously referred to as Gibbs phenomena. Gibbs described an overshoot

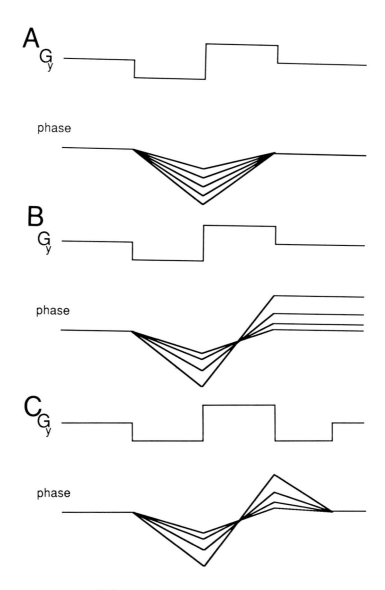

FIG 4–26.
Gradient moment nulling strategies. **A,** stationary protons are suc-
cessfully rephased with simple
bipolar gradient. **B,** laminar flow in-
troduces phase errors not corrected
with these gradients. **C,** additional
gradient pulse rephases the laminar
flow case.

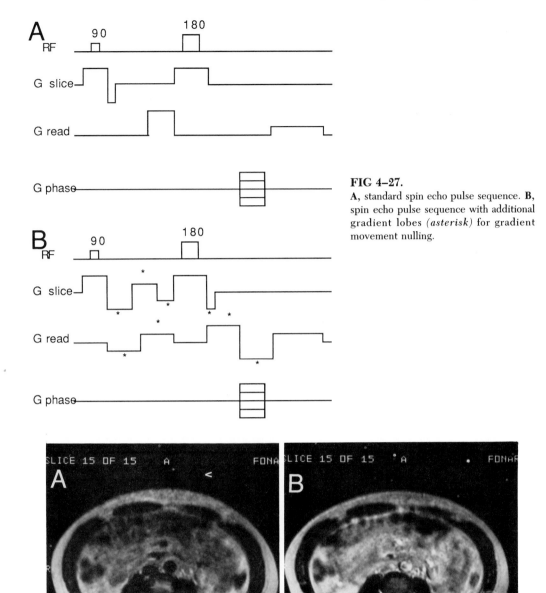

FIG 4–27.
A, standard spin echo pulse sequence. **B,** spin echo pulse sequence with additional gradient lobes *(asterisk)* for gradient movement nulling.

FIG 4–28.
Effect of GMN on normal abdomen motion. **A,** scan (SE/2000/85) without GMN shows significant motion artifact *(arrowhead).* **B,** scan with GMN significantly reduces motion artifacts.

FIG 4–29.
Truncation errors. **A,** tissue discontinuity to be encoded with Fourier series. **B,** single sine wave poorly approximates the boundary. **C,** more terms improve the approximation. **D,** even with many terms a brightness oscillation persists at the boundary due to truncation of the Fourier series. The 8.95% overshoot described by Gibbs *(arrow)* does not account for the major truncation image artifacts.

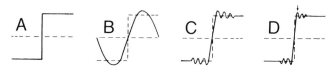

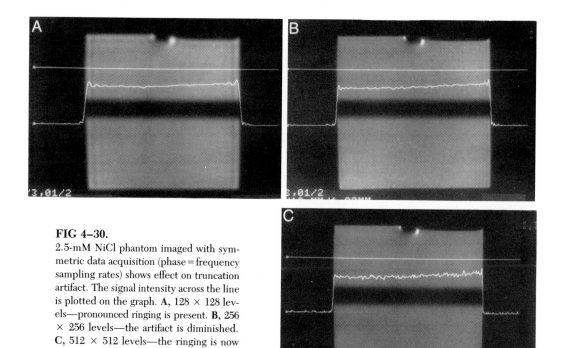

FIG 4–30.
2.5-mM NiCl phantom imaged with symmetric data acquisition (phase = frequency sampling rates) shows effect on truncation artifact. The signal intensity across the line is plotted on the graph. **A,** 128 × 128 levels—pronounced ringing is present. **B,** 256 × 256 levels—the artifact is diminished. **C,** 512 × 512 levels—the ringing is now almost lost in background noise.

equal to 8.95% of the discontinuity amplitude at either end of boundaries with Fourier analysis of incomplete data sets.[35] The Gibbs error is thus a single spike on either side and different from truncation errors.

In addition to degrading the image, truncation artifacts can obscure normal anatomy and be mistaken for pathology.[36] Several strategies are possible for diminution of the effect of truncation artifacts on an image. If more phase and frequency terms are added during data collection, the ringing will have a higher frequency, decay more rapidly, and be generally less noticeable. Unfortunately, since the sampling frequency in the phase axis, or number of phase levels acquired, determines the overall scan time, increasing this results in longer patient examination times. Most manufacturers already implement asymmetric data sampling rates with 128 to 256 phase levels and 256 to 512 levels obtained in the non-time-dependent frequency axis. Thus, the artifact is usually most noticeable in the phase axis because of the

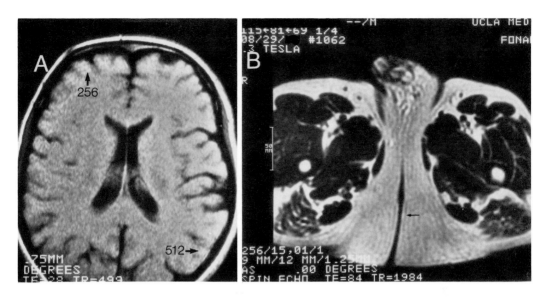

FIG 4–31.
Clinical examples of truncation errors. **A,** normal brain (SE/500/30) 256 × 512 acquisition. The ringing artifact is more pronounced along the phase encoded (256) axis. **B,** truncation artifacts produce dark bands along the gluteal crease *(arrow).*

lower data sampling rates. When the structures being imaged have many edges that tend to occur in one axis, the effects of truncation can be diminished if the patient is positioned so that the edges lie along the frequency axis (which usually has the higher sampling frequency).

High spatial frequency information may be removed from the signal data, which will eliminate most of the ringing due to truncation effects by adding a low-pass filter to the data, however, this will also remove a great deal of the image sharpness. The ringing can also be reduced by modification of the phases of the complex data samples. Although more data processing is required to perform this modification, the technique results in less blurring than occurs in simple low-pass filtering.

MAGNETIC FIELD DISTORTION

Another type of MR artifact that does not necessarily occur at edges results from distortions of the magnetic field. These have a characteristic appearance of geometric distortion of the image that should suggest abnormalities in the magnetic fields—either the null field, the gradients, or some effect due to magnetic material in the patient.

Consider, for example, the situation when a ferromagnetic clip is present in the patient. When the null field is applied, instead of being a uniform field there is a distortion where the iron magnetizes to a higher field than the surrounding diamagnetic tissues in the field. When linear gradients are applied over this null field the linear gradients become nonlinear. When the image is formed with these nonlinear gradients there is nonlinearity or geometric distortion of the image. The null field may be thought of as the canvas on which the MR image is painted. The distortion of the null field deforms the canvas and thus the final image.

Although the appearance of magnetic field distortions is often characteristic, it can occasionally be confusing.[37] Such appearances can occur from metal imbedded in the patient, and usually the artifact is considerably larger than the material causing it. In fact, these artifacts may be produced from small amounts of metal that are invisible on CT or plain film examination following the use of bone drills and saws at surgery.[38] Geometric distortions can also occur from materials outside the patient (such as a paper clip inadvertently left in the magnet).[39] Failure of gradient amplifier power supplies will also result in geometric distortion of the image along one axis, creating pseudoscaphocephaly or causing the image to have a bizarre appearance of some other kind.

The field distortion artifacts are worse with metals with high magnetic susceptibility. Titanium or high nickel content alloys have little artifact. Nickel converts the magnetically susceptible face-centered cubic metal crystal structure to one with more diamagnetic body-centered geometry (Fig 4–32).

The artifact is more pronounced along the readout axis. By changing axes, the artifact in some cases may be repositioned to uncover areas of important anatomy. Gradient echo images tend to make the artifacts worse than spin echo images due to higher T2* sensitivity (Fig 4–33). Finally, for all pulse sequences the artifacts are worse at higher field strengths. Using a mid- or low-field instrument will decrease the artifact size (see Fig 4–33).

ALIASING OR WRAPAROUND

Aliasing is a phenomenon seen in MR images related to sampling of data and the fact that it is not practical to sample an infinite number of levels. This noncontinuous discreet sampling means that it is not possible to unambiguously determine frequencies in the image.

There are at least two frequencies that will appear exactly the same for a given sampling rate (Fig 4–34). The scanners are usually designed so that all the frequencies within the imaging space are unambiguously sampled. However, problems occur when any part of the body extends outside the imaging volume. These higher frequencies outside the imaging volume may appear exactly the same as frequencies within the image. When the image is reconstructed both sets of frequencies and the corresponding image parts are superimposed. This is called *wraparound* or *aliasing* (Fig 4–35).

Fortunately, aliasing can be prevented in the frequency axis by putting high-pass and low-pass filters on either side to remove the out-of-band frequencies. Aliasing is therefore primarily a problem in the phase axis. Phase is continuous—a 370 degree phase angle is

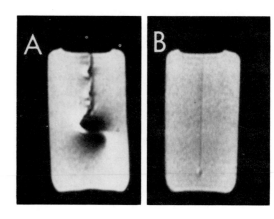

FIG 4–32.
Effect of nickel content on ferromagnetic artifact created by needle suspended in phantom. **A,** large artifact is present in low-nickel (9%) needle. **B,** the artifact is greatly reduced in the higher-nickel (49%) alloy needle.

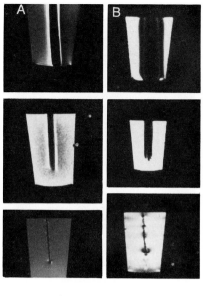

FIG 4–33.
Effect of field strength and pulse sequence on image artifact of needle in phantom. The artifact increases with increasing field strength (.3 T, .5 T, and 1.5 T, *bottom to top*) and is worse on field echo sequences (**B**) compared to spin echo(**A**).

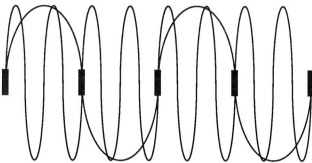

FIG 4–34.
Aliasing. Two different frequencies can appear identical for a given sampling window (*solid rectangles*).

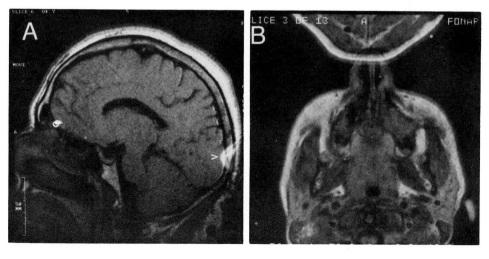

FIG 4–35.
Clinical examples of aliasing artifacts. **A,** sagittal view includes the nose (*arrowhead*) projected over the occiput. **B,** axial view shows similar wraparound.

ALIASING OR WRAPAROUND   SURFACE COILS TO AVOID ALIASING

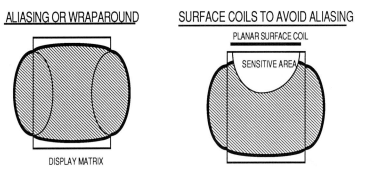

DISPLAY MATRIX

FIG 4–36.
Strategies to avoid aliasing.

OVERSAMPLING TO AVOID ALIASING   PRESATURATION TO AVOID ALIASING

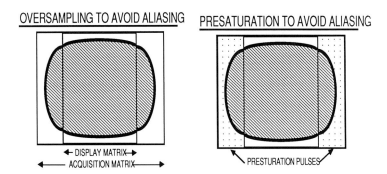

indistinguishable from a 10 degree phase angle. There is no simple way to filter phase as is possible with frequency.

In the phase axis it is possible to minimize aliasing by trying to make the field of view large enough so that the entire patient is included (Fig 4–36). Surface coils can also minimize aliasing by excluding the signal from the portion of the patient that is aliased. Another approach is to oversample the image. Oversampling acquires a larger image than is actually displayed. Finally, presaturation pulses can saturate the signal from portions of the patient that will be subject to wraparound and thus minimize aliasing.

REFERENCES

1. Bradley WG, Waluch V: Blood flow: Magnetic resonance imaging. *Radiology* 1985; 154:443–450.
2. Crooks LE, Mills CM, Davis PL, et al: Nuclear magnetic resonance. Visualization of cerebral and vascular abnormalities by NMR imaging. The effects of imaging parameters on contrast[1]. *Radiology* 1982; 144:843–852.
3. Axel L: Blood flow effects in magnetic resonance imaging. *AJR* 1984; 143:1157–1166.
4. Mills CM, Brant-Zawadski M, Crooks LE, et al: Nuclear magnetic resonance: Principles of blood flow imaging. *AJNR* 1983; 4:1161–1166; *AJR* 1983; 142:165:170.
5. Wendt RE, Murphy PH, Ford JJ, et al: Phase alterations of spin echoes by motion along magnetic field gradients. *Magn Reson Med* 1985; 2:527–533.
6. Bradley WG Jr, Waluch V, et al: The appearance of rapidly flowing blood of magnetic resonance images. *AJR* 1984; 143:1167–1174.
7. Bradley WG, Kortman KE, Burgoyne B: Flowing CSF in normal and hydrocephalic states; appearance on MR images. *Radiology* 1986; 159:611–616.

8. Felmlee JP, Ehman RL: Spatial presaturation: A method for suppressing flow artifacts and improving depiction of vascular anatomy in MR imaging. *Radiology* 1987; 164:559–564.

9. Waluch V, Bradley WG Jr: NMR even echo rephasing in slow laminar flow. *J Comput Assist Tomogr* 1984; 8:594–598.

10. Singer JR: NMR diffusing and flow measurements and an introduction to spin phase graphing. *Phy E Sci Instrum* 1978; 11:281–291.

11. Wedeen VJ, Mueli RA, Edelman RR, et al: Projective imaging of pulsatile flow with magnetic resonance. *Science* 1985; 230:946–948.

12. Valk PE, Hale JD, Kaufman L, et al: MR imaging of the aorta with three-dimensional vessel reconstruction: Validation by angiography[1]. *Radiology* 1985; 157:721–725.

13. Hale JD, Valk PE, Watts JC, et al: MR imaging of blood vessels using three-dimensional reconstruction: Methodology. *Radiology* 1985; 157:727–733.

14. Ruszkowski JT, Damadian R, Giambalvo A, et al: MRI angiography of the carotid artery. *Magn Reson Imaging* 1986; 4:497–502.

15. Ruggieri P, Laub G, Masaryk TJ, et al: Intracranial circulation: Pulse sequence considerations in 3-D volume angiography. *Radiology* 1989; 171:785–791.

16. Axel L, Morton D: MR flow imaging by velocity compensated/uncompensated difference images. *J Comput Assist Tomogr* 1987; 11:31–34.

17. Dumoulin CL, Hart HR: Magnetic resonance angiography. *Radiology* 1986; 161:717–720.

18. Pusey E, Lufkin RB, Brown RKJ, et al: MRI artifacts: Mechanisms and clinical significance. *Radiographics* 1986; 6:891–911.

19. Bellon EM, Hacke M, Coleman P, et al: MRI artifacts: A review. *AJR* 1986; 147:1271.

20. Soila KP, Viamonte M, Starewicz PM: Chemical shift misregistration effect in magnetic resonance imaging. *Radiology* 1984; 153:819–820.

21. Weinreb JC, Brateman L, Babcock EE, et al: Chemical shift artifact in clinical magnetic resonance images at 0.35 T. *AJR* 1985; 45:183–185.

22. Lufkin R, Crues J, Anselmo M, et al: Chemical shift misregistration errors in MRI: Effect of field strength. *Computerized Radiology* 1988; 12:89.

23. Babcock EE, Libby B, Weinreb JC, et al: Edge artifacts in MR images. Chemical shift effect. *J Comput Assist Tomogr* 1985; 9:252–257.

24. Dwyer AJ, Knop RH, Hoult DI: Frequency shift artifacts in MR imaging. *J Comput Assist Tomogr* 1985; 9:16–18.

25. Bertino RE, Porter BA, Stimac GK, et al: Imaging spinal osteomyelitis and epidural abscess with short TI inversion recovery (STIR). *AJNR* 1988; 9:563–564.

26. Wehrli FW, Perkins TG, Shimakawa A, et al: Chemical shift-induced amplitude modulations in images obtained with gradient refocusing. *Magn Reson Imaging* 1987; 5:157–158.

27. Schultz CL, Alfidi RJ, Nelson AD, et al: The effect of motion on two-dimensional Fourier transformation magnetic resonance images. *Radiology* 1984; 152:117–121.

28. Stark DD, Hendrick RE, Hahn PF, et al: Motion artifact reduction with fast spin echo imaging. *Radiology* 1987; 164:183–191.

29. Westcott JL, Henschke CI, Berkmen Y: MR imaging of the hilum and mediastinum: Effects of cardiac gating. *J Comput Assist Tomogr* 1985; 9:1073–1078.

30. Ehman RL, McNamara MT, Pallack M, et al: Magnetic resonance imaging with respiratory gating: Techniques and advantages. *AJR* 1984; 143:1175–1182.

31. Runge VM, Clanton JA, Partain CL, et al: Respiratory gating in magnetic resonance imaging at 0.5 Tesla. *Radiology* 1984; 151:521–523.

32. Bailes DR, Gilderdale DJ, Bydder G, et al: Respiratory ordered phase encoding (ROPE): A method for reducing motion artifacts in MRI. *J Comput Assist Tomogr* 1985; 9:835–838.

33. Pattany PM, Phillips JJ, Chiu LC, et al: Motion artifact suppression technique-(Mast) for MR imaging. *J Comput Assist Tomogr* 1987; 11:369–377.

34. Lufkin RB, Pusey E, Stark DD, et al: Boundary artifact due to truncation errors in MR imaging. *AJR* 1986; 147:1283–1287.

35. Bracewell RN: *The Fourier Transformation and Its Applications.* New York, McGraw-Hill, 1978.

36. Daniels DL, Czervionke LF, Breger RK, et al: "Truncation" artifact in MR images of the internal auditory canal. *AJNR* 1987; 8:793–794.
37. New PFJ, Rosen BR, Brady TJ, et al: Potential hazards and artifacts of ferromagnetic and non ferromagnetic surgical and dental materials and devices in nuclear magnetic resonance imaging. *Radiology* 1983; 147:139–148.
38. Mechlin M, Thikman D, Kressel HY, et al: Magnetic resonance imaging of postoperative patients with metallic implants. *AJR* 1984; 143:1281–1284.
39. Ludeke KM, Roschmann P, Tischler R: Susceptibility artifacts in NMR imaging. *Magn Reson Imaging* 1985; 3:329–343.

Chapter 5 _____

Magnetic Resonance Instrumentation

Robert Lufkin, M.D.

In this chapter, all the concepts that have been previously covered including magnetic resonance (MR) signal generation, contrast, and image formation will be combined in a discussion of the physical implementation of the MR hardware. Despite the variety of magnetic resonance imaging (MRI) systems that are currently available, all MR instruments have the same basic subsystems. If the computer, data storage, image display, and keyboard [which are similar to those found in other cross-sectional imaging machines such as those used in computed tomography (CT)] are excluded MRI instrumentation can be divided into three main component subsystems

1. Main magnetic field
2. Gradient magnetic field generators
3. Radiofrequency (RF) transmitter and receiver

For each of these components there are specific performance parameters and options available. For each choice close attention must be paid to the equipment and performance tradeoffs. Any improvement in signal-to-noise, contrast, or spatial resolution is usually offset by longer scan times, increased cost, or increased sensitivity to artifacts. To fully understand choices available in MR instrumentation, design and performance compromises associated with each decision must be considered.

MAIN MAGNETIC FIELD

The key element in any MR imager is the main magnet.[1] The function of this component is to produce a uniform static magnetic field (also known as the B_0 field) on which is superimposed magnetic field gradients and radio frequency pulses as necessary for imaging.

It is interesting to note that most MR systems are described according to the type of main magnet design. In addition to the type of a magnet the field strength is also generally specified. The assumption that magnetic field type or strength totally defines the performance of an MR system is erroneous. Although the type of magnet does affect machine performance, the other subsystems may have an equal or greater contribution in some situations.

Four different techniques are presently available for the generation of the main magnetic field (Fig 5–1). These are permanent air core resistive, iron core resistive, and superconductive magnets (Table 5–1). The type of magnet that is employed to generate the B_0 field is in many ways irrelevant as far as the individual protons are concerned. Just as the electric current that flows from a wall outlet is the same whether it is generated from a nuclear, hydroelectric, or coal burning electric power plant, the protons respond to B_0 field of the magnet regardless of the type of magnet used to produce it.

There are however, considerable differences in site considerations, operating costs, main field axis, and other factors with the different types of magnets. In fact, it has become clear with modern MR instruments that the main magnet type and field strength are only two of many factors (e.g., gradient and RF coils, and other electronic factors) that all contribute to the ultimate quality of the MR image.

The effect of the magnet on the environment depends to some extent on the type of magnet. The extension of magnetic field into the environment is known as the *fringe field*. The degree to which this occurs depends on the field strength as well as the type of magnet. The fringe fields produced by all magnet types increase more or less with increasing magnetic field strength. Magnets with iron flux return paths (i.e., permanent and iron core resistive systems) have minimal fringe fields. This is because this magnet design allows the magnetic field lines to travel through the iron return path rather than extending into the environment. The limitation of this design is that the upper theoretical field strength limit in iron core flux return magnet systems is around 1.0 T because iron saturates above this field strength.

The use of air (which does not saturate) as a flux return path allows the use of magnet field strengths greater than 1.0 T. This is employed in air core resistive and superconducting magnet systems. The disadvantage of air as a flux return path is that it results in the fringe fields extending out into the environment to a much greater extent. The large fringe fields of air flux return systems can be reduced with the use of large amounts of magnetic field shielding. This is usually accomplished by using large amounts of steel plate. In addition to adding expense, this approach also requires critical readjusting or "shimming" the main magnetic field.

FIG 5–1.
Four types of MR magnets and the field strengths that they can achieve currently. Only superconductive magnets can operate at high (>1.0 T) field.

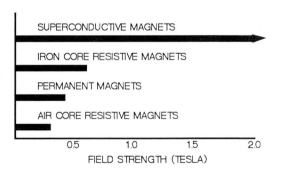

FIELD STRENGTH VERSUS MAGNET DESIGN

SUPERCONDUCTIVE MAGNETS

IRON CORE RESISTIVE MAGNETS

PERMANENT MAGNETS

AIR CORE RESISTIVE MAGNETS

0.5   1.0   1.5   2.0
FIELD STRENGTH (TESLA)

TABLE 5–1.
Magnet Types

Magnet	Field Axis	Installation	Upper Limit	Cost	Fringe Fields
Permanent	Vertical	Component	0.3 T	Low	Low
Air core resistive	Horizontal	Preassembled	0.2 T	Medium	Medium
Iron core resistive	Vertical	Component	0.6 T	Medium	Low
Superconductive	Horizontal	Preassembled	2.0 T+	High	High

Related to the fringe fields is the phenomenon known as the "missile effect." This is the tendency for large ferromagnetic objects to be accelerated into the bore of the magnet. Because of the contained flux return path and thus small fringe fields with permanent and iron core resistive systems, this effect is greatly reduced with these magnet types. Air return flux pathway systems with large fringe fields such as air core resistive and superconductive magnet systems can create powerful missile effects and occasionally may create significant safety hazards, for the patient and staff.

No matter what the field strength, the physical requirements for whole body clinical MR instrument are that a human being along with additional RF and gradient instrumentation must fit inside its bore. In most cases a magnet bore of at least 1 m is necessary.

In addition to the physical size of the magnet, the field that is produced must also have a high degree of both spatial and temporal uniformity. *Temporal uniformity* is the stability of the field over time. Imaging may be accomplished with a spatial field uniformity as low as several hundred parts per million (ppm) over a 50 cm^3 volume although spectroscopic applications may require spatial uniformity as fine as 0.1 ppm over a 10 cm^3 volume.

Permanent Magnets

The permanent magnet design is the simplest approach to creating a magnetic field. Permanent magnets are made up of large blocks of ferromagnetic materials similar to that used in simple horseshoe magnets (Figs 5–2 and 5–3). The magnetic field is generated between the two poles of the magnet without the use of any additional power supply or cooling requirements. As such this design is the most efficient of the four magnet configurations to be discussed.

The term *permanent* is an appropriate description of the magnetic field. Although the magnetic field is permanent the magnet is removable if necessary. Systems using permanent magnets may be disassembled for upgrade or eventual replacement. While the permanent design is efficient in that no power is required to turn on the magnetic field, it is also impossible to turn these systems off. This actually turns out to be only a minor inconvenience. The fear

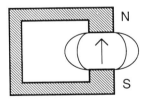

FIG 5–2.
Permanent magnet. The vertical field is produced between the two magnet endplates.

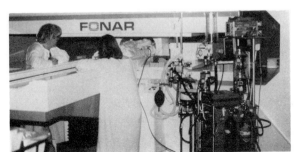

FIG 5–3.
Permanent magnet system. The vertical field and contained flux return path allow the use ferromagnetic life support equipment in close proximity to the magnet.

that increasing numbers of metal objects would be stuck to the magnet forever has proven to be unfounded and small ferromagnetic objects placed in the magnet can easily be removed by hand in most cases.

Installation of permanent magnet systems is simple because, unlike superconducting systems, permanent magnets are assembled on site and most system components can be wheeled in through standard size door frames. While it is easy to install the components of permanent magnets, they tend to be very heavy so that an assembled ferrite permanent magnet system capable of generating 0.3 T may weigh up to 200,000 lb. Newer exotic permanent magnet materials (neodymium-iron-barium [Nd-Fe-Ba]) overcome this weight limitation.

One advantage of the permanent design is that the system is largely self-shielding and an iron return path for the magnetic flux is provided by the magnet frame. The fringe magnetic fields extending out around the magnet are greatly reduced with this type of system. The 5-gauss isoflux line for a 0.3-T imager will be only a few feet from the bore of the magnet.

The endplates in most permanent magnets are oriented so that the field produced between these plates is in the vertical direction. This has important ramifications in the design of RF coils as well as the configuration of fringe fields. As will be discussed shortly, the vertical axis of the main magnetic field allows the use of efficient solenoidal design RF coils for the majority of imaging applications. The vertical field orientation also means that the tendency for metal objects to be accelerated into the bore of the magnet (and patient) is greatly reduced.

Reduction of this phenomena is a significant safety advantage for vertical field systems in general and especially in situations where patients with extensive life support equipment are examined. Patients with accompanying metal "crash" carts, gurneys, intravenous (IV) poles, and ventilators who could not be studied with air core resistive and superconducting systems without substitution of special aluminum equipment, can be easily scanned with permanent and iron core resistive magnet systems.

A limitation of this permanent magnet technology is that the upper practical field strength is around 0.3 T for purely permanent magnet design whole-body imagers. The theoretical problems of field stability with temperature change are not a problem with permanent magnets, presumably due to the significant thermal inertia associated with such a large mass. The field strength and uniformity of current permanent systems also do not allow spectroscopy.

Air Core Resistive Magnet

The second type of magnet is based on the phenomenon that wires carrying electrical current create magnetic fields proportional to the amount of current. If a wire carrying current is wrapped into the form of a coil the magnetic field will be generated along the axis of the coil. This is known as an *electromagnet* and is the basis for the air core resistive as well as superconductive magnet designs.

Air core resistive and superconductive magnets are sometimes referred to as solenoidal design magnets because the field is generated from loops of wire forming a solenoid. This is based on the theoretical ideal design for an electromagnet necessary to produce a perfectly uniform field, which is a wire conductor wound around a sphere (Fig 5–4).

This pure form is not a practical approach for medical imaging because their is no way for the patient to get in or out of the sphere. A workable approximation is to simulate the sphere with four coils of wire that form a solenoid that allows patient access. The term *solenoid magnet* should not be confused with the term *solenoid RF coils* which will be discussed in Superconductive Magnets, below.

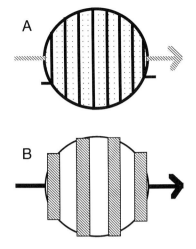

FIG 5–4.
Electromagnet design. **A,** ideal electromagnet with wire conductors forming a sphere prevents patient access to the field. **B,** practical approximation of the sphere with coils allow patient access yet still has good spatial uniformity.

Air core resistive magnets are thus typically made up of four coaxial coils of copper or aluminum with associated cooling water jackets. Because current must be maintained in the wire to generate the magnetic field, this type of magnet has a fairly significant electrical power requirement (20 kW at 0.12 T). Since current flowing in the wire at normal temperatures encounters resistance and produces heat, there is also a significant water cooling requirement in order to remove this thermal load.

These factors determine an upper limit of field strength possible with this design since the strength of the magnetic field generated is dependent on the current in the magnet wire. Because the energy to be dissipated increases as the square of the current, doubling the current (and field) quadruples the cooling needs. Therefore, in order to produce a 0.3-T field over 200 kW of heat are generated which have to be dissipated, which is very impractical. This limits the use of air core resistive systems to generating fields up to 0.2 T or so. An advantage of air core resistive systems is that, of the four magnet designs, they may be purchased at the lowest cost.

Because the field temporal stability is critically dependent on a stable source of electrical current, early systems were plagued by power supply instability problems. Power supplies stable to 1 ppm over time are now available for imaging and this problem is no longer significant. Air core resistive systems, however (like permanent systems), cannot meet the field strength and uniformity demands necessary for most chemical shift spectroscopy applications.

Most, if not all, air core resistive systems are oriented so that the patient lies along the bore of the magnet with a horizontal main field axis (Figs 5–4 and 5–5). This requires the

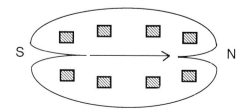

FIG 5–5.
Air core resistive magnet. Most installations are oriented so that a horizontal magnetic field axis is produced.

use of a saddle RF coil design for most imaging applications. This configuration also has significant fringe fields that extend a considerable distance around the magnet compared to permanent designs. The horizontal field also results in a higher tendency for metal objects to be accelerated into the bore of the magnet (missile effect) than vertical field design systems.

Iron Core (Hybrid) Resistive Magnets

A new type of hybrid magnet called the iron core resistive system may be created by combining features of permanent and air core resistive magnet systems. This is done by forming blocks of iron or other more exotic materials into large magnetic endplates on poles like the permanent magnet and then adding coils of wire to each endplate as in the air core resistive magnets. This third type of magnet designed combines many of the advantages of the first two types with relatively few disadvantages (Figs 5–6 and 5–7).

Because of the iron core resistive component, there are lower power and cooling requirements than with an air core design system of similar field strength. This savings results in lower operational costs. Because the iron core aspect of the system is supplemented with resistive components, iron core resistive magnets can be made much smaller and lighter than pure permanent magnet systems of the same field strength. Since the magnetic field does require power to be maintained, the field may be turned off as is the case with air core resistive magnets.

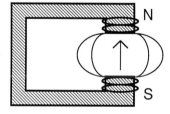

FIG 5–6.
Iron core resistive magnet. As is the case with the permanent magnet, the vertical field is produced between the magnet end plates.

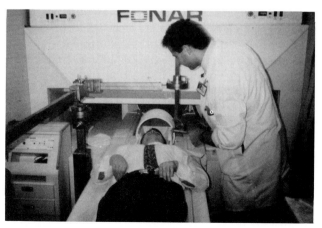

FIG 5–7.
Iron core resistive (hybrid) system. The metal stereotactic system is being used for an MR guided needle aspiration biopsy.

Iron core resistive systems also maintain many of the advantages of permanent magnet systems. The component construction of iron core resistive magnets allows most systems to be assembled on site. This eliminates many of the site access problems associated with delivery of preassembled magnets.

The large iron component acts as a built in shielding and flux return path so that the fringe magnetic fields are minimized as in the case of permanent magnet systems. Most iron core resistive magnets are oriented so that the main field axis is vertical. This allows the use of solenoidal design RF coils. The vertical axis along with the minimal fringe fields also results in minimal missile effect and generally improved safety conditions when working around the magnet with ferromagnetic materials.

The iron core resistive design allows the production of field strengths for human whole body that are higher than that possible with either permanent or air core-resistive designs alone. At the present time iron-core resistive systems are operating at field strengths up to 0.6 T although several researchers feel that a 1.0-T hybrid magnet is not out of the realm of possibility.

Because of the components involved, the purchase price for this type of magnet design is generally higher than that for similar air core resistive systems and similar to that for permanent magnet system.

Superconductive Magnets

Superconductive magnets are similar to air core resistive magnets in that they are electromagnets of the solenoidal design. Both types use large coils of wire which are needed to generate the electromagnetic field. Unlike the air coil resistive design which uses water to remove heat generated by the resistance encountered by the current, superconducting magnets exploit the fact that the electrical resistance of most metals is proportional to their temperature. Thus it is possible to dramatically reduce the resistance by cooling the wires to near absolute zero ($-459.67°F$) with liquid helium in order to maintain a superconducting state. The current in a superconductive wire not only encounters practically no resistance but also circulates nearly indefinitely.

This is practically implemented in a large vacuum cryostat or dewar (similar to a thermos bottle) which contains the conducting wires. Instead of simple copper, niobium, and titanium or similar alloys (which are superconductive at 10 to 20°K) are combined in a copper matrix to create the superconducting environment (Figs 5–8 and 5–9).

Unlike the air core resistive electromagnet system where only four coils are used to approximate the ideal sphere in order to minimize heat production, superconductive magnets do not have this constraint. Most superconductive magnets are instead wound around aluminum or fiberglass cylinders, with the ideal spherical condition simulated by varying numbers of turns of the coils (see Fig 5–8).

A jacket of liquid helium maintains the temperature of the wires at near absolute zero (4.2°K). Since liquid helium is expensive, boiloff of the helium is reduced with an insulating layer of less expensive liquid nitrogen (which boils at around 70°K). The liquids placed in the cryostat to maintain superconduction are referred to as *cryogens*.

This system can fail if either the temperature or current density becomes too high. At that point the magnet goes from superconductive to resistive mode and is said to "quench." Quenching results in the rapid collapse of the magnetic field and the release of heat and sudden boiling off of the cryogens. The collapse of the field usually occurs over 20 to 60 seconds and apparently does not represent a significant risk to the patient. In addition to being an expensive loss of cryogens, the sudden release of gas can result in a safety problem for the patient because of the rapid displacement of breathable oxygen. For this reason most

FIG 5–8.
Ideal spherical electromagnet is simulated by varied spacing of the
magnetic coils. As with other solenoidal electromagnets, a horizontal
field axis is produced.

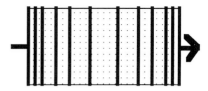

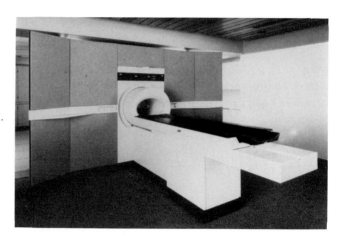

FIG 5–9.
Superconductive system. (Courtesy of M.
Anselmo, M.D.)

superconductive magnet scanner suites have a large space over the magnet for gas collection
in the event of a quench.

In 1986 a revolution occurred in superconducting technology. At that time the IBM
research group in Zurich announced the discovery of ceramic metal oxides that are superconductive at higher temperatures than absolute zero. Since that time other researchers have
pushed this limit up to near room temperature. At present there are still major problems
with achieving high enough current density for magnets used in superconducting imagers.
However, implications of this new technology are certainly dramatic.

Since current flowing in a properly functioning superconducting magnet meets very little
resistance, the power requirements for operating of this system are low. The overall operating
costs are high, however, because of the slow but steady boiloff of cryogens. The cryogens
are stored in large dewars and periodically added to the cryostat. The rate of loss has a weak
correlation with the operating field strength but increases with magnets in mobile or trans-
portable MR units which encounter a large amount of vibration. Closed refrigeration systems
are available to capture and recondense the expensive helium but tend to have significant
power requirements (5 to 20 kW).

The field axis of superconducting magnets is along the bore of the magnet similar to that
of an air-core resistive system. Therefore, RF coils of a saddle configuration are most often
used for the RF system. Significant fringe fields are present with superconducting magnets.
This combined with the horizontal main field axis results in significant missile effects for
ferromagnetic objects.

In addition to having a high operating cost, superconductive magnets are generally the
most expensive magnet to purchase of the four magnet designs. The complex technology
used in the manufacture of superconductive magnets also means that most magnets of this
kind are assembled in the factory and shipped in one piece which can create access problems

for magnet placement at some sites.

The real advantage of superconducting magnets is in high field imaging. This is presently the only choice of magnet design for whole body imaging over 1.0 T. In fact, large core superconducting magnets have been used for imaging at 4.7 T and even higher field strengths.

GRADIENT MAGNETIC FIELD GENERATORS

Although the main magnetic field has a north and south pole it should be as uniform as possible (i.e., the same strength throughout the imaging volume). The purpose of the magnetic field gradient subsystem is to create linear variations in the uniform main magnetic field to allow spatial localization of the MR signal. This is accomplished by superimposing relatively weak gradient magnetic fields on a stronger uniform main magnetic field. The resulting field experienced by the patient's protons is due to the sum of the two applied fields. Although the main magnet type is important in machine performance, the gradient subsystem in many ways defines the limits of imaging performance.

Important performance parameters of the gradient coils and associated power supplies are that they are linear, strong, reproducible, and have a rapid rise time. Both amplitude and change of the gradients must be finely controlled. Linearity is important for accurate mapping of the MR signal. The uniformity of the main field and linearity of the gradients both create a smooth canvas on which the MR image is painted. Nonlinearity of gradients or nonuniformity of the main magnetic field result in geometric distortion of the image and loss of spatial resolution.

The *rise time* is the finite amount of time that is required for the gradient to reach its full amplitude after the power is applied (Fig 5–10). Rapid rise times (less than 1 msec for some high-speed pulse sequences) allow the use of high-gradient amplitudes in order to produce thin sections or high-in-plane spatial resolution. These high-gradient amplitudes cannot be used with slow rise times without significantly limiting the use of short echo time (TE) studies.

Fast pulse sequences such as gradient echo and echo planar place even greater demands on the gradient system than with spin echo imaging. Rapid rise times are also essential for fast scanning applications.

For the majority of pulse sequences, the gradient amplitude is relatively small compared to the main field strength because gradients merely modify the field created by the primary magnet. Gradient fields must be strong enough to overcome nonuniformity of the main magnetic field and to keep chemical shift misregistration errors at an acceptable level. This turns out to be approximately two to three orders of magnitude lower than the main field strength. Gradients are measured in units of mT/m (millitesla per meter) so that a typical

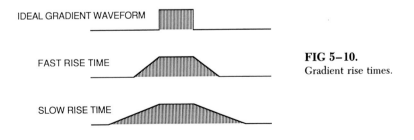

FIG 5–10.
Gradient rise times.

strength gradient for a 0.5-T system is 10 mT/m (1.0 gauss/cm) for spin echo imaging and 50 mT/m for echo planar imaging.

The advantages of steeper gradients, in addition to minimizing field inhomogeneities and chemical shift errors, is to produce higher spatial resolution images. This is offset by higher power supply requirements, longer rise times, increased eddy currents, and lower image signal-to-noise with increasing gradient amplitude.

The gradients are produced in all types of MR imagers by current flowing in wires in the form of electromagnets. Typical gradient systems consist of three coaxial sets of coils corresponding to the three physical gradients Gx, Gy, and Gz. The imaging software later assigns one or more of the physical gradients to the image formation functions of slice selection, phase encoding, and frequency encoding.

The gradients are produced along the axis of the patient (Z axis) by two loops of wire (Fig 5–11). The current flows in opposite directions in each loop to create the field gradient. The field created by one current loop adds slightly to the main field on one end and subtracts slightly at the other end with zero effect in the middle.

The remaining two orthogonal gradients are produced with slightly more complex wire coil arrangements (Figs 5–12 and 5–13). In this case the field gradient is generated across

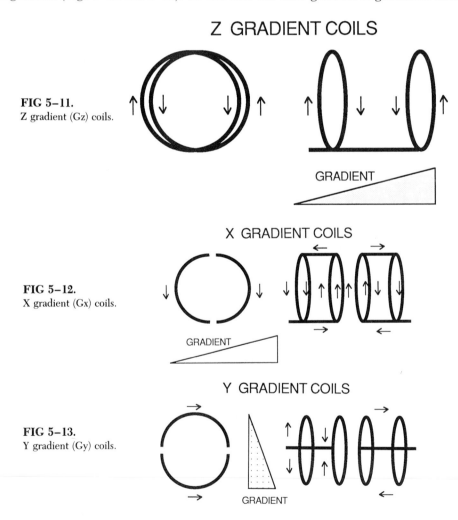

FIG 5–11.
Z gradient (Gz) coils.

FIG 5–12.
X gradient (Gx) coils.

FIG 5–13.
Y gradient (Gy) coils.

the axis of the patient by current flowing in opposite directions in each half of the loops. By combining all three gradients' coil systems it is possible to generate linear gradients in each of three orthogonal axes (Fig 5–14).

Since the gradients are electromagnets, they have some similarities to the magnets in audio speakers. In fact, when the gradients are rapidly pulsed on and off with current as they are in normal MR image production they may produce a slight click or thump. With steep gradients in the higher-strength field used in some systems this sound may be quite loud. Manufacturers now go to great lengths to acoustically shield the gradient coils to avoid this problem. In some machines with particularly loud pulse sequences patients are routinely given ear plugs to avoid damage to the ears.

The magnetic effects of the gradients may also interact with surrounding structures and result in the formation of eddy currents. These degrade image quality and become worse with more robust gradient actions. New specially designed gradients are now in use to minimize these effects.

COMBINED X-Y-Z GRADIENT SYSTEM

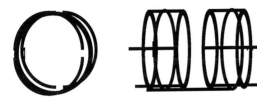

FIG 5–14.
Combined x-y-z gradient system.

RADIOFREQUENCY SUBSYSTEM

Although the hardware devices producing the gradients are sometimes referred to as coils, they must be distinguished from the third type of hardware that will be discussed which is known as the RF coil subsystem. The purpose of this system is to deliver RF pulses (at the Larmor frequency) to the patient as well as to detect signal from the transverse magnetization in the form of a free induction decay (FID) or echo.

The first function of the RF subsystem is to synthesize and transmit the RF signal to the patient at the resonant frequency. In general, transmitter coils are large with high RF uniformity for excitation. Since fine control of frequency is not necessary for transmission it is possible to use high amplifier gains. In general, transmitter coils have a low quality factor (Q) which is ideal for broad excitation.

After the signal is detected by the receiver coils it passes to a preamplifier to increase its strength. A demodulator then subtracts the detected signal from a reference signal at the Larmor frequency so that the image signal information may be processed in the kilohertz rather than megahertz range.

The receiver coil (unlike the transmitter coil) has as dramatic effect on SNR of the system and is therefore important to optimize for image quality. One of the major sources of noise in MR imagers is the patient. Therefore, it is critically important to optimize that interface between the machine and the patient, the RF receiver coil. Surface coils accomplish this with resulting improvements in signal-to-noise anywhere from four- to tenfold compared to standard head or body coils (Fig 5–15).

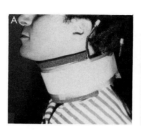
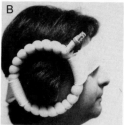

FIG 5–15.
Surface coils. **A,** solenoidal surface coils fits around the neck for studies of the cervical spine or larynx. **B,** planar surface coil in use for temporal bone examination. (Courtesy of John Robert.)

Coil loading and filling factors are a measure of how well the patient is matched to and fills the coils. In routine brain imaging, these factors, which determine the signal-to-noise for the standard head coil, are generally high because of the favorable anatomy of the region. However, for many areas of the body, such as the knee or neck, it is difficult to maneuver RF coils close to the body part being imaged. Thus, the SNR of many areas imaged with standard head and body coils is often poor. With the ability to be positioned close to a patient, surface coils dramatically improve this situation.

Signal-to-noise (SNR) is a critical factor in MR image quality. An improvement in image signal to noise may translate to shortened scan times (fewer excitations), improved spatial resolution (steeper gradients and smaller pixels), or decreased volume averaging errors (thinner slices). The SNR in MR receiver coils is represented by the following equation:

$$\text{SNR} \approx \sqrt{Q_L * n} \tag{1}$$

where Q_L is the quality factor of the coil loaded with a patient and n is the filling factor of the coil (which also depends on the relationship of the patient to the coil).[2] The quality factor of the coil is described by the following equation:

$$Q = (\text{frequency})/(a + b\sqrt{\text{frequency}} + d*\text{frequency}^2) \tag{2}$$

where a is proportional to the direct current (DC) resistivity of the coil material (copper), b is proportional to the RF resistivity of the coil material, and d is dependent on coil loading by the patient. At the higher frequencies currently used for imaging of 12.8 MHz (0.3 T) and greater, the frequency-squared term (and therefore the effects of coil loading by the patient) dominates in the denominator of Equation (2) and consequently determines the SNR in these coils. This is true for coils whose design has been optimized such that the noise due to coil materials is minimized ($Q_{empty} >> Q_{loaded}$).

Surface coils are designed to improve these two important terms that affect the signal-to-noise ratio (SNR), the filling factor, and coil loading by the patient. In addition, surface coils have other benefits due to their localizing design. Unlike conventional body or head coils with broad regions of sensitivity in the body, surface coils generally have a markedly limited region of sensitivity. This localized sensitivity is often maximal for superficial or surface structures and thus the coils are termed *surface coils*. Most images obtained with surface coils have a characteristic dropoff in signal ($1/r^2$) beyond the surface of the coil. Despite this unusual intensity appearance, surface coil MR images are useful clinically (Figs 5–16 and 5–17).

The controlled region of sensitivity possible with surface coils results in further improvement in image quality for several reasons. First, thermal noise is eliminated from parts of

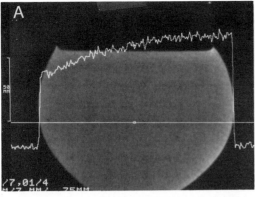
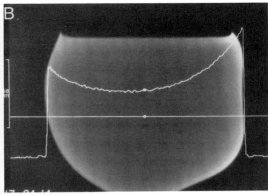
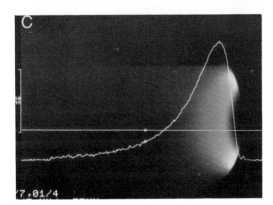

FIG 5–16.
Comparison of signal detection of planar, sole-noidal surface coils and standard body and head coils applied to a uniform 2.5 mM NiCl solution phantom. The curves are plots of signal intensity through the midportion of the phantom. All images are SE/500/28, axial, 4 mm thick, with 0.75 × 0.75 mm pixels obtained with four signal averages. **A,** the body coil (55.9 × 32.4 cm) shows the greatest amount of noise (as indicated by the mottled image appearance and irregular baseline plot) but fairly good deep signal detection. **B,** the 14.5-cm circumferential surface coil shows slightly less deep signal intensity but markedly less image noise. **C,** the 14-cm planar surface coil shows low noise and high superficial signal detection but rapid signal dropoff with increasing distance from the coil surface.

the body outside of the sensitive region. Other artifacts due to patient motion from bowel peristalsis, respiration, or blood flow are also reduced if they are outside the localized imaging region. Second, the limited field of view of most surface coils allows the use of steep imaging gradients while minimizing certain types of associated image artifacts known as wraparound or aliasing.

Despite these major changes in image appearance, signal-to-noise, and reduced artifacts that occur with surface coils, the remainder of imaging options available remain largely the same. Most manufacturers allow all standard pulse sequences to be used with surface coils. Since the magnetic field gradients are not affected by the coils, all gradient options (field of view and slice thickness change), as well as nonorthogonal imaging are available while using surface coils.

Surface coils were initially used for in vivo phosphorus spectroscopy to localize the volume of tissue to be studied.[3, 4] Now surface coils are being applied to an increasing variety of clinical MR imaging situations with dramatic results and are already considered essential for certain studies.[5–12]

A major constraint of RF coil application is that, because of Faraday's law, the only component of the coil that is sensitive to the transverse magnetization of the NMR signal is that portion that is orthogonal to the direction of the applied main magnetic field (B_0). Therefore, the simplest form of a surface coil is a loop of wire placed orthogonal to B_0 such

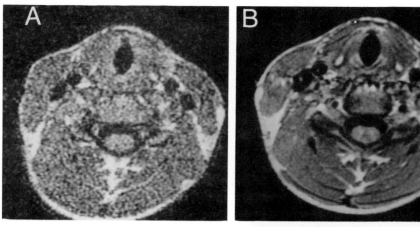

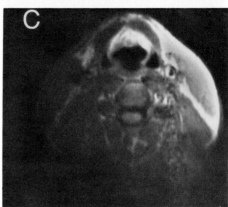

FIG 5–17.
Normal neck with body coil, solenoidal surface coil, and planar surface coil. The same imaging parameters were used as in Figure 5–16. **A,** the images obtained using the body coil have good signal uniformity but rather poor signal-to-noise. **B,** using the circumferential surface coil, the signal-to-noise is dramatically improved while reasonable signal uniformity is maintained. **C,** images produced using the 9-cm planar surface coil resulted in even better signal-to-noise near the coil surface but marked loss of signal from deep structures.

that the entire loop of wire contributes to the signal reception. This is known as a *planar* or *terrhoidal coil.* Planar coils are very useful for studies of superficial structures such as the orbit, parotid gland, and temporal bone.

The rate of planar surface coil signal drop-off depends on the coil dimension. Very little useful signal is present beyond one radius from the center of the coil $(1/r^2)$.[13] By plotting signal intensity vs. depth for several coils of various sizes, it is apparent that as deeper structures are imaged larger coils are necessary.

At the point where depth equals radius of the structure being imaged, the coil may be placed around the object in a circumferential fashion to form a solenoid. Circumferential coils provide good signal response across the image because all points are within one radius from the edge of the coil. Two general configurations are possible with circumferential coils: solenoidal and saddle.

The solenoidal design is a simple loop of conductor around the patient. It is an ideal configuration because the majority of the coil satisfies the condition of orthogonality to B_0 and thus has very good SNR. Solenoid coils also have the advantage that they are simple to apply and may be wrapped around the structure to be studied like a belt or collar. They work best in permanent and iron core resistive magnet systems that have a vertical main magnetic field. In this situation, they may be used to image the neck, knee, ankle, and pediatric chest.

Systems using a solenoidal magnet design (superconducting and air core resistive) have a horizontal main magnetic field and thus cannot use the solenoidal design for most RF coils. These coils cannot be easily positioned around a patient so that the criteria of being orthogonal to the main field can be satisfied. Solenoidal magnet-based systems are forced to use a slightly less efficient circumferential coil design known as a saddle coil.[14, 15]

One obvious disadvantage of planar surface coils is that because of the loss of signal with depth, the coils work best for superficial structures. Deep structures are best imaged with circumferential coils (Fig 5–17). In addition, the marked dropoff in signal with depth from the surface results in images that have a large dynamic range of signal intensities. This large dynamic range may make displaying and photography of the images difficult in certain situations. Strategies for dynamic range compression are being developed to eliminate this problem.[16]

An important consideration in surface coil use is coil decoupling. Whether the surface coil is used passively for receiving only vs. being used actively as both a transmitter and receiver, has several effects on coil performance. By using separate coils for transmission and reception, it is possible to optimize the function of each coil type. The surface receiver coil is designed to have a high Q for high SNR response. The transmitter coil, on the other hand, is usually the standard body coil in this situation. It is has a lower Q which is actually better for transmission because the RF is more homogeneous and therefore tip angles are more uniform. Most systems are now using this decoupled configuration.

Despite the problems of the active transmitter-receiver coil situation, the one situation where this may be advantageous is in high-field strength systems. In high-field systems where RF heating is a concern, transmission through the surface coil will lower the overall heat deposition in a patient for a given study. In some cases, the advantages in this situation will outweigh the RF inhomogeneity problems.

REFERENCES

1. Lufkin R, Hanafee W: Comparison of superconductive, resistive, and permanent magnet MR imaging systems, in Viamonte M (ed): *NMR Update Series.* Princeton, NJ, Continuing Education Center, 1984.
2. Lufkin R, Votruba J, Reicher M, et al: Solenoid surface coils in magnetic resonance imaging. *AJR* 1986; 146:409–412.
3. Ackerman JJH, Grove TH, Wong GG, et al: Mapping of metabolites in whole animals by ^{31}P NMR using surface coils. *Nature* 1980; 283:167–170.
4. Gadian DG: *Nuclear Magnetic Resonance and Its Applications to Living Systems.* Oxford, Clarendon Press, 1982.
5. Bernardo ML, Cohen AJ, Lauterbur PC: Radiofrequency coil designs for nuclear magnetic zeugmatographic imaging, in *IEEE Proceedings of the International Workshop on Physics and Engineering in Medical Imaging.* March 1982, pp 277–284.
6. Schenck JF, Foster TH, Henkes JL, et al: High field surface coil MR imaging of localized anatomy. *AJNR* 1985; 6:181–186.
7. Edelman RR, McFarland E, Stark DD, et al: Surface coil MR imaging of abdominal viscera. Part I. Theory, technique, and initial results. *Radiology* 1985; 157:425–430.
8. Lufkin R, Hanafee W: Application of surface coils to NMR anatomy of the larynx. *AJNR* 1985; 6:491–497.
9. Axel L: Surface coil magnetic resonance imaging. *J Comput Assist Tomogr* 1984; 8:381–384.
10. Fitzsimmons JR, Thomas RG, Mancuso AA: Proton imaging with surface coils on a 0.15-T resistive system. *J Magn Reson Med* 1985; 2:180–185.
11. Lufkin R, Wortham D, Hoover L, et al: Surface coil MRI of the tongue and oropharynx. *Radiology* 1986; 161:69–75.

12. Schenck JF, Hart HR, Foster TH, et al: Improved MR imaging of the orbit at 1.5 T with surface coils. *AJNR* 1985; 6:193–196.
13. Smyth WR: *Static and Dynamic Electricity.* New York, McGraw-Hill, 1968.
14. Hoult DI, Richards RE: Signal to noise ratio of nuclear magnetic resonance experiment. *J Magn Reson* 1976; 24:71–85.
15. Arakawa M, Crooks LE, McCarten B, et al: Comparison saddle-shaped and solenoidal coils for magnetic resonance imaging. *Radiology* 1985; 154:227–228.
16. Lufkin RB, Sharpless T, Flannigan B, et al: Dynamic-range compression in surface-coil MRI. *AJR* 1986; 147:379–382.

PART II _____

Clinical Aspects of Magnetic Resonance Imaging

Chapter 6

Magnetic Resonance Imaging of the Brain

John R. Bentson, M.D.
Robert B. Lufkin, M.D.

In this chapter, the role of magnetic resonance imaging (MRI) in the diagnosis and management of brain disorders is considered. In this regard, MRI must be compared with computed tomography (CT), its main competitor in the imaging of this region. Because of superior soft tissue contrast resolution, multiplanar imaging capabilities, and lack of ionizing radiation, MRI has replaced CT as the study of choice for the majority of abnormalities of the central nervous system.

In central nervous system tissue, water is by far the greatest contributor to the MR signal. This is due both to the high concentration of water in nerve tissue and the fact that the protons of water are "available" to generate signal, unlike those of other components of the central nervous system. Myelin, for example, contains hydrogen that is bound in such a manner that it generates little signal.[1, 2]

In MRI, all water does not give the same signal, because of differences in T1 and T2 related to its environment and because of flow factors. Relatively pure water, such as cerebrospinal fluid (CSF) has long T1 and T2 relaxation times, is of low signal on T1-weighted sequences, and produces high signal on T2-weighted sequences. The addition of protein to water decreases the T1 relaxation time, resulting in a higher signal. It may, therefore, be possible to differentiate lesions containing CSF, such as arachnoid cysts or hydromyelia, from proteinaceous fluids within tumors or infected lesions.

The high sensitivity of MRI to tissue water allows brain edema to be demonstrated very effectively. All types of edema — vasogenic, cytotoxic, and interstitial — will result in altered signals. Edema is best seen on T2-weighted images, which frequently yield such a bright signal that underlying abnormalities may be obscured. It may not be possible to detect a tumor in the midst of the edema. In addition to tumors, brain edema is caused by many other conditions, such as infarction, trauma, inflammation, degeneration, and bleeding. Because these may also not be distinguishable at MRI, other types of information, such as the size and location of the lesion, its appearance and mode of spread, and clinical information are needed to help one make a specific diagnosis.

One consequence of the marked difference in relaxation constants between water and brain tissue is that small structures that are bathed in CSF such as cranial nerves are well demonstrated by MRI, whereas they are not shown by CT. Based on this ability to demonstrate normal cranial nerves, MRI has proved to be superior in showing tumors or other abnormalities of these structures, such as acoustic neuromas and lesions involving the optic chiasm.

The sensitivity of MRI to paramagnetic substances such as iron is also very important clinically. Regions of increased iron deposition in the brain, such as the globus pallidum, substantia nigra, red nucleus, and dentate nucleus, show a lower signal than the remainder of the brain on T2-weighted studies, particularly on high-field units. This opens up a new avenue of research into disorders of these areas, such as Parkinson's disease and other degenerative disorders.[3]

Even more significant clinically is the role of iron imaging in the depiction of hemorrhage. Compounds such as methemoglobin, hemosiderin, and ferritin, formed from hemoglobin after hemorrhage, shorten T1 and/or T2 values to varying degrees, resulting in complex and changing appearances of hematomas on MRI. These substances allow a more definite diagnosis of chronic or subacute hematomas by MRI, but there are some problems in the MRI detection of acute hematomas.

Magnetic resonance imaging is much less sensitive to calcium than CT, and this remains a significant drawback of the former technique. While dense calcifications may result in sufficient signal loss to be visible at MRI, many are not detected because volume-averaging obscures the low-signal region.

Flow effects are very important in MRI of the central nervous system: both blood flow and CSF flow. Although flow generally results in signal loss, there may also be increased signal associated with flow because of such factors as pseudogating, entry slice enhancement, and even-echo rephasing.[4, 5] Magnetic resonance imaging may provide considerable information regarding blood flow, but these data may be confusing if the factors determining signal change from blood flow are not understood.

Flow phenomena of the CSF are similar and may be clinically useful in showing abnormalities of flow related to ventricular obstruction. For example, an abnormal degree of signal loss has been described in the aqueduct in cases of normal pressure hydrocephalus, probably related to decreased compliance of the ventricles.[6] Artifacts related to CSF flow may mimic pathologic lesions, particularly in high-strength MR units, and these must be recognized. Gating, based on pulse rate monitoring, may be necessary to diminish these artifacts.

Finally, MRI is unique in the great variety of programmable parameters that may be selected during imaging. The imaging factors chosen will alter T1 and T2 effects, will change the effects of flow on image strength, and will therefore alter the contrast between normal and diseased tissue. The complexity of sequence selection makes MRI highly versatile and, for the operator, increases the importance of understanding not only the technical factors but also the preferable methods of studying various anatomic areas and disease processes.

VASCULAR DISEASE

Cerebrovascular accidents may be visible within hours after onset on MR images because of changes in water concentration and distribution that result in T2 prolongation. Computed tomographic studies, with or without intravenous contrast material enhancement, may be equivocal or negative within the first 24 hours to 48 hours. In the subacute and chronic stages of ischemic stroke, MRI continues to provide information superior to that of CT regarding

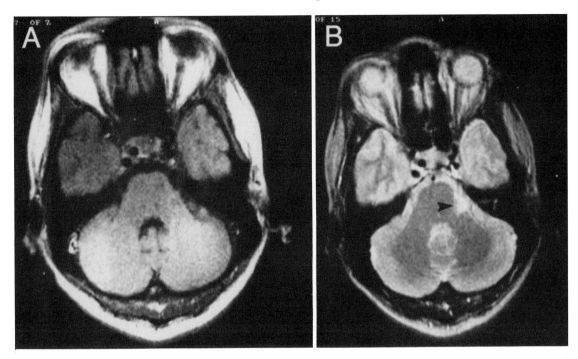

FIG 6–1.
Presumed ischemic stroke in a 44-year-old woman who presented with sudden-onset left-sided seventh and eighth nerve deficits. **A,** axial T1-weighted image (SE 500/30) is unremarkable. **B,** T2-weighted image (SE 2000/85) shows focal increased signal (*arrowhead*) consistent with ischemia or infarction.

blood-brain barrier abnormalities and eventual conversion to microcystic encephalomalacia and gliosis.

Thus, MRI is able to show abnormalities earlier than CT in cases of cerebral ischemia because of its high sensitivity to cerebral edema. One may see T1 and T2 prolongation within 4 to 6 hours in experimental situations.[7, 8] Small infarcts or areas of gliosis that may escape detection by CT will often be demonstrated by MRI.[9] Infarcts involving posterior fossa structures are best demonstrated by MRI (Fig 6–1). Computed tomographic scanning of the posterior fossa suffers from beam hardening artifacts and lack of sensitivity in detecting relatively small ischemic lesions such as those involving the brain stem.

One clinical problem that arises when MRI is used in evaluation of acute ischemic disease is that it may not be possible to demonstrate acute hemorrhagic infarcts as well as CT.[10] This is a very significant disadvantage, as the question of whether or not bleeding has occurred into an infarcted area is often the main reason to obtain an imaging study in the patient with acute stroke. Acute hematomas may be difficult to differentiate from surrounding brain.[11, 12] In the first 24 to 48 hours following a cerebrovascular accident, intracranial hemorrhage is better demonstrated by CT than by MRI because of the high protein content of the blood. Gradient refocusing strategies that improve the detectability of acute hemorrhage because of T2 sensitivity may improve the situation with MRI somewhat (Table 6–1).

Hematomas are better seen on MRI images 72 to 90 hours following infarction, when the periphery of the hematoma becomes hyperintense on T1-weighted images, and later on T2-weighted images, as a result of progressive formation of methemoglobin. Subacute hemorrhage is better defined at MRI than CT scanning because of the presence of paramagnetic methemoglobin.

Chronic hemorrhage is also better seen on MRI when part of the hematoma has been converted to hemosiderin. A ring of hypointensity appears about the margin of the hematoma, related to hemosiderin that has been taken up by macrophages. The strong contrast that results between the hematoma and adjacent brain tissue allows superior demonstration of subacute and chronic hematomas, and this detectability persists longer than abnormalities on CT. At this point CT scanning may be negative for disease. Unenhanced MRI is necessary in the evaluation of the patient with hemorrhage to avoid confusion of enhancement due to gadolinium DPTA (diethylene-triamine pentaacetic acid) with enhancement due to paramagnetic methemoglobin.

The problems in early detection of acute bleeding by MRI decrease its usefulness in the imaging of acute ischemic episodes, as the detection of bleeding is probably more important in planning therapy than the ability to see the area of early infarction. For this reason, as well as the fact that it is normally simpler to scan an acutely diseased patient by CT when monitoring is needed and patient motion is common, CT remains the imaging method of choice in the diagnosis of most acute ischemic disease.

Although vascular malformations and flow in vascular tumors are detected equally well by MRI and CT, MRI gives better resolution of the abnormal vessels, and better shows areas of previous bleeding (Fig 6–2).[13] Magnetic resonance imaging will also better demonstrate abnormal signal from tissue in the vicinity of the mass that is affected by edema or gliosis. Thus, MRI is preferred over CT for evaluating the results of embolization. On MRI, occluded

TABLE 6–1.

Protocols* in Neurologic Magnetic Resonance Imaging

Standard Brain	
Sagittal	SE 300/30
Axial	SE 800/30
Axial	SE 3000/84
Sella turcica	
Coronal	SE 600/28
Sagittal	SE 300/28
Coronal	SE 3000/84
Temporal lobe	
Axial	SE 800/28
Coronal	SE 500/28
Coronal	SE 3000/84

The head coil is used in acquiring all images. Gradient moment nulling motion compensation is added to all T2-weighted sequences. On high-field instruments, cardiac gating may be necessary in order to diminish flow and motion artifacts in some cases. Gadolinium DTPA is used in selected cases for identification of blood-brain barrier disruption or leptomeningeal disease processes. Gradient echo sequences are employed to improve sensitivity to flow and T2 changes with hemorrhage in selected cases.

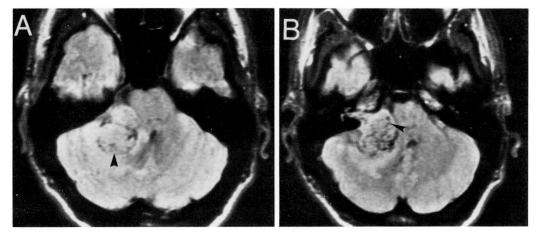

FIG 6–2.
Extremely vascular acoustic neuroma in a 24-year-old woman. Two operations were required for its removal because of difficulties with hemostasis. **A,** axial proton density image (SE 2000/28) shows the extra-axial mass (*arrowhead*) and distortion of the adjacent fourth ventricle. **B,** slightly lower slice shows extension into the internal auditory canal and curvilinear low-signal structures (*arrowhead*) consistent with blood vessels.

vessels can be identified by increased intraluminal signal, and the reaction of the surrounding tissue can be monitored.

Cryptic vascular malformations are better shown on MRI because of its sensitivity in the detection of chronic hemorrhage.[14] On T2-weighted imaging, a small lesion with central high intensity and peripheral low intensity is typically seen. The most common causes of these small hematomas are true cryptic (small) arteriovenous malformations and cavernous hemangiomas.

Venous angiomas (malformations) appear to be demonstrated equally well by MRI and CT.[15] In each, the enlarged and penetrating vein of drainage is the prominent feature, and the multiple smaller venous tributaries may or may not be visible. On MRI, the draining vein may either be hypointense or hyperintense, depending on the rate and direction of blood flow, sequence selection, and factors such as entry slice phenomenon and even-echo rephasing. Most often, it is hypointense.

Aneurysms are also better demonstrated by MRI (Fig 6–3). Newer imagers have adequate resolution to demonstrate small aneurysms, which are seen as rounded areas of flow void. Other aneurysms may contain areas of different density, related either to clot within the aneurysm or to flow effects. Blood within the center of a large aneurysm may remain in the field sufficiently long to provide a high signal, whereas more peripheral blood has higher velocity and gives little if any signal. Changing sequence parameters may show a change in the relative proportions of high and low signal if signal variation is caused by flow effects. Giant aneurysms often have a layering of different intensities, representing various stages of blood clotting.[16] In this way, they are similar to parenchymal hematomas. The aneurysm lumen is seen as a signal void and is often eccentric.

TRAUMA

The efficacy of CT has been established in the diagnosis of acute trauma, as a result of rapid scan times; relative tolerance of patient motion; and ability to show areas of bleeding, fracture, and brain tissue displacement. When MRI is used in patients with acute trauma, it will show most areas of bleeding, although small amounts of blood, such as may occur in the subarachnoid space, are not seen as well as with CT. However, MRI better demonstrates areas of shearing injury, contusions, and infarcts.[17] Early results of comparisons between CT and MRI in imaging acute injuries suggest that the additional information provided by MRI may not be of great advantage in patient management.[18]

While it appears that CT remains the preferred imaging modality for evaluation of acute head trauma, MRI does have advantages in evaluating patients with subacute and chronic trauma.[19] Its better ability to show areas of brain parenchymal damage and regions of chronic bleeding aids the understanding of the extent of injuries and helps provide an accurate prognosis.[20]

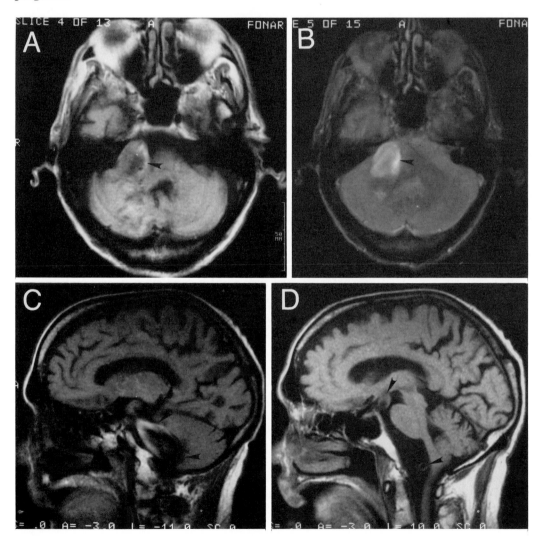

FIG 6–3.
Fusiform basilar artery aneurysm in an 81-year-old man presenting with ipsilateral sensorineural hearing loss. **A,** axial T1-weighted image (SE 500/30) shows an extra-axial mass (*arrowhead*) centered over the internal auditory canal with heterogeneous signal. **B,** T2-weighted image in the same plane again shows the heterogeneous-signal mass (*arrowhead*). **C,** sagittal T1-weighted image better defines the craniocaudal extent (*arrowheads*). **D,** slightly lateral sagittal view shows the proximal and distal vessels (*arrowheads*) joining the aneurysm.

NEOPLASIA

It is difficult to generalize regarding the role of MRI in brain tumor imaging because there is such variation of results for various tumors and for various anatomic locations[21, 22] (Figs 6–4 through 6–8). In general, MRI is effective in the detection of tumors because it is so sensitive to cerebral edema, which accompanies most tumors. It therefore has an advantage in the detection of small lesions, such as metastases, which are found in greater numbers by MRI than by CT.[23] It also has an advantage in the detection of small extra-axial tumors such as acoustic neuromas.

If bleeding into a tumor has occurred, this may be better appreciated by MRI than by CT, both because the abnormal signal from blood persists longer on MRI and because there is no problem in distinguishing hemorrhage from calcification by MRI. Cysts within tumors are visible on MRI, as they are by CT, and more information may be available regarding the contents of the cysts as seen on MRI, because the intensity of fluid varies with its protein content.

There are disadvantages in using MRI in tumor detection. The tumor itself is frequently obscured by the high signal from the surrounding edema. Using a variety of sequences may allow the tumor to be seen in such cases. Magnetic resonance imaging also profits from the use of paramagnetic contrast media that pass into regions without an effective blood-brain barrier, and will highlight tumors. Injection of the paramagnetic substance, Gd-DTPA results in clear demonstration of most neoplasms by MRI.[24, 25]

Another deficiency of MRI that is overcome by using Gd-DTPA is in the detection of small meningiomas, which may be difficult to see because their T1 and T2 values are close to those of brain parenchyma. Without this contrast agent, one relies mainly on detecting the distortion of brain tissue to recognize these neoplasms. Prior to the use of gadolinium, this difficulty in detecting benign tumors such as meningiomas was a principal reason why the sensitivity of MRI in detecting intracranial lesions, mainly tumors, was lower than that of CT in a carefully constructed blinded clinical comparison performed by Haughton et al.[26]

Initially it was hoped that it would be possible to perform tissue characterization of brain tumors by determining T1 and T2 values. However, there appears to be such wide overlap of these values that neither tumor type nor the degree of malignancy can be predicted.[27] The inability of MRI to demonstrate calcification is also a disadvantage in the characterization of brain neoplasms. However, MRI probably gives a better representation of the extent of a primary infiltrating brain tumor than does CT, since it is known that primary tumors actually extend beyond the apparent outline of the mass as demonstrated by either CT or MRI, and it may be safer to consider that the tumor may have spread throughout the zone of edema, which is more clearly delineated by MRI.[28]

A search for the occasionally present structural lesion causing seizures should be performed with the most sensitive tools available. At this time, MRI and positron-emission tomography appear to be the most sensitive, with MRI showing a significant increase in lesions detection over CT.[29] Besides being able to better delineate small tumors and vascular malformations in the temporal lobe, MRI provides superior anatomic resolution of that region, which is a problem area for CT because of bone artifacts. Some centers are using MRI to monitor placement of MR-compatible deep electrodes for the investigation of refractory partial complex seizures (see Fig 6–6).

At present, it appears that both MRI and CT are quite effective in the demonstration of brain tumors. Magnetic resonance imaging has the advantage of greater sensitivity for detecting edema as well as the potential for demonstrating a lesion in several projections. With the use of Gd-DTPA, MRI is now also better able to show meningiomas and is presently better in characterizing neoplasms.

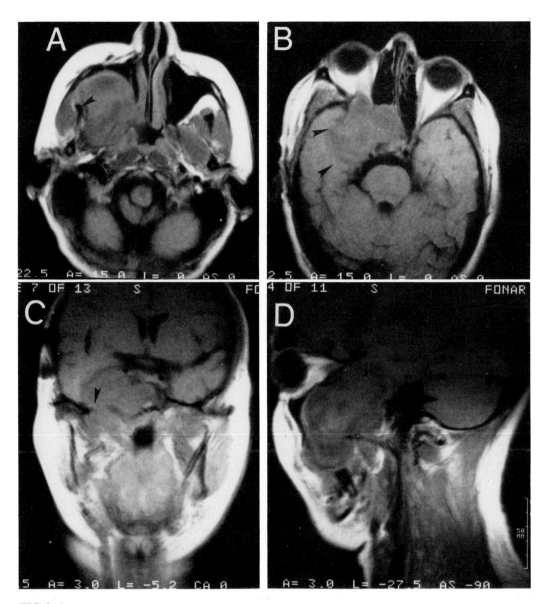

FIG 6–4.
Neurofibroma arising from the fifth nerve. All pulse sequences are T1 weighted (SE 800–300/30). **A,** axial views through the maxillary antrum reveal a large homogeneous mass filling the sinus and displacing infratemporal fossa structures. Note remodeling of bone (*arrowhead*), suggesting relatively slow growth. **B,** axial view through the cavernous sinus shows extension of the mass along the course of the fifth nerve into the orbit, associated with proptosis, as well as laterally into the middle cranial fossa (*arrowheads*). **C,** coronal view defines the course of the mass extending through an enlarged foramen ovale (*arrowhead*) into the region of Meckel's cave. **D,** the sagittal view completes the three-dimensional appearance of the lesion by showing direct extension from the infratemporal fossa, displacing the temporal lobe of the brain (*arrowhead*).

Gliomas are well demonstrated by MRI. Particular complications of the tumors — such as mass effect, herniation, and hydrocephalus — are generally better seen with multiplanar MRI than with CT scanning. Tumor boundaries may be obscured in either technique by extensive edema. Contrast enhancement is valuable for the delineation of blood-brain barrier abnormalities and subarachnoid spread[30] (see Fig 6–7).

A solitary metastasis may be difficult to differentiate from a glioma. However, multiplicity of lesions strongly suggest metastatic disease. Magnetic resonance imaging is particularly valuable for evaluating common complications of bleeding in metastases, especially those seen with melanoma, choriocarcinoma, and oat cell carcinoma of the lung.

Computed tomographic scanning better defines calcification and the associated hyperostosis of meningioma. Both CT and MRI easily demonstrate the lesions following intravenous contrast material enhancement. Magnetic resonance imaging consistently demonstrates smaller acoustic tumors with greater detail than does CT scanning. This eliminates the need for intrathecal air or other contrast material. Acoustic neuromas show striking contrast enhancement on both CT and MRI.

It appears that MRI provides superior information concerning the precise extent of

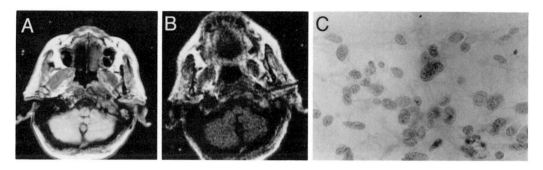

FIG 6–5.
Glomus jugulare. This 45-year-old man presented with multiple unilateral cranial nerve deficits referable to the jugular foramen. **A,** axial image (SE 800/30) reveals a mass centered in the jugular foramen region descending into adjacent soft tissues (*arrowhead*). They are associated with a mastoiditis presumably secondary to the eustachian tube dysfunction. **B,** axial spin echo image (SE 500/30) shows MRI-directed needle in place (*arrowhead*). The image is noisy as a result of the rapid imaging time (138 seconds). **C,** cytologic picture of the aspirated cells is consistent with glomus jugulare (photograph courtesy of Dr. Lester Layfield.)

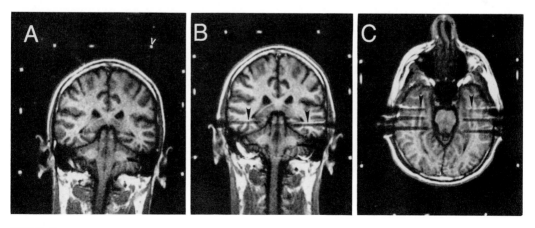

FIG 6–6.
Deep electrode placement (MRI guided) in a 38-year-old man with refractory partial complex seizures undergoing evaluation for possible temporal lobectomy. All pulse sequences are T1 weighted (TR 1276/300). **A,** scout coronal view with external fiducial markers in place (*arrowhead*). **B,** following bilateral electrode placement, signal void is present along the course of the electrodes (*arrowheads*). **C,** axial view defines the extent of the electrode array (*arrowheads*).

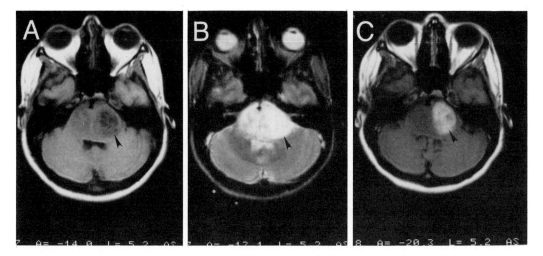

FIG 6–7.
Brain stem glioma in a 20-year-old woman. **A,** axial T1-weighted image (SE 505/22) shows a well-defined intra-axial mass arising in the mid pons (*arrowhead*). **B,** T2-weighted image at the same level shows a generalized increase in signal secondary to edema and tumor (*arrowhead*). **C,** axial T1-weighted image with gadolinium shows focal enhancement in the region of the blood-brain barrier abnormality within the tumor (*arrowhead*), which is distinct from edema.

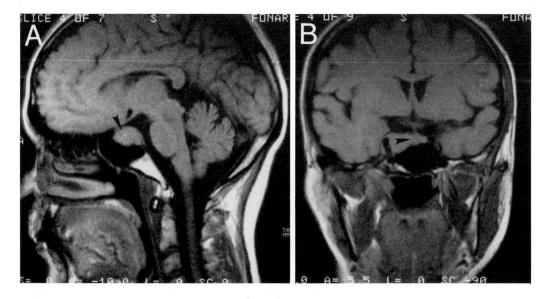

FIG 6–8.
Pituitary adenoma in a 43-year-old woman. **A,** sagittal T1-weighted image (SE 480/30) shows a pituitary mass (*arrowhead*). No significant suprasellar extension is present. **B,** coronal view shows lateral extension to the right with displacement of the pituitary gland (*arrowhead*) and infundibulum to the left.

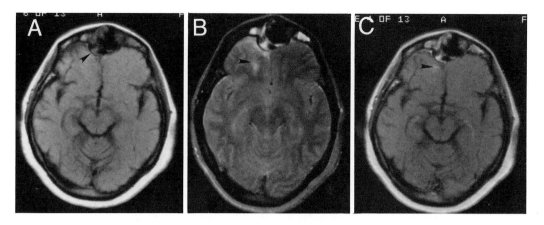

FIG 6–9.
54-year-old patient with osteoma of the frontal sinus, mucocele, and associated meningoencephalitis. **A,** T1-weighted image (SE 800/30) before gadolinium administration shows the osteoma and expansion of the frontal sinus (*arrowhead*). **B,** T2-weighted image (SE 2000/85) shows associated areas of edema in the underlying brain (*arrowhead*). **C,** postgadolinium image identifies areas of blood-brain barrier disruption associated with the mass as high-signal regions. (*arrowhead*). No ring enhancement or central low signal is present to suggest a frank abscess.

pituitary lesions as well as the effect on surrounding structures (see Fig 6–8). Further studies suggest that MR may be superior in the detection of intrasellar microadenomas. It also appears to be superior in the evaluation of parasellar lesions because it lacks bone artifacts and has multiplanar imaging capability.

INFLAMMATION

The respective roles of MRI and CT in the diagnosis of infection of the brain are similar to their roles in the study of brain tumors.[31] Magnetic resonance imaging is highly sensitive in detecting infection within the brain parenchyma, again related to early detection of white matter edema. Contrast material-enhanced MRI is necessary for showing meningeal involvement, such as in the case of tuberculous meningitis. Magnetic resonance imaging is also readily capable of demonstrating subdural and epidural empyemas.

The higher sensitivity of MRI for detection of edema makes it the study of choice in the diagnosis of early encephalitis. The specificity of MRI is increased by using paramagnetic contrast agents to demonstrate breakdown of the blood-brain barrier (Fig 6–9). The rims of abscesses are enhanced, and it may be possible to recognize a multiplicity of lesions that are in close proximity. It is now possible to determine if a lesion is active or inactive on MRI, as indicated by the presence of blood-brain barrier abnormalities. While CT and MRI are in a limited sense complementary studies, MRI with the addition of paramagnetic contrast agents now replaces CT in the investigation of infectious disease.[32]

In multiple sclerosis and other disease resulting in demyelination, MRI has replaced CT as the study of choice (Fig 6–10). It is much more sensitive in showing subtle white matter abnormalities of any type. This is a group of conditions in which demonstration of blood-brain barrier breakdown is both less common and not as diagnostically helpful as in other brain diseases. For the same reason, MRI is the study of choice in showing vascular disease of the deep white matter.

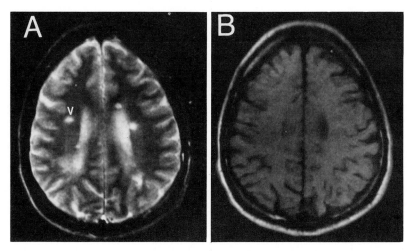

FIG 6–10.
Multiple sclerosis in a 32-year-old man with visual changes and weakness of the right hand. **A,** axial T2-weighted image (SE 3000/85) shows multiple focal areas of high signal intensity in the periventricular white matter (*arrowhead*). **B,** axial T1-weighted image (SE 649/22) at the same area at the same level is largely unremarkable.

CONCLUSION

It is apparent that MRI has the attributes of a superior imaging tool, with high resolution, high contrast, high sensitivity, and a wide range of selectable scanning parameters that allow one to study flow as well as tissue characteristics of central nervous system abnormalities. Many of the past deficiencies of MRI are now eliminated with the introduction of a blood-brain barrier contrast agent. Magnetic resonance imaging has clearly become the dominant imaging tool for the detection of most diseases of the brain.

REFERENCES

1. Wehrli F, Breger R, MacFall J, et al: Quantification of contrast in clinical MR imaging at high magnetic field. *Invest Radiol* 1985; 20:360–369.
2. Kjos B, Brant-Zawadzki M, Kucharczyk W, et al: Cystic intracranial lesions: Magnetic resonance imaging. *Radiology* 1985; 155:363–369.
3. Drayer B, Burger P, Darwin R, et al: MRI of brain iron. *AJR* 1986; 147:103–110.
4. Bradley W, Waluch V: Blood flow: Magnetic resonance imaging. *Radiology* 1985; 154:443–450.
5. Waluch V, Bradley W: NMR even echo rephasing in slow laminar flow. *J Comput Assist Tomogr* 1984; 4:594–598.
6. Bradley W, Kortman K, Burgoyne B: Flowing cerebrospinal fluid in normal and hydrocephalic states: Appearance on MR images. *Radiology* 1986; 159:611–616.
7. Brant-Zawadzki M, Pereira B, Weinstein P, et al: MR imaging of acute experimental ischemia in cats. *AJNR* 1986; 7:7–11.
8. Levy R, Mano I, Bristo A, et al: MR imaging of acute experimental cerebral ischemia: Time course and pharmacologic manipulations. *AJNR* 1983; 4:238.
9. Bradley WG Jr, Waluch V, Brant-Zawadzki M, et al: Patchy periventricular white matter lesions in the elderly: A common observation during NMR imaging. *Noninvasive Med Imaging* 1984; 1:35–41.
10. Hecht-Leavitt C, Gomori J, Grossman R, et al: High-field MRI of hemorrhagic cortical infarction. *AJNR* 1986; 7:581–585.

11. De La Paz R, New P, Bunonanno F, et al: NMR imaging of intracranial hemorrhage. *J Comput Assist Tomogr* 1984; 8:599–607.

12. Gomori J, Grossman R, Goldberg H, et al: Intracranial hematomas: Imaging by high-field MR. *Radiology* 1985; 157:87–93.

13. Lee B, Herzberg L, Zimmerman R, et al: MR imaging of cerebral vascular malformations. *AJNR* 1985; 6:863–870.

14. Gomori J, Grossman R, Goldberg H, et al: Occult cerebral vascular malformations. High-field MR imaging. *Radiology* 1986; 158:707–743.

15. Augustyn G, Scott J, Olson E, et al: Cerebral venous angiomas: MR imaging. *Radiology* 1985; 156:391.

16. Atlas S, Grossman R, Goldberg H, et al: Partially thrombosed giant intracranial aneurysms: Correlation of MR and pathologic findings. *Radiology* 1987; 162:111–114.

17. Zimmerman R, Bolanink L, Hackney D, et al: Head injury: Early results of comparing CT and high-field MR. *AJNR* 1986; 7:757–764.

18. Snow R, Zimmerman R, Gandy S, et al: Comparison of magnetic resonance imaging and computed tomography in the evaluation of head injury. *Neurosurgery* 1986; 18:45–52.

19. Moon KL, Brandt-Zawadzki M, Pitts LH, et al: Nuclear magnetic resonance imaging of CT isodense subdural hematomas. *AJNR* 1984; 5:319–323.

20. Kelly AB, Zimmerman RD, Snow RB, et al: Head trauma: Comparison of MR and CT — experience in 100 patients. *AJNR* 1988; 9:699–708.

21. Muller-Forell W, Schroth G, Egan PJ: MR imaging in tumors of the pineal region. *Neuroradiology* 1988; 30:224–231.

22. Yuh WT, Barloon TJ, Jacoby CG, et al: MR of fourth-ventricular epidermoid tumors. *AJNR* 1988; 9:794–796.

23. Lee B, Kneeland J, Cahill P, et al: MR recognition of supratentorial tumors. *AJNR* 1985; 6:871–878.

24. Graif M, Bydder G, Steiner R, et al: Contrast-enhanced MR imaging of malignant brain tumors. *AJNR* 1985; 6:855–862.

25. Felix R, Schnorner W, Laniado M, et al: Brain tumors: MR imaging with gadolinium-DTPA. *Radiology* 1985; 156:681–688.

26. Haughton V, Rimm A, Sobocinski K, et al: A blinded clinical comparison of MR imaging and CT in neuroradiology. *Radiology* 1986; 160:751–755.

27. Komiyama M, Yaguro H, Baba M, et al: MR imaging: Possibility of tissue characterization of brain tumors using T1 and T2 values. *AJNR* 1987; 8:65–70.

28. Shuman W, Griffin B, Haynor D, et al: The utility of MR in planning the radiation therapy of oligodendroglioma. *AJNR* 1987; 8:93–98.

29. Latack J, Abou-Khalil B, Siegel G, et al: Patients with partial seizures: Evaluation by MR, CT, and PET scanning. *Radiology* 1986; 159:159–163.

30. Krol G, Sze G, Malkin M, et al: MR of cranial and spinal meningeal carcinomatosis: Comparison with CT and myelography. *AJR* 1988; 151:583–588.

31. Ramsey RG, Geremia GK: CNS complications of AIDS: CT and MR findings. *AJR* 1988; 151:449–454.

32. Post M, Sheldon J, Hensley G, et al: Central nervous system disease in acquired immunodeficiency syndrome: Prospective correlation using CT, MR imaging, and pathologic studies. *Radiology* 1986; 158:141–148.

Chapter 7

Magnetic Resonance Imaging of the Spine

John R. Bentson, M.D.

Eric Spickler, M.D.

Robert B. Lufkin, M.D.

Magnetic resonance imaging (MRI) is now firmly entrenched as a major method of imaging the spine and surrounding soft tissues. This modality is often superior to computed tomography (CT) and myelography in imaging this region. The wide range of selectable techniques in MRI makes it possible to tailor an examination to derive maximum information in both specific anatomic regions and pathologic conditions. The technique is sufficiently comprehensive that contrast material is not needed in the majority of cases. In certain instances, such as leptomeningeal abnormalities and in the differentiation of scar tissue from recurrent disks, the addition of gadolinium provides more information than had previously been given by any imaging modality.

TECHNIQUE

It is not possible to specify a technique that is optimal for imaging all portions of the spine in all patients. Many technical factors must be considered, such as repetition time (TR) and echo time (TE) parameters, thickness of slices, matrix size, number of excitations, the flip angle when gradient echo techniques are used, and surface coils. Patient-related factors that must be taken into account include the type of abnormality one may encounter, the level of patient cooperation and tolerance of the examination, and a consideration of which projections are most likely to be helpful. The characteristics of the MR instrument must also be considered. For example, if an instrument has a superior signal-to-noise performance, the number of excitations required to obtain satisfactory resolution may be decreased. It may be possible to obtain images of superior quality by increasing the number of excitations or by using the standard T2-weighted spin echo technique as opposed to gradient echo technique, but the increase in time required may adversely affect both patient tolerance of the examination and patient throughput. To help optimize the signal-to-noise ratio and to allow the desirable use of thin slices, surface coils should be used whenever possible in MRI of the spine.[1]

In general, T1-weighted spin echo images are the mainstay of spinal MRI examinations. Resolution tends to be superior, and anatomic detail is better appreciated. Most spines are scanned for disk-related or other degenerative conditions, and T1 images given excellent information regarding both the appearance of disks and vertebra, the adequacy of intervertebral foramina, and even the state of facet joints. The outlines of the spinal cord are best shown by T1-weighted sequences, but abnormalities of the internal structure of the cord are better demonstrated by T2-weighted spin echo techniques. Typical T1-weighted techniques would include TR values of 300 to 600 msec, and TEs of 20 to 30 msec. It may be necessary to lengthen the TR to accommodate a larger number of sections.

Sequences that emphasize the T2 effect are essential in looking for problems within the spinal cord such as tumor, demyelination, post-traumatic myelopathy, and vascular malformation, and also in evaluating abnormalities of the bones, especially in suspected osteomyelitis. Best results with the fewest artifacts can generally be obtained by using traditional T2-weighted spin echo techniques, such as a TR of 2,000 to 3,000 msec, and a TE of 80 to 120 msec. An alternative method of obtaining the T2 effect is by the use of gradient echo imaging, which significantly reduces imaging time. However, signal-to-noise ratio and intrinsic T2 contrast are inferior to those obtained with true T2-weighted images.

One advantage of T2-weighted sequences is to produce a high-density cerebrospinal fluid (CSF), giving the "myelographic effect."[2, 3] This can be done either by using standard T2-weighted techniques or by using gradient echo technique, with flip angles in the 10° to 20° range. Such techniques emphasize the contrast between the disks and ligaments and the subarachnoid space.

NORMAL ANATOMY

On T1-weighted spin echo images, the vertebrae appear as low-signal strips of cortical bone surrounding the higher signal areas of cancellous bone (Fig 7–1). The fat in the marrow results in marrow having a signal between that of normal muscle and fat. Small areas of higher signal within the marrow may represent regions of fat deposition. The basivertebral vein complex in the mid-posterior vertebral body has a high signal, due either to surrounding fat or to the slow flow of blood within the vein. With aging, the marrow may have a higher fat content and be less homogeneous. On T2-weighted images, vertebral bodies have a lower signal.

Disks are composed of cartilaginous end plates, a peripheral annulus fibrosis, and the central nucleus pulposus. On T1-weighted images, the nucleus pulposus, with its higher water content, is slightly darker than the annulus. On T2-weighted images, the contrast between the nucleus and annulus is increased, but now the nucleus is of higher intensity. A thin zone of higher intensity parallel to the vertebral end plates may be seen bisecting the nucleus pulposus on T2-weighted sagittal images because of the fibrous bands that extend centrally from the annulus. The posterior longitudinal ligament, just posterior to the disks, is difficult to distinguish from the adjacent annulus or the CSF on T1-weighted images, as each gives little signal. On T2-weighted images, differentiation of this ligament from the annulus is often possible, and the distinction of the ligament from the CSF is clear because of the high signal of the CSF.

Posterior to the posterior longitudinal ligament is the epidural space, which may be seen as a region of higher intensity because of the fat present in the space. The rich epidural

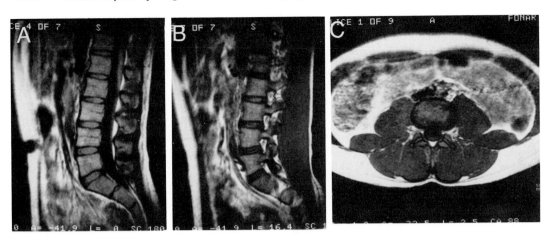

FIG 7–1.
Normal lumbar spine. **A,** midsagittal T1-weighted image. **B,** parasagittal T1-weighted image through the intervertebral foramina, demonstrating the exiting lumbar nerves (*arrow*) surrounded by fat. **C,** axial section through L3-4. Note the cauda equina in the posterior part of the subarachnoid space, the fat in the intervertebral foramina and surrounding the nerves that have exited above this section (*arrow*), and the normal facet joints.

venous plexus may have varing intensity, depending upon rate of blood flow and imaging factors.

The spinal cord is best outlined using T1-weighted images because of the excellent contrast between it and the low intensity of the CSF. The anterior and posterior roots may be visible on T1-weighted images in the cervical region, and differentiation between gray and white matter may sometimes be seen.[4]

The neural foramina of the spine may be shown on either sagittal or axial images (see Fig 7–1,B). On T1-weighted images, the fat within the foramina outlines the exiting nerve roots. Oblique imaging of cervical foramina has been used, but is not generally necessary.

On sagittal views, the spinal cord is seen to gradually decrease in its anteroposterior diameter as it descends through the cervical area, then becomes quite small in the thoracic region, only to again enlarge at the T-12 and L-1 levels, the region of the conus. The roots making up the cauda equina may lie in close proximity in the posterior part of the subarachnoid space in the lumbar region, resembling the cord. However, no cord outline is apparent in the axial projection, and the enlargement of the conus at the normal level is a good clue to the true nature of the cauda equina.

Imaging the facet joints is of most significance in the lumbar spine. These are often seen quite well on axial T1-weighted images. The joint spaces are seen as regions of higher intensity between the darker cortical bone surfaces of the articular processes (see Fig 7–1,C).

Coronal imaging may provide good views of the nerve roots in the neural foramina but is seldom used except in patients with scoliosis or in pediatric patients who have relatively straight spines.[5]

ARTIFACTS

In order to interpret MR images of the spine, one should understand potentially confusing artifacts. One common artifact is the chemical shift artifact, which occurs in the direction of the frequency encoding axis and which is proportional to field strength.[6] This artifact is seen as black or white lines adjacent to fat-water interfaces, commonly on sagittal T1-weighted images. This artifact is based on the fact that fat and water protons resonate at different frequencies as a result of their local magnetic environment effects. Another type of chemical shift artifact relates to cancellation between fat and water signals and is found primarily when using flip angle gradient echos, as a result of the differential refocusing of fat and water protons because of their different Larmour frequencies. This may occur both along the phase and frequency axes on gradient echo images.

Motion and flow may result in propagation of image harmonics along the phase encoding axis. A common example of this artifact is seen in the thoracic region, when the phase encoding axis is perpendicular to the spine. The movement of the heart results in artifacts across the spinal canal. By switching the phase and frequency encoding axes, one can effectively project the cardiac motion artifact away from the spine.

A more complex approach to motion artifact suppression involves cardiac gating, in which the repetition time selected is dependent upon the R wave to R wave interval, as seen on the ECG. This dependency lengthens image acquisition time. Recently, more sophisticated approaches to motion suppression can remove artifacts caused by velocity and acceleration by using special compensatory or nulling gradients. This generally causes no constraint on the TR time. This is especially helpful in high-field instruments and when using sequences with long TE times, in which motion artifacts tend to be particularly troublesome.[7]

Another common artifact seen in spine imaging is a black line that projects over the cord, simulating a syrinx. This is called the truncation artifact, and it occurs at highly contrasting interfaces due to truncation of the image data set prior to Fourier transformation.[8]

One further artifact is an iatrogenic one produced by the presence of residual Pantopaque within the thecal sac. On T1-weighted imaging, Pantopaque gives a bright signal relative to the low signal of the CSF. On T2-weighted imaging, the CSF becomes bright, and the Pantopaque assumes an isointense appearance.[9]

DEGENERATIVE DISEASE

Degenerative conditions of the intervertebral disks and the spinal column are very common and are of great social and economic importance. Disk degeneration is the common denominator of these conditions. With repeated stress and aging, there is loss of water content of the nucleus pulposus and fragmentation and fissuring of the annulus fibrosis. This may result in protrusion of the disk or in herniation of the nucleus pulposus through the degenerated annulus. This leads to further degeneration of the thinned disk, which cannot adapt to the loads placed upon it, and to secondary changes in the vertebral bodies and the facet joints. On MRI, bulging disks are usually recognized by their relatively uniform extension beyond the borders of the adjacent vertebral bodies, and by not having the focality that is seen with herniated disks.[10, 11] Loss of height and signal intensity are typically seen in bulging disks, and the continued degeneration may lead to the vacuum disk phenomenon, in which prominent areas of low signal are seen within a disk.

The majority of lumbar disk herniations occur at the L4-5 or L5–S1 levels. In herniation, part of the nucleus pulposus extends through a tear in the annulus fibrosis but usually does not extend through the posterior longitudinal ligament. The lesion is characteristically focal, usually posterolateral with respect to the vertebral body (Fig 7–2). The herniated disk may extend into an intervertebral foramen. However, there is often no direct evidence of nerve compression, even though there is clinical evidence of radiculopathy.

Herniated disks may be well seen on both axial and sagittal MR images. However, the axial images are more likely to demonstrate the focal nature of the disk lesion, which is considered so characteristic. In general, the signal intensity of the herniated portion of the disk resembles that of the remainder of the disk. However, in T2-weighted imaging, the herniated portion may have a higher signal intensity. A black line may be seen bordering the posterior margin of the herniation related to the posterior longitudinal ligament, which has not been crossed. Secondary signs of disk herniation include obliteration of epidural fat and indentation of the thecal sac.

In the cervical region, herniated or protruding disks may displace the epidural venous plexus, giving high signal adjacent to the disk itself on T1-weighted sagittal images.[12] (Fig 7–3).

Occasionally, the herniated nucleus pulposus may extend through the posterior longitudinal ligament to produce a sequestered fragment.[13] Signs favoring this are lack of continuity of the fragment with the remainder of the disk, distancing of the fragment from the level of the disk space, and absence of the dark line of the posterior longitudinal ligament from the posterior margin of the disk fragment.

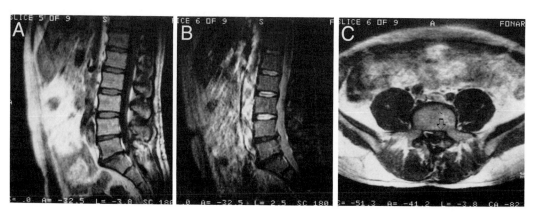

FIG 7–2.
Herniated L4-5 disk. **A**, this midsagittal T1-weighted image shows some posterior displacement of the thecal sac by the L4-5 herniation. **B**, midsagittal T2-weighted image better shows the posterior margin of the herniated disk as contrasted with the high intensity of the spinal fluid. Note the decreased intensity of the degenerated L4-5 and L-5 to S-1 disks. **C**, axial view at the L4-5 level shows the herniation is posterolateral on the left (*arrow*).

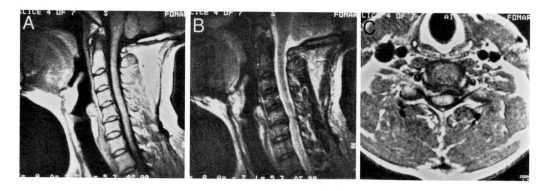

FIG 7–3.
Herniation at the lateral C5-6 level. **A**, note posterior displacement of the disk, some increased intensity just above the disk representing venous plexus displacement, and mild cord displacement. **B**, T2-weighted image shows similar findings. **C**, axial T1-weighted image shows the herniation filling the left foramen and distorting the cord.

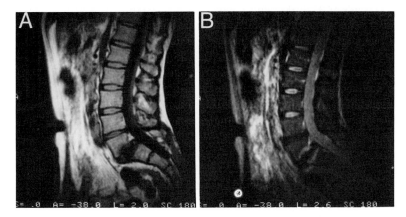

FIG 7–4.
Changes (Modic type 1) in the vertebral bodies adjacent to a degenerated L-5 to S-1 disk, caused by spondylolisthesis. **A,** decreased signal intensity is seen adjacent to the disk on the T1-weighted image. **B,** there is increased signal intensity of bodies on the T2-weighted image.

It has been very difficult to distinguish between recurrent disk herniation and postoperative fibrosis prior to MRI. Postoperative scar in the lumber spine may be identified as an area of signal intensity that is lower than that of normal epidural fat on T1-weighted images. When this change is seen posterior to the subarachnoid space, its nature is obvious. If the main findings are between the subarachnoid space and the vertebral body, this is a more difficult diagnostic problem. This postoperative scar is sometimes of high intensity on the T2-weighted images, resembling herniated disk fragments. The use of gadolinium is proving to be very helpful in this differentiation.[14] When imaging is performed immediately after gadolinium injection, epidural fibrosis will enhance in a relatively uniform fashion, but herniated disks will not enhance. Some enhancement of disks may occur more than 30 minutes following injection. In some cases, there is enhancement of the margin of a disk fragment, probably representing some fibrosis occurring around the herniated fragment.

It is common to see changes in the intensity of the vertebral bodies adjacent to chronically degenerated disks. Modic et al. have described three forms.[15] In type I, there is decreased signal intensity on T1-weighted images and increased signal intensity on T2-weighted images, correlating with pathologic evidence of vascularized fibrotic response within the marrow (Fig 7–4). In type II, there is increased signal intensity on T1-weighted images and mild hyperintensity or isointensity on T2-weighted images, correlating with the replacement of marrow elements with fat in the involved portions of the vertebral bodies. The type II changes appear to follow type I changes. In type III, signal intensity is decreased on both T1- and T2-weighted images, corresponding to extensive bony sclerosis adjacent to a chronically degenerated disk.

Spinal stenosis is of two general types. The first is congenital stenosis, generally idiopathic but also seen in such conditions are achondroplasia and bony dysplasias. The MR images in this type will demonstrate thick pedicles and decreased size of the spinal canal. The more common form is acquired spinal stenosis, which is a common condition in elderly people and is generally associated with long-standing degenerative disk disease. There are some limitations in the diagnosis of spinal stenosis with MRI, as the bony structures and ligamentous calcifications are not as clearly seen as on CT scans. However, MRI is generally successful in demonstrating the presence of stenosis, showing reduction in the size of the spinal canal, enlargement of the ligamentum flavum, bony hypertrophy associated with degenerative face joint disease, bulging of disks, and the presence of spondylolisthesis.[16] The epidural fat is reduced or obliterated in the presence of significant spinal stenosis, and this is a valuable sign of stenosis on T1-weighted images. Stenosis of the lateral recess, which is posterior to the vertebral body and anterior to the superior articular facet, may be apparent on axial MR images of good quality. The neural foramina may also be diminished in spinal stenosis, and can be evaluated on either sagittal or axial projections, and occasionally through oblique projections. Satisfactory imaging of these foramina is not always possible in MRI. Degenerative spondylolisthesis is readily detected on MR images, and the presence or absence of pars defects can usually be determined. In evaluating patients for spinal stenosis, one should remember that both MRI and CT scanning of the supine relaxed patient may not show stenoses that are revealed by hyperextension during myelography.

In evaluations of cervical stenosis of the cervical region, MRI has a considerable advantage over CT scanning because deformities of the cord are readily apparent without the use of intrathecal contrast material. There is a positive correlation between deformity of the spinal cord and the presence of a clinically apparent myelopathy. On T2-weighted images, a region of the cord that has been chronically compressed may demonstrate abnormally high signal.

TRAUMA

The initial examination following spine trauma continues to be plain film radiography, which allows detection of most fractures and subluxations. Sectional imaging is then done in selected cases. Computed tomography is superior in demonstrating fractures, particularly those involving the posterior elements, and is also preferred for the detection of bone fragments within the spinal canal or foramina. However, MRI may be superior in demonstrating ligamentous injuries and is certainly better at showing spinal cord trauma.[17–19] First, the MRI study will demonstrate the relationship of fractured or subluxed vertebral bodies to the cord, and will show a significant stenosis. Second, areas of signal abnormality demonstrated within the cord can be used in identifying the degree of trauma. Areas of bleeding within the cord may initially be seen as hypointense areas because of the presence of deoxyhemoglobin, particularly seen on high field strength MRI. Beginning a few days after the trauma, degradation of deoxyhemoglobin to methemoglobin results in peripheral hyperintensity of the area of hemorrhage on the T1-weighted images. Eventually, both T1- and T2-weighted images will show increased intensity. If, on the other hand, cord contusion is present without significant bleeding, MRI will demonstrate low or normal signal on T1-weighted images and increased signal on T2-weighted images. Prognosis with contusion is better than in cases in which bleeding has occurred.

In determining whether someone suffering acute spine trauma should undergo an MRI examination, one must consider whether traction or stabilization devices are ferromagnetic, as iron may cause image distortion or hazardous movement in the imager.[20] Problems related to monitoring of acutely injured patients and the use of ventilators must also be considered.

Another important use of MRI in respect to trauma is in the detection of post-traumatic cyst formation.[21, 22] Development and expansion of such cysts may be catastrophic in patients with permanent neurologic deficits. These cysts may occur either above or below the original site of cord trauma, and are readily detected by MRI.

NEOPLASIA

Magnetic resonance imaging provides an excellent method of demonstrating tumors involving the spine, the spinal canal, and the spinal cord, both because of its high resolution capabilities and its sensitivity to different types of tissue. Normally, the vertebral bodies are quite homogeneous in their signal intensities. Local areas of inhomogeneity, such as those caused by fat deposits in marrow or by benign cystic lesions, are easily recognizable. Metastases involving the vertebral bodies are easily recognizable, as the replacement of marrow fat results in decreased signal on T1-weighted imaging[23] (Fig 7–5). There may be also some increased signal on T2-weighted images, although this is variable and generally not as obvious as the changes seen on T1-weighted studies (Fig 7–6). When metastases are blastic, decreased signal may be seen on both image sequences. Involvement of the posterior elements of the

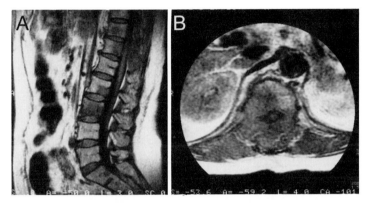

FIG 7–5.
Metastatic breast carcinoma. **A,** sagittal T1-weighted image shows hypointensities in several vertebral bodies representing marrow replacement by tumor. Note canal narrowing at T-12. **B,** axial T1-weighted image at T-12 shows tumor in laminae as well as the body, with some stenosis of the spinal canal and early cord compression.

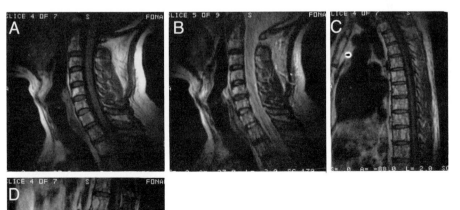

FIG 7–6.
Multiple myeloma. **A,** sagittal T1-weighted image (SE 500/30) shows diffuse mottling of cervical vertebrae. **B,** T2-weighted view (SE 2000/85) does not demonstrate the mottling as well. **C,** similar appearance of the thoracic spine (SE 500/30). **D,** the appearance of the lumbar spine is equally abnormal.

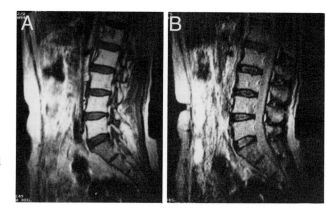

FIG 7–7.
Marrow changes following radiation therapy. **A,** sagittal view (SE 480/30) shows abnormally bright signal from the lumbar vertebral bodies relative to signal from the sacrum. **B,** the alterations in intensity are not as obvious on the T2-weighted image (SE 2000/85).

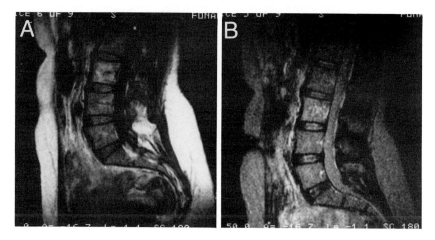

FIG 7–8.
Vertebral body hemangioma. **A,** T1-weighted image shows high intensity involving most of the L-3 body. **B,** the intensity is also high on the T2-weighted view.

vertebrae may be more difficult to recognize and is best studied by examining multiple projections. Extension of vertebral metastatic disease to involve the spinal canal is readily apparent on MRI, and the degree of cord compression can usually be assessed. When there is a complete block, one may see increased signal from the CSF below this block as a result of the dampening effect of the block on CSF pulsations and also the increased protein content of the fluid. Because of this ability to demonstrate extradural involvement, MRI is replacing myelography in the assessment of acute spine-related symptoms in patients with metastatic disease. In evaluating the spine for evidence of metastatic disease, one must recognize the hyperintensity of vertebral bodies indicating past radiation therapy (Fig 7–7).

Hemangiomas of the vertebral bodies also result in changes of signal intensity, but these differ from metastases in that bright signals are visible on both T1- and T2-weighted images (Fig 7–8). This higher signal on T1-weighted images has been considered a result of the fat adjacent to the thickened bony trabeculae, although slow flow of blood in these lesions may also have an effect.[24] Chordomas mainly occur at the sacrococcygeal area or from the clivus, but some are found elsewhere in the spine. These characteristically cause erosions of the posterior margins of one or more vertebrae. The signal intensity of chordomas on T2-weighted images tends to be high. Wherever they occur, these tumors are characterized by marked local bone destruction.[25]

Extramedullary intradural tumors are a relatively large group of masses occurring within the spinal canal, and consist mainly of meningiomas and nerve sheath tumors[26] (Fig 7–9). These tumors are readily recognizable on MR images as relatively well-demarcated masses outlined by CSF within the spinal canal, compressing and displacing the spinal cord. Meningiomas may have intensity characteristics similar to those of the spinal cord, whereas nerve sheath tumors tend to have a higher signal intensity on T2-weighted images. These tumors are seen to enhance strongly with intravenous gadolinium injection.

Intramedullary tumors are also clearly shown by MRI.[27] On T1-weighted images, the cord will be seen to be enlarged, and cysts may be recognizable within the cord. Nearly half of intramedullary tumors have associated cysts. On T2-weighted images, increased signal will be seen in the tumor and also in related cysts, relative to the signal of the spinal cord. Astrocytomas and ependymomas are among the more common spinal cord tumors. Astrocytomas may be very extensive, and often have multiple cystic spaces. The tumors may seem to blend gradually with the normal cord. Ependymomas are more likely to be lobulated masses.

INFLAMMATORY DISEASE

Inflammatory diseases of the spine and disks are best evaluated using T1- and T2-weighted imaging in the sagittal plane. Similar imaging in the axial plane is also helpful. Disk space infections are usually accompanied by osteomyelitis in the adjacent portions of the vertebral bodies.[29] Both areas will be seen to have decreased signal intensity on T1-weighted images when compared with signal from normal structures. On T2-weighted images, both the involved portions of the vertebral bodies and the intervening disk will have higher than normal signal intensity. There may also be a decrease in the height of the disk. In some cases, the vertebral bodies will be partially compressed. Extension of the infectious process into the paraspinal soft tissues may be apparent on both sagittal and axial projections. Infection may also spread into the epidural space, with formation of an epidural abscess. These may present as neurological emergencies. Typically, epidural abscesses spread widely. On T1-weighted

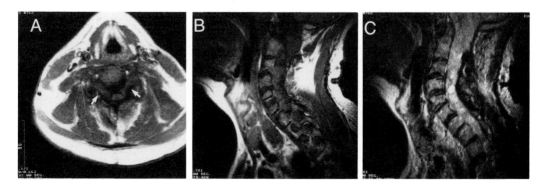

FIG 7–9.
Multiple neurofibromas in a patient with neurofibromatosis. **A,** axial image (SE 708/20) shows bilateral enlargement by tumor-filled intervertebral foramina (*arrows*). **B,** parasagittal T1-weighted view also demonstrates the tumors within the foramina (*arrows*). **C,** T2-weighted sagittal image shows regions of high intensity within the spinal canal representing the tumors (*arrows*).

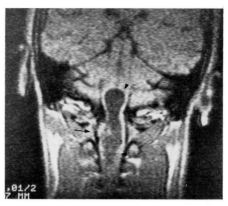

FIG 7–10.
Cystic hemangioblastoma. Coronal T1-weighted image shows an intramedullary cyst extending into the medulla oblongata (*arrowheads*). There is a mural nodule at the lateral margin of the cyst (*arrow*).

images, they are generally of higher signal intensity than the CSF. On T2-weighted images, these abscesses have high signal intensity.

In patients with rheumatoid arthritis, MRI may be used to evaluate atlantoaxial subluxation, abnormal upward dislocation of the dens, stenosis of the spinal canal, and the presence of soft tissue abnormalities (pannus) posterior to the dens.[30] As in other conditions of the spine, MRI is very effective in demonstrating compression of the spinal cord. On the other hand, MRI does not have significant advantages over plain films and tomograms in the detection of subluxations, bony erosions, and facet joint changes.

When multiple sclerosis involves the spinal cord, some cord widening may be shown by MRI. This is most likely to occur in the cervical area. On T2-weighted images, increased signal may be seen in the lesion. Frequently, these are not homogeneous. It is rare to find cord lesions without finding other demyelinating plaques in the white matter of the brain.[31] Other processes such as amyotrophic lateral sclerosis, cord infarction, sarcoidosis, and toxic demyelination may also be seen by MRI, particularly with T2-weighted imaging.[32]

DEVELOPMENTAL ANOMALIES

Downward displacement of the cerebral tonsils, as seen in the Chiari I malformation, is readily detectable with MRI.[33] It seems that the tonsils may lie at the level of the foramen magnum, or even 1 to 2 mm below, in healthy individuals. If the tonsils dip lower than this, Chiari malformation should be suspected. It is important to look for associated abnormalities, particularly syringomyelia. Myeloceles and myelomeningioceles are characteristically associated with Chiari II malformation, in which there is descent of cerebellar vermian tissue as well as tonsils.

Most of the features of spinal dysraphism, with the exception of bony changes such as spinal bifida, are better detected by MRI than by other imaging means. The location of a low, tethered cord is obvious on T1-weighted images. The thickened filum terminale may be identified. Intradural lipomas are commonly associated with low-tethered cords, and are seen as high-intensity fat deposits within the spinal canal on T1-weighted views. In other cases, dermal sinuses may be seen to extend posteriorly from the spinal canal. In diastematomyelia, the cord is split for a variable distance. Frequently there is a bone spur between the two halves of the cord; in other cases, there is a fibrous band instead of a bony spur; in some cases, neither occurs. While MR images well demonstrate the split in the cord, the finer anatomy of the area is better appreciated on CT scans with the use of intrathecal contrast material.

CONCLUSION

In recent years, there has been remarkable improvement in the capabilities of MRI of the spine and its contents. These changes have first allowed MRI to compete with myelography and CT scanning, and by now have demonstrated its superiority in certain situations. It seems likely that the future will bring even better sensitivity, higher resolution, and greater efficiency in MRI of the spine. Refinements in pulse sequences may provide new physiologic data as well as increased resolution. The use of gadolinium and other paramagnetic agents is likely to increase. The future of MRI of the spine is indeed very exciting.

REFERENCES

1. Lufkin R, Votruba J, Reicher M, et al: Solenoid surface coils in MR. *AJR* 1986; 146:409.
2. Rubin JB, Enzmann DR: Optimizing conventional MR imaging of the spine. *Radiology* 1985; 163:777–783.
3. Mararilla KR, Lesh HP, Weinreb JC, et al: Magnetic resonance imaging of the lumbar spine with CT correlation. *AJNR* 1985; 6:237–245.
4. Flannigan BD, Lufkin RB, McGlade C, et al: MR imaging of the cervical spine: Neurovascular anatomy. *AJNR* 1987; 8:27–32.
5. Barnes PD, Lester PD, Yamanashi WS, et al: Magnetic resonance imaging in infants and children with spinal dysraphism. *AJNR* 1986; 7:465–472.
6. Pusey E, Lufkin R, Brown R, et al: Magnetic resonance imaging artifacts: Mechanisms and significance. *RadioGraphics* 1986; 6:891.
7. Patany PM, Phillips JJ, Shiu LC, et al: Motion artifact suppression technique (MAST) for MR imaging. *J Comput Assist Tomogr* 1987; 11:369–377.
8. Czervionke LF, Czervionke JM, Daniels DL, et al: Characteristic features of MR truncation artifacts. *AJNR* 1988; 9:815–824.
9. Manourian AC, Briggs RW: The appearance of Pantopaque on MR images. *Radiology* 1986; 158:457–460.
10. Modic MT, Masaryk TJ, Ross JS, et al: Imaging of degenerative disc disease. *Radiology* 1988; 168:177–186.
11. Edelman RR, Shoukimas GM, Stark DD, et al: High-resolution surface-coil imaging of lumbar disk disease. *AJR* 1985; 144:1123–1129.
12. Flannigan BD, Lufkin RB, McGlade C, et al: MR imaging of the cervical spine: Neurovascular anatomy. *AJNR* 1987; 8:27–32.
13. Masaryk TJ, Ross JS, Modic MT, et al: High-resolution MR imaging of sequestered lumbar intervertebral disks. *AJR* 1988; 150:1155–1162.
14. Huefte M, Modic MT, Ross JS, et al: Lumbar spine: Postoperative MR imaging with Gd-DTPA. *Radiology* 1988; 167:817–824.
15. Modic MT, Steinberg PM, Ross JS, et al: Degenerative disk disease: Assessment of changes in vertebral body marrow with MR imaging. *Radiology* 1988; 166:193–199.
16. Modic MT, Masaryk T, Boumphey F, et al: Lumbar herniated disk disease and canal stenosis: Prospective evolution by surface coil MR, CT and myelography. *AJNR* 1986; 7:709–717.
17. Tarr RW, Drolshagen LF, Kerner TC, et al: MR imaging of recent spinal trauma. *J Comput Assist Tomogr* 1987; 11:412–417.
18. Chakeres DW, Flickinger F, Bresnahan JC, et al: MR imaging of acute spinal cord trauma. *AJNR* 1987; 8:5–10.
19. Mirvis SE, Geisler FH, Jelinek JJ, et al: Acute cervical spine trauma: Evaluation with 1.5 T MR imaging. *Radiology* 1988; 166:807–816.
20. New PJ, Rosen BR, Brady TJ, et al: Potential hazards and artifacts of ferromagnetic and nonferromagnetic surgical and dental materials and devices in nuclear magnetic resonance imaging. *Radiology* 1983; 147:139–148.

21. Gebarski SS, Maynard FW, Gabrielsen TO, et al: Posttraumatic progressive myelopathy. *Radiology* 1985; 157:379–385.

22. Quencer RM, Sheldon JJ, Donovan Post MJ, et al: MRI of chronically injured cervical spinal cord. *AJNR* 1986; 7:457–464.

23. Smoker WRK, Godersky JC, Knutzon RK, et al: The role of MR imaging in evaluating metastatic spinal disease. *AJNR* 1987; 8:901–908.

24. Ross JS, Masaryk TJ, Modic MT, et al: Vertebral hemangiomas: MR imaging. *Radiology* 1987; 165:165–169.

25. Sze G, Vichanco LS, Brant-Zawadzki MN, et al: Chordomas: MR imaging. *Radiology* 1988; 166:187–191.

26. Scotti G, Scialfa G, Colombo N, et al: MR imaging of intradural extramedullary tumors of the cervical spine. *J. Comput Assist Tomogr* 1985; 9:1037–1941.

27. Gay AMC, Pinto RS, Raghavendra BN, et al: Intramedullary spinal cord tumors: MR imaging with emphasis on associated cysts. *Radiology* 1986; 161:381–386.

28. Dormont D, Gelbert F, Assouline E, et al: MR imaging of spinal cord arteriovenous malformations at 0.5 T: Study of 34 cases. *AJNR* 1988; 9:833–838.

29. Modic MT, Feiglin DH, Piraino DW, et al: Vertebral osteomyelitis: Assessment using MR. *Radiology* 1985; 157:157–166.

30. Bundschuh C, Modic MT, Kearney F, et al: Rheumatoid arthritis of the cervical spine: Surface coil MR imaging. *AJNR* 1988; 9:565–571.

31. Edwards MK, Farlow MR, Stevens JC: Cranial MR in spinal cord MS: Diagnosing patients with isolated spinal cord symptoms. *AJNR* 1986; 7:1003–1005.

32. Kelly RB, Mahoney PD, Cawley KM: MR demonstration of spinal cord sarcoidosis: Report of a case. *AJNR* 1988; 9:197–199.

33. DeLaPaz RL, Brady TJ, Bunoanno PF, et al: Nuclear magnetic resonance imaging of Arnold-Chiari type I malformation with hydromyelia. *J Comput Assist Tomogr* 1983; 7:126–129.

Chapter 8

Magnetic Resonance Imaging of the Pediatric Central Nervous System

Rosalind B. Dietrich, M.B., Ch.B.

The ability of magnetic resonance imaging (MRI) to produce multiplanar images of any body region without ionizing radiation, extensive patient preparation, or invasive techniques makes it a potentially advantageous modality with which to evaluate children. Pediatric patients suffer a spectrum of diseases different from that of adults and experience a higher proportion of congenital anomalies, a differing group of neoplasms, and a lower incidence of metastatic and degenerative disease. Because of this, pulse sequences and techniques used routinely to evaluate disease processes in adults are often inappropriate to optimally demonstrate and characterize disease in children.

TECHNIQUE

As children may be apprehensive about the imaging study, parents should be encouraged to stay with the child to give reassurance if necessary. Children under 7 years of age frequently require sedation. At the University of California, Los Angeles, children under 18 months of age are given chloral hydrate, 50 to 75 mg/kg body weight orally 30 minutes before imaging. Children over 18 months of age are initially given thiopental, 25 mg/kg, administered rectally 5 minutes before imaging.[1] If sedation is not achieved by 15 minutes, a repeat half-dose is also given.

Devices are now available for respiratory, cardiac, and temperature monitoring that cause minimal or no image degradation when used in conjunction with the MR imager.[2, 3] In sedated patients who are medically stable, usually all that is necessary is respiratory monitoring with an apnea monitor. Of course, more extensive monitoring is usually required when imaging intensive care patients or premature infants.

It may be necessary to adapt the MR instrument patient bed for pediatric use, as these beds have been designed for adults. Extra pads can be used to ensure that the child is positioned in the center of the coil. Some instruments are also equipped with cradle devices to help position and immobilize children optimally during imaging.

When evaluating the spine of a pediatric patient, it is necessary to use either solenoid

FIG 8–1.
Anatomy of the premature brain at 34 weeks' gestation. **A**, axial spin echo (SE) (700/30) (repetition time/echo time). T1-weighted image demonstrates a thin high-signal-intensity cortical rim (*arrow*) surrounding the lower-signal-intensity white matter. A paucity of sulci and gyri are present at this age. **B**, parasagittal SE (700/30). The paucity of sulci and gyri are seen, particularly over the frontal regions, with increased cerebral spinal fluid spaces seen over the parietal lobes (*arrow*).

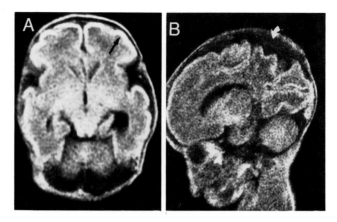

band coils or planar surface coils in order to increase the signal-to-noise ratio.[4, 5] Surface coils may also be useful in the evaluation of the neonatal brain.

When imaging young children, it is imperative that the initial imaging sequences yield maximal information, as the study may have to be terminated if the child awakens or is unable to remain still.[6] Because of this it is important to tailor the study to detect the abnormalities most suspected from the clinical history. It may be necessary to use interleaved sequences or sequences that generate slices thinner than those routinely obtained when especially small structures are being evaluated. This is particularly true with instruments that cannot produce contiguous cuts on all sequences. Images obtained in nonorthogonal planes may also be useful for better defining the relationships of adjacent structures and for demonstrating structures and lesions in an oblique orientation.[7]

NORMAL APPEARANCES AND MYELINATION

Before abnormalities of the pediatric brain can be identified, it is essential to have a thorough knowledge of the normal age-related appearances of the pediatric brain on the pulse sequences routinely used when screening for abnormalities. The transition of the cortex in the developing preterm brain from a relatively smooth appearance with no or few convolutions to the extensively and compactly infolded cortex seen in the healthy term infant can be well demonstrated by MRI.[8–10] The sequential MR appearances illustrating the increasingly complex arrangement of sulci and gyri in the developing brain can be well seen on T1-weighted sequences[8, 10] (Fig 8–1). The exact age of premature neonates can thus be determined.

The neonatal brain has a higher water content in both the gray and white matter than does the adult brain. During the infant's 1st year of life, the water content of the brain decreases rapidly, from 88% at birth to 82% at 6 months of age.[11, 12] After 1 year of age, this decrease in water content continues but at a much slower rate. Relatively more is lost from the white matter than from the gray matter at this time. Concomitantly, hydrophobic myelin is being laid down within the white matter, and the lipid and protein content of the brain increase.

As MRI is so highly sensitive to the differences in water and lipid content of gray and white matter, it offers a unique opportunity to study white matter maturation in vivo both sequentially and relative to a known standard.[13, 14] Myelination is a process that greatly enhances the functional efficiency of neurons by increasing the speed of conduction, and because this dynamic process starts in some sites during intrauterine life and continues after the child's birth, it can be an extremely useful index of brain maturation during infancy. There is evidence to suggest that the myelin sheaths continue to undergo remodeling throughout life,[15] but the changes are most visible during the first 2 years when they occur most rapidly. Care has to be taken, however, when interpreting myelination changes in studies obtained on imagers of different field strengths and with different sequence parameters.[16] To optimally visualize the myelin present within the white matter of the brain, T2-weighted spin echo or heavily T1-weighted (either inversion recovery, or short repetition time, short echo time spin echo) pulse sequences should be obtained, as these maximize inherent tissue contrast differentiation.

Although developmentally normal children show a spectrum of relative intensities of gray and white matter, their gray-white matter patterns fall into three distinct groups: "infantile," "isointense," and "early adult."[13] At birth and generally for the first 8 months, the "infantile" pattern shows reversal of the normal adult pattern seen on T2-weighted images, that is, in neonates the white matter is more intense that gray matter (Figs 8–2 and 8–3). Children between the ages of 8 and 12 months demonstrate the transient "isointense" phase in which there is poor differentiation of gray and white matter (Fig 8–4). The "early adult" pattern, in which gray matter has a higher intensity than white matter, is seen in all healthy children over 12 months (Fig 8–5) and may be seen as early as 10 months of age. The transient isointense pattern is rarely seen throughout the entire brain at one time. Patients more frequently show an infantile-isointense pattern or an isointense-adult pattern. In some children all three patterns may be seen concomitantly. When more than one pattern is seen in different areas of the brain of the same child, the more immature pattern is always present in the areas of later myelination.

As the process of myelination progresses, the previously nonmyelinated, high-intensity, infantile white matter develops lower signal intensity on T2-weighted sequences following established patterns.[13, 14, 17] At birth some myelin is already present supratentorially in the thalamus and infratentorially in the inferior cerebellar peduncles (see Fig 8–2). In children over 1 month of age, myelin can be seen in the region of the posterior limb of the internal capsule (see Fig 8–3). As myelination continues, areas of lower signal intensity are also identified sequentially in the optic radiations (3 months) (see Fig 8–3), the anterior limb of the internal capsule, and radiations to the precentral gyrus (6 months) (see Fig 8–4), the parietal and frontal white matter (8 months) (see Figs 8–4 and 8–5), and the white matter of the temporal lobes (1 year) (see Fig 8–5). After 1 year of age the portion of myelinated central white matter increases progressively as myelination extends more peripherally and causes finer branching of the myelinated subcortical fibers and increased differentiation of the signal intensity of the gray and white matter.

On inversion recovery images, areas of the white matter already myelinated have a high signal intensity compared with that of adjacent nonmyelinated areas.[18] The progression of myelination seen with inversion recovery sequences parallels that seen on spin echo sequences. Although the presence of myelin in any specific tract may be seen earlier on T1-weighted images,[14] the timing of the deposition of myelin as seen on T2-weighted sequences better correlates with that seen on autopsy sections stained for myelin.

In children with clinical developmental delay, MRI usually shows the same sequential appearance of myelin deposition but demonstrates both a delay in the development of myelin in the white matter and in the transition from one gray-white matter differentiation pattern to another.[13]

DEMYELINATING AND DYSMYELINATING DISEASES

Although MRI is sensitive in the demonstration of demyelinating and dysmyelinating processes, the appearances among this group of diseases are relatively nonspecific, and they usually cannot be differentiated. Most demyelinating diseases presenting during childhood are diagnosed using a combination of clinical data, biochemical tests, and brain biopsy results. The major roles of MRI are therefore in demonstrating the presence of disease and in documenting its possible progression with time. The pattern of discrete patchy areas of high

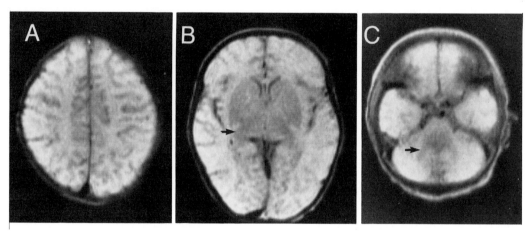

FIG 8–2.
Neonatal brain of a healthy infant at 6 days of age. **A,** at the level of the centrum semiovale. Axial SE (2000/84). The white matter demonstrates high signal intensity compared with adjacent gray matter. **B,** at the level of the basal ganglia. Axial SE (2000/84). A small amount of myelin is already present in the region of the thalami bilaterally (*arrow*). A septum cavum pellucidum is also present. **C,** at the level of the posterior fossa. Axial SE (2000/84). A small amount of low-signal-intensity myelin is already present (*arrow*).

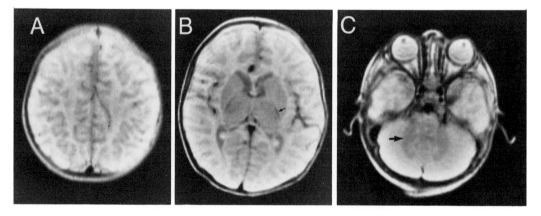

FIG 8–3.
Neonatal brain of a healthy infant at 3 months of age. **A,** at the level of the centrum semiovale. Axial SE (2000/84). The white matter maintains higher signal intensity than the adjacent gray matter. **B,** at the level of the basal ganglia. Axial SE (2000/84). Myelin is now present in the region of the posterior limb of the internal capsule (*arrow*) and is now beginning to be laid down within the white matter of the occipital lobe. **C,** at the level of the posterior fossa. Axial SE (2000/84). More myelin has been laid down within the posterior fossa at this age (*arrow*) than in the 6-day-old child in Figure 8–2.

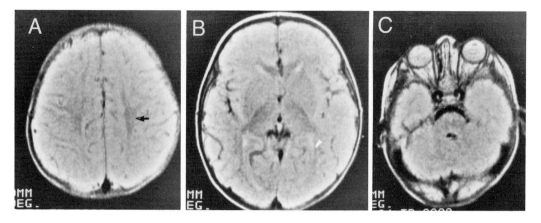

FIG 8–4.
Neonatal brain of a healthy infant at 8 months of age. **A**, axial SE (2000/84). There is a small amount of myelin present within the white matter of the parietal lobes (*arrow*). The gray-white matter demonstrates relative isointensity. **B**, at the level of the basal ganglia. The gray and white matter demonstrate little difference in signal intensities. Myelin is present within the thamalus, posterior limbs of the internal capsule, the occipital white matter, and in the anterior limb of the internal capsule. **C**, at level of the posterior fossa. Axial SE (2000/84).

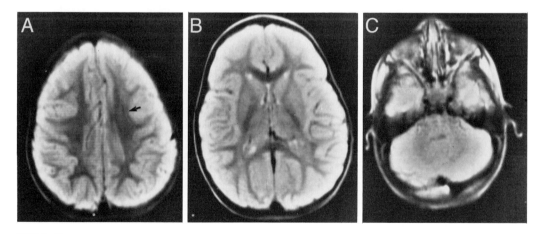

FIG 8–5.
Brain of a healthy infant at 2 years of age. **A**, at the level of the centrum semiovale. Axial SE (2000/84). The white matter (*arrow*) demonstrates lower signal intensity than the adjacent gray matter. **B**, at the level of the basal ganglia. Axial SE (2000/84). The area of white matter myelinated is progressing peripherally toward the subcortical U-fibers. Very little secondary branching is present at this time. **C**, at the level of the posterior fossa. Axial SE (2000/84).

signal intensity so characteristically seen in adult patients with multiple sclerosis is rare in children. More frequently, children demonstrate diffuse supratentorial involvement of white matter and sometimes infratentorial involvement associated with various degrees of atrophy.[19, 20] Both inherited disorders—such as metachromatic leukodystrophy (Fig 8–6)—and postviral causes of demyelination—such as subacute sclerosing panencephalitis—demonstrate this pattern, though the latter frequently demonstrates more severe atrophy. Adrenoleukodystrophy, however, is the exception and may demonstrate a more characteristic appearance with white matter involvement extending anteriorly from the occipital lobes for a variable extent correlating with the pathologic distribution of this disease (Fig 8–7). Conditions such as Pelizaeus-Merzbacher disease are described as having a more patchy distribution patho-logically; however, more patients with this and similar disease processes will have to be imaged before knowledge of the ability of MRI to demonstrate and differentiate these entities is known.

CONGENITAL BRAIN MALFORMATIONS

The nervous system has a higher incidence of congenital malformations than any other organ system in the body. The advent of computed tomography (CT) and MRI allowed visualization of the cross-sectional anatomy of the brains of living children with congenital anomalies. Because sequential studies can be obtained noninvasively, these modalities can give valuable information regarding the evolution of abnormalities.

Different congenital anomalies result from noxious events occurring at one of the different

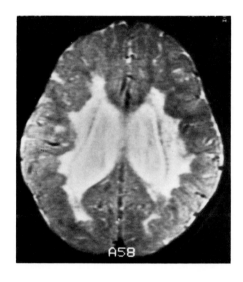

FIG 8–6.
Metachromatic leukodystrophy. Axial SE (3000/85). High signal intensity is seen diffusely throughout the white matter associated with some dilation of the lateral ventricles.

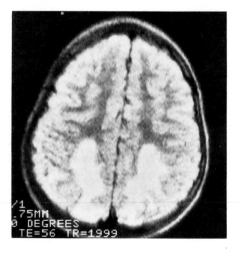

FIG 8–7.
Adrenoleukodystrophy. Axial SE (2000/84). High signal intensity is seen in the white matter extending from the occipital lobes anteriorly into the parietal region.

TABLE 8–1.

Congenital Anomalies Associated With Different Stages of Brain Development

Stage	Gestational Time	Anomalies Produced
Dorsal induction	3–4 wk	Anencephaly
		Encephalocele
		Myelomeningocele
		Chiari malformation
		Spinal dysraphism
Ventral induction	5–10 wk	Holoprosencephaly
		Septo-optic dysplasia
		Cerebellar hypoplasia
		Dandy-Walker malformations
Neuronal migration	2–5 mo	Schizencephaly
		Lissencephaly
		Pachygyria
		Polymicrogyria
		Neural heterotopias
		Aphasia of Corpus callosum
Neuronal proliferation	2–5 mo	Macrencephaly
		Micrencephaly
		Congenital vascular malformations
		Congenital tumors
		Hydranencephaly
Neuronal histiogenesis	2–5 mo	Tuberous sclerosis
		Neurofibromatosis
		Sturge-Weber syndrome
		von Hippel-Lindau disease

From Van der Knapp MS, Valk J: Classification of congenital abnormalities of the CNS. *AJNR* 9:315–325, 1988. Used with permission.

stages of brain development.[21] Chronologically, these stages are dorsal induction, ventral induction, neuronal proliferation, neuronal migration, neuronal organization, and myelination. The more common abnormalities resulting from problems occurring at these times are listed in Table 8–1.

As MRI enables one to visualize in multiple planes without the need to reposition the patient, it is an ideal modality with which to evaluate the structural anatomy of congenital anomalies.[21–24] Short TR, short TE sequences—with their superior resolution and shorter imaging times—are best for the depiction of displacement of structures, and for evaluation of the gyral-sulcal pattern and the size and shape of the ventricles and the extracerebral space, as the cerebrospinal fluid (CSF) has lower signal intensity than the adjacent gray and white matter on these sequences. When evaluating children with suspected anomalies, T1-weighted sequences should be obtained in at least two planes. T2-weighted sequences are useful to give additional information, demonstrating associated abnormalities of myelination, areas of heterotopic gray matter, or the presence of additional hamartomatous or malignant lesions.

Children with holoprosencephaly show a failure of normal development of the cerebral hemispheres, thalamus, and hypothalamus because of a defect of midline cleavage. There is fusion of the lateral ventricles, which have failed to separate, and a lack of development of the sagittal fissure and falx.[25] In more severe forms (alobar prosencephaly) there is a large single ventricular cavity with a saucer-like rim of cerebral tissue anteriorly and a large dorsal cyst. In less severe forms (semilobar prosencephaly) there is a partial separation into cerebral lobes, and the frontal horns of the lateral ventricles are fused but separate occipital horns are visible. The interhemispheric fissure and the falx are only partially developed and may be seen posteriorly. The roof of the monoventricle is indented downward in the midline. In lobar prosencephaly the interhemispheric fissure is usually present from the occiput to the anterior portion of the frontal lobes. There may be only a small portion of cortex fused just ahead of the anterior corpus callosum. The bodies of the lateral ventricles have a narrowed appearance with fusion of the anterior horns.

Septo-optic dysplasia is a syndrome first described by de Morsier, consisting of blindness, hypoplasia of the optic discs, and absence of the septum pellucidum in females. These girls frequently have hypopituitarism. Magnetic resonance studies show small optic nerves, absence of the septum, and enlargement of the chiasmatic cistern. The falx and interhemispheric fissure are normal.[26]

Congenital anomalies of the posterior fossa structures such as Dandy-Walker malformations, cerebellar hypoplasia, and Chiari malformations can be well seen using T1-weighted images. Sequences obtained in the sagittal plane are particularly useful in defining the full extent of the anomaly and showing associated abnormalities such as absence of the corpus callosum.

When abnormalities of migration occur the cortex develops abnormal thickness, folding, and disorganization. Early disturbances in migration produce changes that are more severe and more nearly symmetric; those occurring later produce changes that are milder and less symmetric.[27] In these children MRI clearly defines the surface anatomy of the brain[28, 29] showing the paucity of gyri and sulci in such conditions as lissencephaly and pachygyria. In the most severe cases, agyria or lissencephaly occurs with complete absence of gyri (Fig 8–8). Migrating neurons are unable to reach the superficial layers of the cortex, which becomes thickened, and the white matter is "reduced in size"; these changes are seen on T2-weighted images, with their superior differentiation of gray and white matter. Normal gyral formation does not occur, so the surface of the brain remains flat. In cases of pachygyria, T1-weighted images show that the broad, flat gyri are separated by shallow sulci and that the temporal and frontal lobes are hypoplastic and separated by shallow sylvian fissures. The lateral ventricles are moderately dilated.

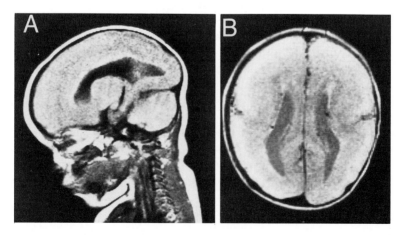

FIG 8–8.
Lissencephaly. **A,** parasagittal SE (500/30). There is a total absence of sulci and gyri present along the surface of the brain on this T1-weighted sequence. **B,** axial (3000/40). There is a remarkably thickened cortex with a small amount of periventricular white matter present. There is mild dilation of the lateral ventricles.

In polymicrogyria, multiple small abnormal gyri, with either histologically incomplete or absent intervening sulci and lack of secondary branching, are present. These abnormal gyri may be seen especially on sagittal images.[28]

In children with schizocephaly, who have clefts lined on either side by gray matter traversing the brain tissue, imaging in multiple planes is necessary to define the full extent of the anomalous anatomy. If images are obtained in only one plane, the cleft may be entirely missed.[30]

Magnetic resonance imaging is particularly valuable in the demonstration of heterotopic gray matter. Gray matter heterotopias are collections of nerve cells that are in abnormal locations as a result of their arrest along the migration pathway from the germinal matrix to the cortex. These areas have the same signal intensity as adjacent gray matter no matter what MR pulsing parameters are used. Those in a periventricular location can be seen as pseudomasses invaginating to the lateral ventricles on both MR images and CT scans. Only MRI, however, enables one to distinguish the areas of heterotopic gray matter that are buried within the white matter of the brain. These are optimally seen on sequences that show good gray-white matter differentiation.[31, 32] Additional MR images to show the pattern of myelination are often helpful in this group of patients, who frequently demonstrate delay in the myelination process.

Images in multiple planes are also useful in evaluating abnormalities of the corpus callosum and associated lesions.[33–35] In such patients sagittal images demonstrate total or partial absence of the corpus callosum, distortion of the cingulate gyrus, radiation of the midline sulci, and the presence of associated lesions such as lipomas, cysts, or posterior fossa anomalies including Dandy-Walker and Chiari malformations. On axial images the characteristic appearance of the lateral ventricles with dilation of the occipital horns of the lateral ventricles and separation of the beaked anterior horns can be seen (Fig 8–9). When partial absence of the corpus callosum occurs it is usually the posterior portion that is absent, as its development occurs from anterior to posterior. In the rare instance when absence of the anterior portion occurs it is usually secondary to a vascular insult occurring in utero.

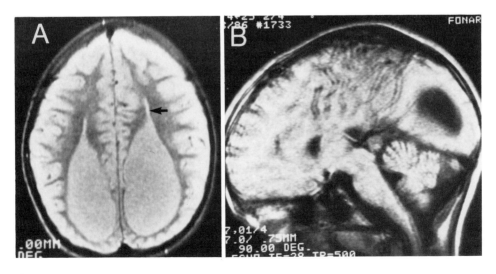

FIG 8–9.
Absence of the corpus callosum. **A,** axial SE (2000/84). There is marked dilation of the posterior horns of the lateral ventricles (colpocephaly), with beaking and separation of the anterior horns (*arrow*). **B,** sagittal SE (500/28). The entire corpus callosum is absent.

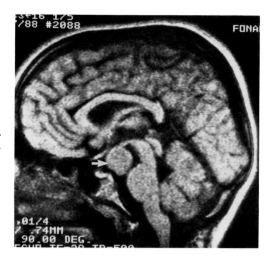

FIG 8–10.
Hamartoma of the tuber cinerum. Sagittal SE (500/28). Isointense mass is seen in the suprasellar region (*arrow*).

Abnormalities of neuronal proliferation occur concomitantly with those of migration and histiogenesis. Hamartoma of the tuber cinereum (Fig 8–10) is a congenital malformation consisting of a tumor-like, ectopic mass of neuronal tissue. Children with this abnormality present with precocious isosexual puberty or neurologic symptoms such as seizures, intellectual impairment, and behavioral problems. Magnetic resonance images reveal a mass in the region of the interpeduncular cistern that does not enhance after administration of contrast agents.[36] Such lesions remain unchanged in size on consecutive studies.

Megalencephaly is a rare anomaly that may be unilateral or bilateral in distribution. Infants with this condition present with early seizures and severe encephalopathy. It is associated with a chaotic hyperplasia and hypertrophy of neuronal elements, resulting in an abundance of disorganized brain parenchyma and cerebral dysfunction. The CT and MRI findings in five children with this anomaly have been recently described and show hemispheric hypertrophy with lateral ventricle dilation, abnormal gyral pattern, and a thick cortex on the enlarged side.[37]

Disorders of histiogenesis or the phakomatoses are hereditary developmental disorders characterized by disordered cell proliferation both in the nervous system and in the skin. In children with this group of abnormalities, administration of gadolinium-DTPA (diethylenetriaminepentaacetic acid; Gd-DTPA) may give additional information[38] and help differentiate the hamartomatous lesions present in these entities from lesions that have undergone malignant degeneration.

In tuberous sclerosis, fibrocellular nodules or tubera are present in the brain cortex and periventricular areas. Nodules may obstruct the foramen of Monro, leading to hydrocephalus, and these may develop into giant cell astrocytomas. Enhancement following administration of Gd-DTPA may be seen in lesions that have developed into giant cell tumors. Magnetic resonance imaging shows the subependymal masses but is less sensitive than CT scanning in the detection of calcification. Despite this, MRI is the study of choice for the evaluation of patients with possible tuberous sclerosis.[39–41] Because of its superior tissue contrast differentiation it is able to demonstrate the plaques in the cortex and white matter that cannot be well identified by CT scanning (Fig 8–11).

Children with neurofibromatosis may demonstrate both peripheral and central nervous system manifestations. Peripherally, multiple subcutaneous nerve sheath tumors may be present. Centrally optic gliomas are frequently seen. For demonstration of the optic nerves both axial and coronal T1-weighted sequences should be used because of their superior anatomic resolution. These images should be obtained contiguously using thin slices with the child's chin tilted so that the entire course of the optic nerves, chiasm, and radiations can be obtained on the same axial slice. T2-weighted sequences are also needed when evaluating children with neurofibromatosis in order to demonstrate possible extension of the gliomas along the optic radiations. T2-weighted sequences may also show areas of high signal intensity within the white matter or basal ganglia regions. These areas are thought to represent hamartomatous lesions or areas of gliosis.[42, 43] In older children and adults, meningiomas and cranial nerve neuromas, particularly those arising from the acoustic nerve, are seen, but these lesions are uncommon in younger children. Occasionally, aqueductal stenosis may also be present.

The osseous dysplasia seen in some children with neurofibromatosis is unilateral involvement of the sphenoid bone. The bony changes present can be demonstrated by MRI but are frequently better seen by CT scanning.

The Sturge-Weber syndrome, in its classic form, consists of facial capillary hemangioma (port wine stain) in the distribution of one or more divisions (usually the upper division) of the fifth cranial nerve, and ipsilateral leptomeningeal angiomatosis. The findings differ depending on the age of the child at the time of imaging. Before 1 to 2 years of age MRI may show the affected hemisphere to be enlarged with small arachnoid spaces and lateral ventricles. There is ipsilateral enlargement of the choroid plexus. Alternatively, the arachnoid spaces and ipsilateral ventricle may appear enlarged. Calcifications may be seen within the angioma. Two recent MRI studies of children in this age range with Sturge-Weber syndrome reported accelerated myelination of the involved hemisphere compared to the contralateral side.[44] In older children, the angioma is progressively excluded from the circulation. Large areas of calcification are seen, and focal or generalized cerebral atrophy develops, probably secondary to chronic ischemia and prolonged seizure activity (Fig 8–12). In patients of this age MR images will show the atrophy, calcifications, and vascular channels of the angioma.

Arachnoid cysts develop when fluid is loculated within arachnoid layers. They most frequently occur adjacent to the temporal horns, in the interhemispheric region, over the

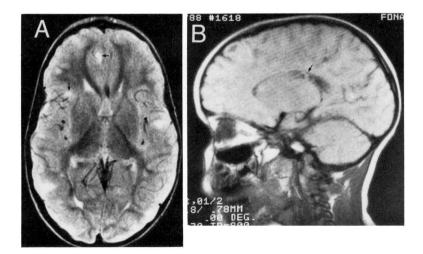

FIG 8–11.
Tuberous sclerosis. **A,** axial SE (2000/85). Patchy areas of high signal intensity present in gray and white matter represent hamartomatous lesions (*arrows*). **B,** sagittal SE (800/30). Periventricular tubera (*arrow*) invaginate into the lateral ventricles.

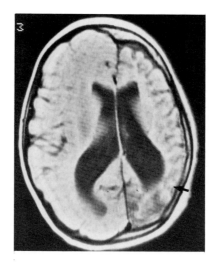

FIG 8–12.
Sturge-Weber syndrome. Axial SE (800/30). Atrophy of
the left cerebral hemisphere and leptomeningeal
angioma involving the posterior parietal lesion.

convexities, and in the cerebellopontine angle or the suprasellar region. Magnetic resonance imaging shows the cysts to have thin walls and to contain fluid. The adjacent brain parenchyma is displaced inward, and the adjacent calvarium may be eroded. Those cysts situated adjacent to the ventricular system may cause hydrocephalus as a result of compression. Magnetic resonance imaging can frequently aid in the differentiation of arachnoid cysts from porencephalic cysts by demonstrating that the former do not communicate with the ventricular system on images obtained in multiple planes.

SPINAL DYSRAPHISM

In children less than 6 months of age, ultrasonography is the initial screening modality of choice for the evaluation of suspected spinal dysraphism. However, MRI should be used in children over this age and in those under 6 months with abnormal ultrasound studies. Images should be obtained in at least two planes (usually sagittal and axial) using sequences with thin, contiguous slices. If this is not possible, then interleaved sequences should be obtained. When imaging children with severe scoliosis, axial images are usually obtained first. Additional coronal or sagittal images are then obtained depending on the degree of kyphosis and lordosis present. Magnetic resonance imaging is able to demonstrate the presence of tethered cord, widened dural sac, dermal sinus, cyst, lipoma, diastematomyelia, meningocele, and hydrosyringomyelia, and is therefore extremely useful to fully define the extent of abnormalities prior to surgery[45–47] (Figs 8–13 and 8–14). At present, MRI is not as helpful as metrizamide myelography at demonstrating thickened fila and thin dural adhesions.

HYDROCEPHALUS

Magnetic resonance imaging is extremely useful in the evaluation of the child with suspected hydrocephalus. T1-weighted sequences obtained in multiple planes will not only demonstrate the presence or absence of ventricular dilatation but also accurately locate the level of the obstruction. And because both the brain substance and the ventricular system are imaged directly, one sees if the obstruction is caused by an adjacent cystic or neoplastic mass lesion and if hemorrhage is also present (Fig 8–15). T2-weighted sequences may better demonstrate tumors causing hydrocephalus and may also show subependymal edema adjacent to ventricular systems under pressure. T_2-weighted spin echo and gradient echo images may also demonstrate evidence of previous hemorrhage into the ventricular system as the cause for the development of the hydrocephalus. In patients with shunts, MRI is also helpful in demonstrating decrease in the size of ventricles; recurring hydrocephalus secondary to mal-

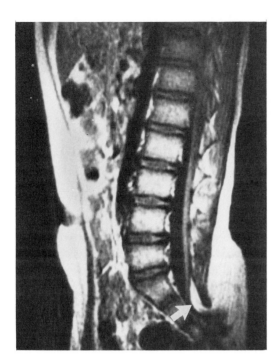

FIG 8–13.
Spinal dysraphism. Sagittal SE (500/30). Spinal cord extends inferiorly into the sacral region where it is tethered by a high-signal-intensity lipoma (*arrow*).

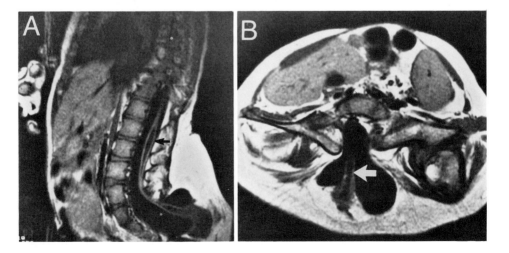

FIG 8–14.
Myelomeningocele. **A,** sagittal SE (500/30). Large septated myelomeningocele. There is dilation of the central canal of the lumbar spinal cord (*arrow*). **B,** axial SE (500/30). Abnormal angulation of the iliac wings. Lower spinal cord (*arrow*) extends into meningocele.

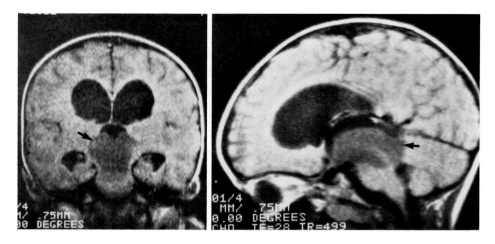

FIG 8–15.
Glioma causing hydrocephalus. **A,** coronal SE (800/28). Low signal intensity glioma (*arrow*) involves the brain stem and hypothalamus and is causing obstruction at the level of the third ventricle. **B,** sagittal SE (500/28). Glioma (*arrow*) compressing and obstructing the third ventricle.

functioning shunts; and such complications as the development of septations within the ventricles, subdural fluid collections, and/or hematomas.

TUMORS

Children demonstrate a different spectrum of tumors than do adults, with a much lower incidence of metastic lesions and a higher preponderance of infratentorial lesions. There are three main roles for MRI in the evaluation of children with brain tumors: (1) demonstrating the presence of a lesion, (2) demonstrating its origin and defining its extent, and (3) evaluating the response to therapy and demonstrating possible recurrence. Because of its multiplanar capability, MRI is an ideal modality for preoperative mapping of tumors. Although differentiation of viable tumor from surrounding edema and necrosis is often difficult, the use of Gd-DTPA as a contrast agent should help overcome this problem and may be particularly useful in demonstrating areas of viable tumor in patients who are to undergo brain biopsy (Fig 8–16; Table 8–2). The majority of tumors demonstrate lower signal intensity than the adjacent healthy brain tissue on T1-weighted sequences and higher signal intensity on T2-weighted sequences; therefore, MRI is not useful in predicting tumor type based on signal characteristics alone. Exceptions to this are lesions such as lipomas, teratomas, and dermoids, which may contain fatty tissue and thus demonstrate high signal intensity on T1-weighted sequences, and hamartomas, which frequently show only slight increase in signal intensity on T2-weighted sequences as compared with adjacent brain tissue. Craniopharyngiomas appear as smooth-walled suprasellar masses and may demonstrate either high or low signal intensity on T1-weighted sequences depending on the nature of the cholesterol within them (Fig 8–17).

When evaluating tumors with a propensity to leptomeningeal spread or the development of drop metastases, it is essential to obtain T1-weighted images both before and after administration of Gd-DTPA. Leptomeningeal disease is extremely difficult to demonstrate on pre-Gd-DTPA images.[48] The contrast agent is also helpful in the differentiation of tumor from postoperative scarring in patients who have had previous surgical resections. Although most

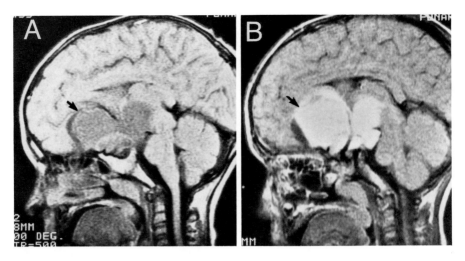

FIG 8–16.
Optic chiasm glioma following partial surgical resection. **A,** sagittal SE (500/30). Glioma (*arrow*) demonstrates lower signal intensity than surrounding healthy brain and contains some cystic areas. **B,** sagittal SE (500/30) post-Gd-DTPA. Tumor enhances after injection of Gd-DTPA (*arrow*). Cystic areas still demonstrate low signal intensity.

tumors are well demonstrated by both CT and MRI, the main advantage of MRI over CT is its improved visualization of lesions in the temporal lobes and posterior fossa[49] as a result of its ability to image in multiple planes and the lack of bony artifacts.

HEMORRHAGE AND HYPOXIC-ISCHEMIC ENCEPHALOPATHY

In both preterm and term babies, hypoxic-ischemic encephalopathy from perinatal asphyxia can result in subsequent chronic neurologic disability, such as cerebral palsy, mental retardation, and epilepsy.[50, 51]

Children who have suffered anoxic-ischemic events in utero may demonstrate hemispheric defects or porencephalies. Porencephaly is a cystic malformation of the brain probably secondary to destruction and subsequent absorption of a portion of the brain parenchyma. This results in one or more cystic cavities that communicate with the ventricles and frequently with the subarachnoid space. Magnetic resonance imaging is able to demonstrate the cystic cavities seen in children with porencephaly. Multiplanar T1-weighted images are likely to

TABLE 8–2.
Indications for the Use of Gadolinium-DTPA

Brain tumors
    Aid in differentiation of viable tumor from edema or necrosis in prebiopsy patients
    Demonstration of leptomeningeal spread or drop metastases
    Aid in differentiation of tumor from postoperative changes in postsurgical patients
Neurophakomatoses
    Demonstration of malignant degeneration
Infections and inflammatory lesions
    Brain abscess
    Meningitis

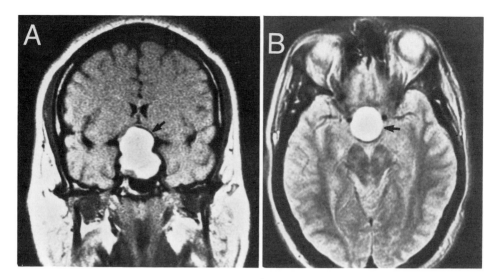

FIG 8–17.
Craniopharyngioma. **A**, coronal (500/30). Suprasellar mass extends inferiorly into the sella and demonstrates high signal intensity on this T1-weighted sequence (*arrow*). **B**, axial (2000/85). Lesion has smooth margins and high signal intensity on this T2-weighted sequence (*arrow*).

be able to demonstrate communication of the cavity with the ventricular system. At times, however, it is not possible to differentiate porencephalic cysts from arachnoid cysts.

Intraventricular and periventricular hemorrhage is a frequent and severe complication of prematurity. Bleeding usually occurs in the subependymal germinal matrix adjacent to the head of the caudate nucleus. The hemorrhage may rupture into the lateral ventricles and can be seen collecting in the occipital horns, the fourth ventricle, and cisterna magne. Clots within the ventricular system may lead to obstruction of CSF flow. More severe cases have associated intraparenchymal hematomas. Ultrasound and CT are superior to MRI in the detection of parenchymal hemorrhage in the first few days after its occurrence. After this time, MRI is the single best modality for visualization of hemorrhage and is superior at all times for the identification of subdural or epidural hemorrhage.[52–54] Magnetic resonance phase mapping techniques have been reported to improve the detection of small areas of hemorrhage in this patient population, but are not routinely used at this time.[55]

Periventricular leukomalacia[56, 57] may develop in premature infants with cardiorespiratory disturbances and less commonly in term infants with congenital heart disease. Ischemic areas develop in the watershed areas bordering the lateral ventricles, particularly around the foramen of Monro or along the course of the optic radiations. In these regions, ischemic necrosis is followed by subsequent development of gliosis. In more severe cases, loss of brain substance occurs. Radiographically, the borders of the dilated lateral ventricles demonstrate irregularity, with a rim of high signal intensity surrounding them on T2-weighted images. In more severe cases, cystic areas may be seen in the periventricular white matter (Fig 8–18).

In term infants, perinatal ischemic injury may lead to massive cerebral infarction. In the acute phase this is usually manifested as diffuse cerebral edema. Compression of the lateral ventricles may be seen, and the cerebral parenchyma may have diffuse edematous density (low signal intensity on T1-weighted images and high signal intensity on T2-weighted images) in comparison with the adjacent nonischemic cerebellum and brain stem. A case has been reported, however, in which the normal high water content of the neonatal brain apparently masked a large acute infarction that was very obviously seen on later studies.[58]

Localized lesions in the brain stem and basal ganglia may result from prenatal or perinatal asphyxia or hypoxic-ischemic encephalopathy and can be identified by imaging modalities if of large enough size. Delayed MRI studies in children with severe hypoxic ischemic episodes may show areas of gliosis in the basal ganglia regions and corticular areas. These areas of gliosis may be associated with areas of low signal intensity in the basal ganglia and/or white matter that are thought to represent areas of iron deposition. In some cases calcification may also be present.[59]

INFECTIOUS DISEASES

Congenital infectious disease entities such as herpes encephalitis and toxoplasmosis frequently have devasting results. Magnetic resonance images obtained at the time of the infection may show diffuse cerebral edema or more localized areas of involvement that demonstrate high signal intensity on T2-weighted sequences (Fig 8–19). Herpes encephalitis often involves the temporal lobe. Later sequelae such as areas of demyelination (Fig 8–20) or areas of porencephaly may be seen on images obtained some time after the initial episode.

Prior to the availability of Gd-DTPA, MRI studies were disappointing in the evaluation of children with meningitis. Recent studies using animal models have shown MRI with Gd-DTPA to be superior to CT with iodinated contrast agents in the evaluation of this disease entity.

Localized brain abscesses are easily defined using MRI and may show diffuse or ring enhancement following administration of Gd-DTPA.

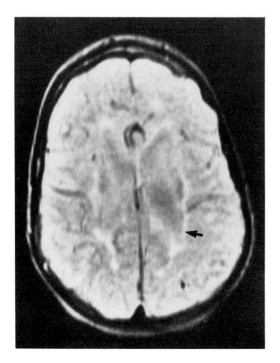

FIG 8–18.
Periventricular leukomalacia. Axial SE (2000/84). The lateral ventricles have a rim of high signal intensity and irregular borders (*arrow*).

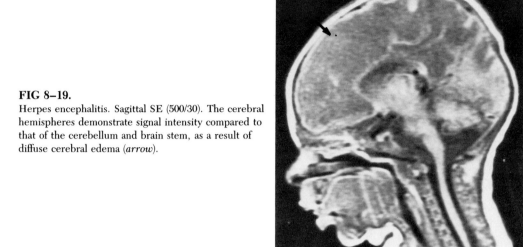

FIG 8–19.
Herpes encephalitis. Sagittal SE (500/30). The cerebral hemispheres demonstrate signal intensity compared to that of the cerebellum and brain stem, as a result of diffuse cerebral edema (*arrow*).

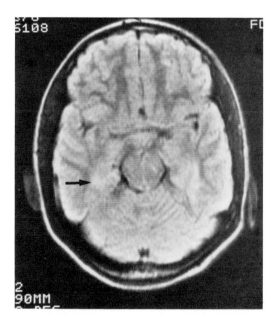

FIG 8–20.
Patient with previous episode of herpes encephalitis. Axial SE (2000/28). Areas of high signal intensity are seen in the temporal white matter bilaterally as a result of demyelination (*arrow*).

USES OF GADOLINIUM-DTPA

Although the uses of Gd-DTPA in the evaluation of the pediatric central nervous system are not yet fully evaluated, early studies have already started to define its role.[38] It is essential for radiologists to be aware of the indications for contrast agent usage in order to fully evaluate patients and to avoid unnecessary administration of the agents in this young population.

Indications for its usage have already been discussed in the appropriate sections. Table

8–2 is a summary of our indications for the use of Gd-DTPA in evaluation of the pediatric brain at the present time.

SUMMARY

In conclusion, the multiplanar imaging capabilities of MRI, together with its superior contrast differentiation, make it an ideal modality with which to screen children for possible central nervous system disease or to fully define disease already known to be present in children of all ages.

REFERENCES

1. Burckart GJ, White TJ, Siegle RI, et al: Rectal thiopental versus an intramuscular cocktail for sedating children before computed tomography. *Am J Hosp Pharm* 1980; 37:222–224.
2. McArdle CB, Nicholas DA, Richardson CJ, et al: Monitoring of the neonate undergoing MRI: Technical considerations. *Radiology* 1986; 159:223.
3. Roth JL, Nugent M, Gray JE, et al: Patient monitoring during magnetic resonance imaging. *Anesthesiology* 1985; 62:80.
4. Lufkin RB, Votruba J, Reicher M, et al: Solenoid surface coils in magnetic resonance imaging. *AJR* 1986; 146:409.
5. Edelman RR, McFarland E, Stark DD, et al: Surface coil MR imaging of abdominal viscera. I: Theory, technique, and initial results. *Radiology* 1985; 157:425.
6. Dietrich RB, Kangarloo H: Pediatric body imaging, in Stark DD, Bradley WG (eds): *Magnetic Resonance Imaging.* St Louis, CV Mosby Co, 1988, pp 1434–1453.
7. Huber DJ, Mueller E, Heubes P: Oblique magnetic resonance imaging of normal structures. *AJR* 1985; 145:843.
8. McArdle CB, Richardson CJ, Nicholas DA, et al: Developmental features of the neonatal brain. Part 1: Gray-white matter differentiation and myelination. *Radiology* 1987; 162:223–229.
9. McArdle CB, Richardson CJ, Nicholas DA, et al: Developmental features of the neonatal brain. Part II: Ventricular size and extracerebral space. *Radiology* 1987; 162:230–234.
10. Mintz MC, Grossman RI, Isaacson G, et al: MR imaging of fetal brain. *J Comp Assist Tomogr* 1987; 11:120–123.
11. Penn RD, Bernadette T, Baldwin L: Brain maturation followed by computed tomography. *J Comput Assist Tomogr* 1980; 4:614–616.
12. Dobbing J, Sands J: Quantitative growth and development of human brain. *Arch Dis Child* 1973; 48:757–767.
13. Dietrich RB, Bradley WG Jr, Zaragosa E, et al: MR evaluation of early myelination patterns in normal and developmentally delayed infants. *AJNR* 1988; 9:69–76.
14. Barkowitz AJ, Kjos BO, Jackson DE, et al: Normal infant maturation of the neonatal and infant brain: MR imaging at 1.5T. *Radiology* 1988; 166:173–181.
15. Fishman MA, Agrawal HC, Alexander A, et al: Biochemical maturation of human central nervous system myelin. *J Neurochem* 1975; 24:689–694.
16. Nowell MA, Hackney DB, Zimmerman RA, et al: Optimal pulse-sequence parameters for MR imaging of the immature brain. *Radiology* 1987; 162:272–273.
17. Holland BA, Haas DK, Norman D, et al: MRI of normal brain maturation. *AJNR* 1986; 7:201–208.
18. Johnson MA, Pennock JM, Bydder GM, et al: Clinical NMR imaging of the brain in children: Normal and neurological disease. *AJR* 1983; 141:1005–1018.
19. Dietrich RB, Bradley WG: Normal and abnormal white matter maturation. *Semin US CT and MR* 1988; 9:192–200.
20. Nowell MA, Grossman RI, Hackney DB, et al: MR imaging of white matter disease in children. *AJNR* 1988; 9:503–509.

21. Van der Knapp MS, Valk J: Classification of congenital abnormalities of the CNS. *AJNR* 1988; 9:315–325.

22. Lee BCP, Lipper E, Nass R, et al: MRI of the central nervous system in neonates and young children. *AJNR* 1986; 7:605–616.

23. Han JS, Benson JE, Kaufman B, et al: MR imaging of pediatric cerebral abnormalities. *J Comput Assist Tomogr* 1985; 9:121.

24. Pennock JM, Bydder GM, Dubowitz LMS, et al: Magnetic resonance imaging of the brain in children. *Magn Reson Imaging* 1986; 4:1–9.

25. Fritz CR: Holoprosencephaly and related entities. *Neuroradiology* 1983; 25:225–238.

26. O'Dwyer AJ, Newton TH, Hoyt WF: Radiologic features of septooptic dysplasia de Morsier syndrome. *AJNR* 1980; 1:443–447.

27. Zimmerman R, Bilaniuk L, Grossman R: Computed tomography in migratory disorders of human brain development. *Neuroradiology* 1983; 25:257–263.

28. Zimmerman R, Bilaniuk L: Pediatric central nervous system, in Stark DD, Bradley WG (eds): *Magnetic Resonance Imaging.* St Louis, CV Mosby Co, 1988, pp 683–715.

29. Barkovich AJ, Chuang SH, Norman D: MR of neuronal migration anomalies. *AJNR* 1987; 8:1009–1017.

30. Barkovich AJ, Norman D: MR imaging of schizencephaly. *AJNR* 1988; 9:297–302.

31. Bairamian D, Di Chiro G, Theodore WH, et al: MR imaging and positron emission tomography of cortical heterotopia. *J Comput Assist Tomogr* 9:1137–1139.

32. Deeb ZL, Rothfus WE, Maroon JC: Case report. MR imaging of heterotopic gray matter. *J Comput Assist Tomogr* 1985; 9:1140–1141.

33. Davidson HD, Abraham R, Steiner RE: Agenesis of the corpus callosum. Magnetic resonance imaging. *Radiology* 1985; 155:371–373.

34. Atlas SW, Zimmerman RA, Bilaniuk LT, et al: Corpus callosum and limbic system: Neuroanatomic MR evaluation of developmental anomalies. *Radiology* 1986; 160:355–362.

35. Kendall BE: Dysgenesis of the corpus callosum. *Neuroradiology* 1983; 25:239–256.

36. Peterman SB, Steiner RE, Bydder GM: Magnetic resonance imaging of intracranial tumors in children and adolescents. *AJNR* 1984; 5:703–709.

37. Kalifa G, Chiron C, Sellier N, et al: Hemimegalencephaly: MR imaging in five children. *Radiology* 1987; 165:29–33.

38. Dietrich RB, Crim J, King W, et al: When is Gd-DTPA essential in the evaluation of the pediatric brain? *Radiology* 1988; 169(p):268.

39. McMurdo SK Jr, Moore SG, Brant-Zawadzki M, et al: MR imaging of intracranial tuberous sclerosis. *AJR* 1987; 148:791–796.

40. Roach ES, Williams DP, Laster DW: Magnetic resonance imaging in tuberous sclerosis. *Arch Neurol* 1987; 44:301–303.

41. Vaghi M, Visciani A, Testa D, et al: Cerebral MR findings in tuberous sclerosis. *J Comput Assist Tomogr* 1987; 11:403–406.

42. Kortman K, Bradley WG: Supratentorial neoplasms, in Stark DD, Bradley WG (eds): *Magnetic Resonance Imaging.* St Louis, CV Mosby Co, 1988, pp 375–413.

43. Braffman BH, Bilaniuk LT, Zimmerman RA: The central nervous system manifestations of the phakomatoses on MR. *Radiol Clin North Am* 1988; 26:773–800.

44. Jacoby CJ, Yuh WC, Afifi AK, et al: Accelerated myelination in early Sturge-Weber syndrome demonstrated by MR imaging. *J Comput Assist Tomogr* 1987; 11:226–231.

45. Barnes PD, Lester PD, Yamanashi WS, et al: MRI in infants and children with spinal dysraphism. *AJR* 1986; 147:339–346.

46. Walker HS, Dietrich RB, Flannigan BD, et al: Magnetic resonance imaging of the pediatric spine. *RadioGraphics* 1987; 7:1129–1152.

47. Han JS, Benson JE, Kaufman B, et al: Demonstration of diastematomyelia and associated abnormalities with MR imaging. *AJNR* 1985; 6:215–219.

48. Davis CD, Friedman NC, Fry SM: Leptomeningeal metastasis: MR imaging. *Radiology* 1987; 163:449–454.

49. Kucharczyk W, Brant-Zawadzki M, Sobel D, et al: Central nervous system tumors in children: Detection by magnetic resonance imaging. *Radiology* 1985; 155:131–136.
50. Volpe JJ: *Neurology of the Newborn,* ed 2. Philadelphia, WB Saunders Co, 1987, pp 311–361.
51. Johnson MA, Pennock JM, Bydder GM, et al: Serial MR imaging in neonatal cerebral injury. *AJNR* 1987; 8:83–92.
52. Gomori JM, Grossman RI, Goldberg HI, et al: High-field spin-echo MR imaging of superficial and subependymal siderosis secondary to neonatal intraventricular hemorrhage. *Neuroradiology* 1987; 29:339–342.
53. McArdle CB, Richardson CJ, Mayder CK, et al: Abnormalities of the neonatal brain. Part 1: Intracranial hemorrhage. *Radiology* 1987; 163:387–395.
54. Pennock JM, Bydder GM, de Vries LS, et al: MRI of intracranial hemorrhage in neonates. Book of Abstracts, Society of Magnetic Resonance in Medicine. Sixth Annual Meeting, New York, August 1987, p 73.
55. Young IR, Khenia S, Thomas DGT, et al: Clinical magnetic susceptibility mapping of the brain. *J Comput Assist Tomogr* 1987; 11:2–6.
56. Wilson DA, Steiner RE: Periventricular leukomalacia: Evaluation with MR imaging. *Radiology* 1986; 160:507–511.
57. De Reuck J, Chatha AS, Richardson EP: Pathogenesis and evolution of periventricular leukomalacia in infancy. *Arch Neurol* 1972; 27:220–236
58. Moore JB, Parker CP, Smith RJ, et al: Concealment of neonatal cerebral infarction on MRI by normal brain water. *Pediatr Radiol* 1987; 17:314–315.
59. Dietrich RB, Bradley WG: Iron accumulation in the basal ganglia following severe ischemic-anoxic insults in children. *Radiology* 1988; 168:203–206.

Magnetic Resonance Imaging of the Head and Neck

Robert B. Lufkin, M.D.

William N. Hanafee, M.D.

Magnetic resonance imaging (MRI) has revolutionized radiographic depiction of the head and neck and has replaced computed tomography (CT) as the study of choice for many lesions of the extracranial head and neck. The notable exceptions in which CT is still essential are inflammatory and congenital lesions of the temporal bone, osteomas of the sinuses, and a few other specific disease entities. Magnetic resonance imaging easily surpasses CT in its ability to reveal subtle differences in soft tissue boundaries and extensions of tumors of the head and neck. The beam hardening artifacts on CT images from dental amalgam and from the dense cortical bone of the mandible, skull base, shoulders, and other areas are also not a problem with MRI. Multiplanar imaging capabilities and lack of ionizing radiation make MRI the preferred imaging study for many head and neck processes that in the past would have required CT scanning.

The role of any imaging modality in most head and neck cancers is to identify deep infiltration of tumors. Mucosal changes are for the most part best evaluated by direct inspection during physical examination. Physiologic studies of motion, fixation, and so forth are beyond the capability of present-day MRI techniques, but blood flow and vascularity determinations can be performed with MRI, eliminating the need of many invasive angiographic procedures.

Probably no where else in the body do anatomic boundaries provide such important clues to the cause of a disease process as in the head and neck. Even when the exact nature of the offending process cannot be determined, disruptions of facial planes and muscle interfaces help to define surgical or radiation therapy management of the patient.

TECHNIQUE

Surface coils greatly increase the signal-to-noise ratio and allow higher spatial resolution of most MRI examinations of the area. While acceptable studies of the sinuses, nasopharynx,

TABLE 9–1.

Protocols* for Magnetic Resonance Imaging of the Head and Neck

Larynx, hypopharynx (performed with neck coil)

Axial	SE 800/30
Axial	SE 2000/84
Coronal	SE 600/30
Sagittal	SE 300/30

Tongue, oropharynx

Axial	SE 800/30
Axial	SE 2000/84
Coronal	SE 600/30

Paranasal sinuses

Axial	SE 800/30
Coronal	SE 600/30
Axial	SE 2000/84

Nasopharynx

Axial	SE 800/30
Coronal	SE 500/30
Sagittal	SE 500/30
Axial	SE 2000/84

Parotid gland

Axial	SE 500/30
Coronal	SE 500/30
Sagittal	SE 500/30
Axial	SE 2000/84

Temporal bone

Axial	SE 500/30
Axial	SE 2000/84

*Gradient moment nulling motion compensation is added to all T2-weighted sequences. On high-field instruments, cardiac gating may be necessary to diminish flow and motion artifacts in some cases. SE = spin echo.

and oropharynx, may be obtained with the standard head coil, the use of surface coils for examination of the larynx and hypopharynx is practically essential.[1]

While specialized surface radio frequency (RF) coils are important factors that make quality MR images of the head and neck possible, perhaps the most significant factors in the superiority of MR over CT scanning in this area is the superior soft tissue contrast resolution of MRI. By changing the pulse sequence parameters [repetition time (TR), echo time (TE), and flip angle (Theta)], MR image contrast can be manipulated in many ways not possible with CT scanning. Unlike the central nervous system, in which virtually no MR signal from fat is present, the abundance of fat-water interfaces in the extracranial head and neck, which literally defines the anatomy of this region, greatly influences the selection of pulse sequences of optimum image contrast.

The high signal levels available on T1-weighted images permit anatomic details to be detected that are often not seen on CT scans. This improved contrast resolution, plus the availability of easy coronal, sagittal, and oblique viewing, greatly enhances the information obtained by axial scanning. The vast majority of head and neck imaging is performed with T1-weighted pulsing sequences. T2-weighted pulsing sequences are used when more information is required regarding tumor infiltration into muscle, fluid collections, and obstructed sinuses (Table 9–I).

The use of CT-guided aspiration cytology studies of deep or clinically occult lesions has improved the work-up of many patients with head and neck tumors. Aspiration cytology is now possible with MRI guidance using specially developed MR-compatible needles (E-Z-EM Corp., Westbury, N.Y.).[2-4]

The role of gadolinium-DTPA (diethylenetriaminepentaacetic acid) in MRI examinations of the head and neck is currently under investigation.[5] Preliminary studies show that although tumor enhancement occurs, little clinically relevant information is added in many cases. When intracranial extension is present, however, the gadolinium can improve the detection of blood-brain barrier and leptomeningeal abnormalities.

TEMPORAL BONE

The technique of MRI of the temporal bone varies greatly depending on the type of MR instrument used and availability of surface coils. For individuals with unilateral disease or symptoms, planar surface coils are very useful (Fig 9–1). For poorly localized, bilateral, or central disease, the limited sensitivity of planar surface coils is unacceptable, and bilateral coils must be used.

For most studies, T1-weighted pulse sequences are used. These maximize contrast at dural-cerebrospinal fluid interfaces as well as showing other anatomy with generally high signal-to-noise. More T2-weighted images are used in limited situations to confirm findings on T1 sequences and to evaluate cystic areas or edema.

High-resolution technique is critically important, and submillimeter pixel resolution is practically mandatory. In instruments that cannot produce contiguous slices, it is necessary to reimage with interleaving to avoid missing small acoustic neuromas. Gadolinium-DTPA may also help in the detection of small tumors.

The axial plane is used so that both internal auditory canals can be followed in the same plane of section. Coronal and sagittal examinations are useful in certain cases such as following the entire course of the facial nerve through the temporal bone.[6, 7]

Abnormalities affecting the temporal bone often result in symptoms that fall into three main groups:

1. Lesions resulting in sensorineural hearing loss; these frequently involve the eighth nerve, cochlea, and vestibular apparatus.

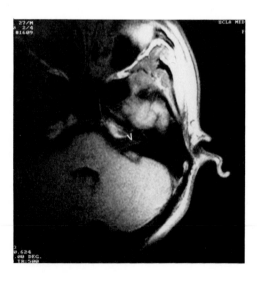

FIG 9–1.
Axial surface coil MR image (SE 500/30) of the normal temporal bone. The individual nerves are visible in the internal auditory canal (*arrowhead*). The variation in signal intensity is the result of RF nonuniformity of the surface coil.

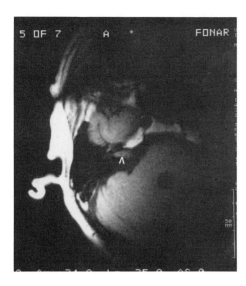

FIG 9–2.
Axial T1-weighted image (SE 500/30) in a patient with sensorineural hearing loss shows a small intracanicular acoustic neuroma (*arrowhead*).

2. Lesions resulting in conductive hearing loss frequently related to the middle ear, tympanic membrane, and external auditory canal. With some inflammatory diseases and their complications, however, the vestibular system may be secondarily involved.

3. Miscellaneous inflammatory processes and tumors affecting the temporal bone but not primarily affecting hearing.

Magnetic resonance imaging is the modality of choice in evaluations of sensorineural hearing loss and to a large extent in evaluating the facial nerve in its course through the petrous temporal bone. Surface coil thin-section MRI now reliably enables one to detect even intracanalicular acoustic tumors without the need for gas CT cisternography (Fig 9–2). Acoustic neuromas, by far the most common neoplasm of the cerebellopontine (CP) angle, account for over 80% of all CP angle tumors; meningiomas and primary cholesteatomas (epidermoids) are much less common .MRI now replaces CT scanning as the imaging study of choice for evaluating all three lesions.

Computed tomography remains the imaging study of choice at present for identifying inflammatory disease and conditions resulting in conductive hearing loss. Important information about the status of the ossicles and bony covering of the facial nerve canal is still best obtained with CT. It can also best visualize tumors and metabolic diseases affecting the middle ear and mastoid air cells. For the remainder of lesions of the temporal bone, CT and MRI will continue to play complementary roles in the imaging work-up. Depending on the location and particular abnormality, each of the imaging modalities will contribute information.

SALIVARY GLANDS

The preferred method of imaging the salivary glands has evolved with new developments in imaging technology as well as clinical needs. While intraductal contrast plain film sialography is still used to evaluate inflammatory lesions of the salivary glands, early CT scanners quickly replaced plain radiography for evaluation of masses. As CT technology improved spatial resolution, intravenous contrast material replaced intraductal contrast for the CT sialogram evaluation of salivary gland masses. Now, MRI has replaced CT scanning for the imaging evaluation of the majority of masses in the major salivary glands.[8–13]

The approach to the study of masses in this area has been to use surface coils whenever possible and to obtain T1-weighted images in the axial plane. These views are supplemented with coronal or sagittal views when there is suggestion of temporal bone involvement. Complex, cystic, or unusual lesions are also evaluated with additional T2-weighted sequences when necessary.

Because 80% of major salivary gland tumors occur in the parotid gland, we will focus our attention on this particular region. The three main clinical goals for examining parotid masses are:

1. Differentiation between benign and malignant tumors.
2. Differentiation between extrinsic parapharyngeal space masses presenting as a parotid mass and actual intrinsic parotid masses.
3. Definition of the relationship of the facial nerve to the parotid tumor. Is the tumor superficial, deep, or combined?

The policy at the University of California, Los Angeles, is to perform fine-needle aspiration cytology on most tumors. This means that the first two goals are often achieved for superficially located tumors with a combination of clinical palpation and cytologic study in the clinic before any imaging studies are requested.

Magnetic resonance imaging can only rarely suggest the histologic character of tumors—such as lipomas, by their characteristic fat appearance, or the possibility of a Warthin's tumor in multilobulated cystic masses of the parotid gland. In the majority of cases, MRI is not any more accurate than CT in predicting the histologic nature of parotid lesions. This is in part due to the unusual histology of salivary gland tumors.

Therefore, the value of MRI in most cases, like that of CT, is to define the gross morphologic characteristics of the tumor outline. Although poor tumor margination may be a clue to malignancy, it is certainly not a reliable finding in MRI (or CT) studies. Deep parapharyngeal space involvement may be demonstrated with CT; however, MRI provides much better soft tissue contrast resolution. The real advantage of MRI in evaluating parotid masses is its ability to more accurately define the extent of the masses, to localize the tumor as extraparotid or intraparotid, and to determine whether the intraparotid tumor is superficial or deep (Figs 9–3 and 9–4).

With CT, only a rough estimate of the relationship of the parotid tumor to the facial nerve can be made. This as well as other imaging techniques prior to MRI has failed to accomplish imaging of the intraparotid facial nerve. T1-weighted MR images acquired with the use of surface coils can be used to demonstrate the major trunk of the facial nerve as it enters the parotid gland. On axial images the facial nerve can be seen as a structure of slightly lower signal intensity lying within the high signal of the fat surrounding the stylomastoid foramen. Its course from the stylomastoid foramen passing laterally to the retromandibular vein is characteristic. Coronal images are sometimes useful in determining the distance of the parotid mass from the stylomastoid foramen.

The relationship of the parotid tumors to the facial nerve, which courses through and divides within the parotid gland, is of obvious value in planning the surgical approach and in more thoroughly appreciating the potential morbidity of operation preoperatively. Malignant tumors in close relation to the facial nerve may require excision of part of that structure and subsequent microsurgical repair or transposition of the facial nerve. Access to larger deeper lesions may require division and reflection of the ramus of the mandible.

PARANASAL SINUSES

At first glance it would appear that MRI would not be suitable for examination of the paranasal sinuses. Because cortical bone and air do not return a signal on MRI, one might assume that CT or other x-ray procedures would be needed to adequately visualize the sinus walls. Actually, most diseases affecting the paranasal sinuses are primarily soft tissue abnormalities of the lining of these cavities rather than of the bones themselves.

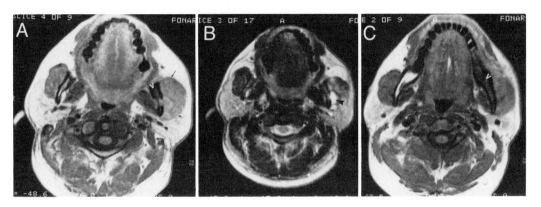

FIG 9–3.
Masticator space infection presenting as a parotid mass. Sialogram and repeat fine-needle aspiration of the parotid gland revealed only inflammatory cells. **A**, axial T1-weighted image (SE 587/30) through the ramus of the mandible reveals swelling of the left masseter muscle (*arrows*) with bony destruction of the mandible and replacement of normal high signal marrow with lower signal (*arrowhead*). **B**, T2-weighted image (SE 3000/85) at the same level reveals similar changes plus a focal area of high signal intensity (*arrowhead*) consistent with fluid collection. **C**, axial T1-weighted images (SE 587/30) through the angle of the mandible again reveals soft tissue changes as well as diffuse marrow replacement on the side of the abnormality (*arrowhead*).

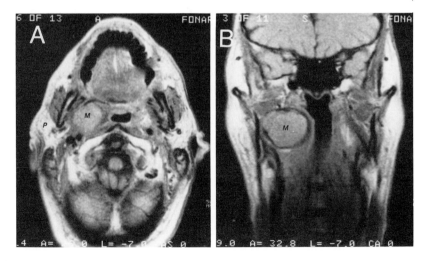

FIG 9–4.
Recurrent adenocarcinoma of the parapharyngeal space. Both sequences are T1 weighted (SE 800/30). **A**, axial view through the level of the palate reveals a soft tissue mass arising in the right parapharyngeal space (*M*) which distorts the pharyngeal airway, but does not invade it. The parotid gland (*P*) is unremarkable. **B**, coronal view also shows the relationships of the mass (*M*) to the adjacent displaced pharyngeal wall and surrounding parapharyngeal space structures.

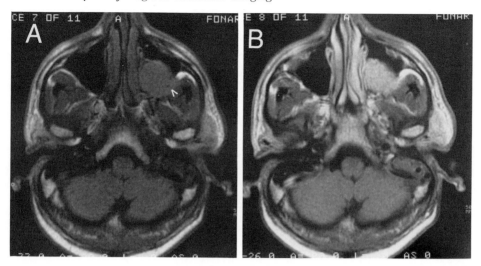

FIG 9–5.
Squamous cell carcinoma of the maxillary sinus in a 41-year-old man. **A,** pregadolinium T1-weighted image (SE 600/20) shows the mass in the maxillary sinus with erosion of the posterior sinus wall (*arrowhead*). **B,** following gadolinium administration, the image shows mild increased signal intensity of the tumor.

Changes in the bony walls of the sinuses are generally secondary manifestations of the mucosal disease. As a matter of fact, the sclerotic thickened margins of the sinuses interfere with visualization of mucosa. If bone destruction is present, it is usually a late manifestation of malignant disease of the mucosa. Deformed and displaced bony septa may contribute to or be the result of disease. In this situation MRI is actually an excellent imaging modality because the bony septa are lined by mucosa, which gives a high signal. The bony septum can be visualized as a negative shadow, that is, a lower signal between the layers of high-signal soft tissue.

It is therefore not surprising that MRI is extremely valuable in evaluating masses of the paranasal sinuses. It allows excellent delineation of solid tissue masses surrounded by secretions within the paranasal sinuses. Erosions of the bony walls are also well demonstrated as the absence of signal void normally present in cortical bone (Fig 9–5). For extensions outside the bony sinuses, MRI is the clear study of choice because it differentiates skeletal muscle from tumor extension, which can be difficult on CT studies (Fig 9–6). In cases where there is a question of extension to the anterior or middle cranial fossa, MRI with gadolinium enhancement remains the study of choice.

Magnetic resonance imaging is also valuable in repeated follow-up studies of diseases in children, such as juvenile angiofibroma, in which multiple studies are required and radiation dose becomes a factor. The flow sensitivity of MRI is also important in imaging these vascular lesions and may provide more information than CT scanning.

The high soft tissue contrast capabilities of MRI in distinguishing low-protein fluids, high-protein fluids, soft tissues, and normal musculature make it ideal for display of benign and malignant paranasal sinus disease. Frequently the very ill patient is just the individual who requires coronal or sagittal projections that are difficult or impossible to obtain with most CT equipment.

While the mainstay for imaging inflammatory paranasal sinus disease will continue to be plain radiographs because of their relative low cost, MRI can now be substituted for CT scanning to evaluate advanced lesions of this type in most cases. With continued development

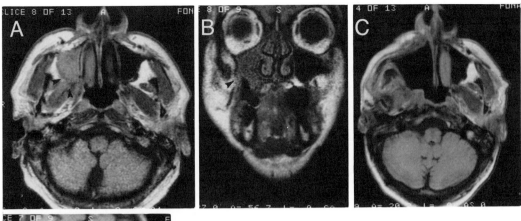

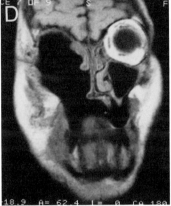

FIG 9–6.
Squamous cell carcinoma of the maxillary sinus. All images are T1 weighted (SE 800–500/30). **A,** axial view through the midantrum shows opacification with bony destruction posteriorly through the pterygoid plates invading the adjacent muscle (*arrowhead*). **B,** coronal view confirms this information and additionally shows involvement of the orbital floor and destruction of lateral maxillary sinus wall (*arrowhead*). **C,** axial view following total resection shows satisfactory removal of the mass. **D,** coronal view also confirms successful gross total removal.

of faster, lower cost MR instrument, it is not impossible that MRI will eventually replace even plain radiography for the evaluation of this area.

NASOPHARYNX

The lack of motion and abundant facial planes of the nasopharynx result in high-quality MRI studies.[14, 15] Retropharyngeal adenopathy, tumor infiltration beyond the pharyngobasilar fascia, and hypertrophic lymphoid tissue are all identified with greater ease on MR images than on CT scans (Fig 9–7).[16] T1-weighted images are usually adequate for examining the nasopharynx because of the abundance of loose areolar tissue between various muscle groups and bundles. Tumors with inflammatory changes can be identified as low-signal regions in these loose areolar planes.

Usually seven axial slices will adequately cover the area from the soft palate up to the skull base and the floor of the middle cranial fossa. An additional seven coronal views may be helpful in giving better coverage of the posteriorly located nodal changes following the jugular vein.

If sagittal projections are obtained, at least seven slices should be acquired so that the lateral extremities of the cavernous sinuses and the foramen lacerum regions can be completely examined. If a patient has symptoms of cranial nerve IX, X, XI or XII involvement, slices in addition to the 7 already acquired will be needed for an adequate evaluation of these more peripheral regions.

In particular, the direct coronal and sagittal MR images are valuable in assessing craniocaudal extension of tumor with skull base involvement. While CT scanning is unquestionably more accurate in detecting small amounts of calcification per se, the MRI examination is adequate to evaluate skull base invasion. Abnormalities of the skull base are detected by replacement of the normal low-signal cortical bone with higher signal neoplasm. Its capability of multiplanar imaging and far superior soft tissue resolution make MRI the clear imaging study of choice in evaluation of the nasopharynx.

The configuration of the nasopharynx is dominated by a very tough fascial membrane called the pharyngobasilar fascia. This tough fascia represents a continuation of a pharyngeal constrictor muscles and extends from the level of the soft palate to the base of the skull. Its function is to maintain the airway as an open channel for breathing during normal activities and during chewing. During the act of swallowing, the soft palate obliterates the lumen produced by the pharyngobasilar fascia.

The pharyngobasilar fascia is pierced anteriorly by the eustachian tube. The eustachian tube, passing from the middle ear cavity, communicates with the nasopharynx through an opening just behind the anterior attachment of the pharyngobasilar fascia to the medial pterygoid plate. Only malignant tumors and very aggressive inflammatory processes such as those caused by *Mucor* will pass from the mucosa of the nasopharynx through the pharyngobasilar fascia to involve the structures within the paranasopharyngeal space. The first anatomic structure to become involved in usually the tensor veli palatini muscle which lies immediately lateral to the medial pterygoid plate and takes its origin from the skull base.

The tensor veli palatini muscle is enveloped in a fascial plane of its own that divides the paranasopharyngeal space into two compartments.[17] The tensor veli palatini muscle fascia passes posterior to the styloid process and divides the space into a lateral compartment (which is spoken of as the prestyloid space) and a medial compartment (which is spoken of as a poststyloid space). This terminology comes from the surgical approaches because the surgeons encounter the more lateral space as they come in from the side and, hence, see this space before the styloid process. The more medially placed space is visualized after the styloid

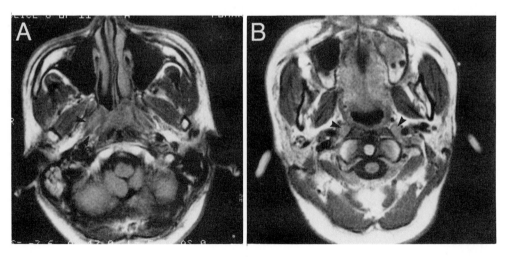

FIG 9–7.
Nasopharyngeal squamous cell carcinoma. **A,** axial view (SE 700/30) through the nasopharynx reveals a mass with obliteration of the surrounding fascial planes and crossing of the pharyngobasilar fascia (*arrowhead*). **B,** axial section with the same parameters obtained through the level of Passavant's muscle shows no evidence of primary tumor; however, large bilateral retropharyngeal lymph nodes (*arrowheads*) are present.

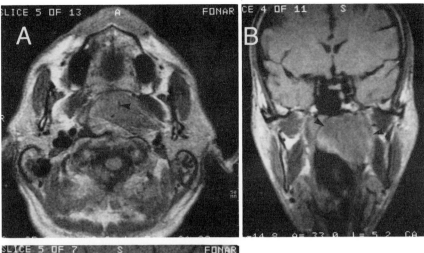

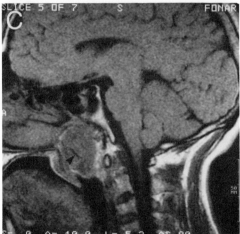

FIG 9–8.
Hamartomatous angiomyolipoma of the nasopharynx.
All images are T1 weighted (SE 800–400/30). **A**, axial
view through the level through the hard palate shows
a soft tissue mass filling the pharynx, with small
curvilinear areas of low signal intensity centrally
(*arrowhead*). **B**, coronal view again shows the mass
(*arrowheads*). Note there is no invasion of skull base.
C, sagittal view shows the mass filling the nasopharynx
and extending downward into the superior oropharynx.
Again note linear low-signal structures (*arrowhead*)
(consistent with high flow in vessels).

process has been seen; hence, it is the poststyloid space. This poststyloid space communicates anteriorly between the pharyngobasilar fascia and the tensor veli palatini fascia; posteriorly it goes back to the carotid artery. In the more lateral compartment (prestyloid compartment) lies the deep lobe of the parotid gland. The amount of parotid tissue in the region between the tensor veli palatini muscle fascia and the fascia covering the medial pterygoid muscle is quite variable. These two fascial planes generally fuse just before their attachment to the base of the skull. Their skull base attachment is immediately medial to the foramen ovale.

The nasopharynx remains an area that is obscure to casual clinical examination. Its proximity to the skull base makes cancers in this region particularly devastating. Most malignancies of the nasopharynx are squamous cell carcinomas with varying degrees of differentiation. The tumors may affect all age groups including children and teenagers. Plasmocytomas, lymphocytomas, and occasionally rhabdomyosarcomas are also encountered (Fig 9–8). These tumors tend to be bulkier and infiltrate more widely than squamous cell carcinoma.

The presenting symptoms of nasopharyngeal carcinoma vary widely. The most common complaints of patients presenting with nasopharyngeal tumors are nasal obstruction, local invasion of cranial nerves, serous otitis media, and cervical lymph node metastases (Fig 9–

9).[18] In general, patients fall into two main categories for nasopharyngeal MRI examination:

1. To delineate the extent of a known malignancy.
2. To search for the presence of the tumor to explain symptoms or clinical findings.

Clinical examination may be extremely difficult as a result of the gag reflex or poor patient cooperation. Visualization of the vault of the nasopharynx and regions surrounding the eustachian tube can be difficult under the best of circumstances. Prominent, chronically inflamed adenoidal tissue may obscure much of the nasopharynx even if the structure is reasonably accessible to inspection. Nasopharyngeal tumors have a tendency to infiltrate beneath the mucosa and extend over the wide areas with little superficial evidence of their presence. This is especially true in recurrent disease following therapy, where the mucosa can return to relatively normal status but where deep infiltrations persist. Magnetic resonance imaging is particularly well suited to compliment the clinical examination in this situation.

UNKNOWN PRIMARY

The patient presenting with the solitary enlarged cervical lymph node presents one of the most interesting challenges in head and neck diagnosis. This is the so-called unknown primary when only the metastasis to the node is clinically evident. Sound surgical principles dictate that the primary tumor should be managed at the same setting as the metastasis. Statistics suggest that failure to follow this principle leads to a logarithmic jump in postoperative complications and treatment failures.

Unfortunately there are no clear-cut signal changes on MRI to indicate malignant adenopathy. The morphologic size criteria used in CT may also be applied to MRI (Fig 9–10).[19–22] Under no circumstances should an open biopsy of the lymph node be performed until all areas of the head and neck have been ruled out as a source of the primary tumor.[23] Since the nasopharynx presents such a difficult area to examine clinically, MRI performs a vital task in showing the presence or absence of a deeply infiltrating tumor.

FIG 9–9.
Diagnosis by MRI guided aspiration cytology of recurrent squamous carcinoma of the parapharyngeal space extending to the skull base. **A,** coronal image (SE 700/30) shows a mass in the high infratemporal fossa (*arrow*). **B,** follow-up fast gradient-echo image after needle placement. Although image quality is diminished with rapid scanning techniques (SE 173/10/60° flip angle), the needle is well visualized (*arrow*), and imaging time is reduced to 48 seconds.

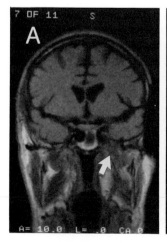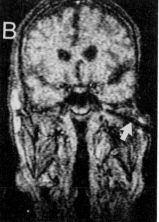

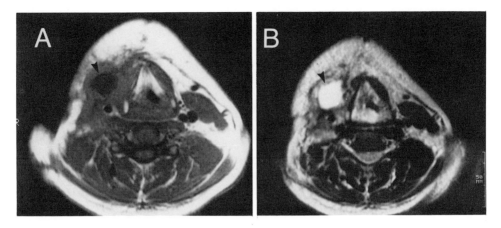

FIG 9–10.
Recurrent squamous cell carcinoma of the neck. Adenopathy with central necrosis and extracapsular extension is seen following partial glossectomy and radical neck dissection. **A,** axial T1-weighted image (SE 649/22) reveals a soft tissue mass lateral to the thyroid cartilage, with obliteration of fascial planes and low-intensity center (*arrowhead*). The sternocleidomastoid muscle and jugular vein are absent following radical neck dissection. **B,** axial T2-weighted image at the same level (SE 2000/85) reveals high signal intensity within the mass, again confirming central necrosis (*arrowhead*).

TONGUE AND OROPHARYNX

Because the information that MRI now provides regarding the tongue and oropharynx is superior to that possible with CT, it is considered the study of choice to evaluate masses in these areas.[24, 25] The tongue is one area in the head and neck for which T2-weighted pulse sequences are extremely valuable. The musculature of the tongue is of low signal on both T1- and T2-weighted images. Tumors produce a very similar signal on T1-weighted images. By prolonging the study to obtain late echoes, the tumors with longer T2 relaxation times give an increased signal relative to the tongue musculature. For this reason we use axial scanning with T2 weighting to obtain image slices from the tongue and soft palate region to a level below the inferior pole of the tonsil to include the pre-epiglottic space of the larynx.

Anatomic details of the midline are best obtained by coronal T1-weighted images. The T1 weighting allows us to survey lymph nodes in the loose areolar tissue surrounding the jugular vein and digastric tendons. This fibrofatty tissue gives a very bright signal on both T1- and T2-weighted images. On T1-weighted images the tumor will stand out as a low-signal structure. On T2-weighted images the tumor increases in signal and becomes difficult to distinguish from the areolar tissue, carotid artery, and jugular vein.

Squamous cell carcinomas account for well over 90% of the malignancies of the tongue.[26] The remaining lesions are lymphomas, leukemic infiltrations, rhabdomyosarcomas, and an assortment of benign tumors and inflammatory processes. Their behavior is largely governed by the location in lymphatic drainage.

Squamous cell carcinomas of the tongue, tonsillar bed, and posterior pharyngeal wall are the lesions most likely to require radiologic imaging. Occasionally an infiltrating tumor of the hard palate may have spread to the nasopharynx, so that additional imaging is needed prior to surgical management. Adenoid cystic carcinomas almost invariably extend along perineural lymphatics, so that some type of imaging can at times be helpful. Unfortunately, as the most central spread of these tumors is microscopic in nature, it cannot be detected reliably by present imaging methods. The remaining anterior lesions of the cheek, retromolar trigone, alveolar ridge, and lips are readily visible by inspection or available to the palpating finger, and imaging studies are seldom necessary.

Tongue and tonsillar fossa tumors can be considered together because the anatomic structures to be visualized are all seen on the same projections. Frequently, the exact site of origin of a lesion cannot be determined and will involve both regions. Posterior pharyngeal wall tumors are quite rare. They infiltrate locally and extend to the retropharyngeal lymphatics and jugular nodes. The primary tumors are easily seen by clinical examination, but at times their extensions may be obscure. Their nodal spreads constitute the principal indication for radiologic investigation. When the nodes show extracapsular spread to adjacent structures, prognosis worsens markedly. Tumor *totally* surrounding the carotid artery is generally considered a contraindication to surgery. A case is not called inoperable if only one side of a carotid artery is involved because the surgeon may be able to find a plane of dissection.

Two anatomic regions need defining in order to plan surgical management. These are (1) the neurovascular bundles that are intimately involved with the muscles comprising the lateral border of the tongue, and (2) the midline fibrous septum that separates the two lateral halves of the tongue. Integrity of these structures is necessary for the surgeon performing a hemiglossectomy. At least one hypoglossal nerve and one lingual artery must be retained. A total glossectomy is a much more involved procedure for selected patients (discussed later) and ideally requires specialized preoperative planning.

Axial sections with T2 weighting will show whether the tumor has spread from the anterior and middle thirds of the tongue into the base (Figs 9–11 and 9–12). The relationship of the tumor to the lingual artery and nerve is easily visible because these lie in intimate relationship to the interdigitation of the styloglossus and hyoglossus muscle. Here the base of the fibrous septum becomes deficient, and tumors have easy access to spreading across to the opposite side. Disruption of fascial planes of the diaphragm of the floor of the mouth (the mylohyoid muscle) in a bilateral fashion clearly indicates a far advanced tumor.

Tumors in the anterior third of the tongue and floor of mouth are readily available to inspection and palpation and seldom require imaging studies. Tumors of the middle third of the tongue, like those of the anterior third, tend to have unilateral nodal drainage. Their incidence of metastases at the time of patient admission is slightly higher than for the anterior tongue because they are usually discovered late. The intimate association of the lateral portion of the tongue with the glossopalatinus muscle and glossopharyngeal sulcus means that these tumors have ready access to the tonsillar beds by direct extension. Frequently it is impossible to state whether the tumor originated in the tongue, the glossopharyngeal sulcus, or the tonsillar bed.

Carcinomas of the posterior third of the tongue are particularly troublesome. Because of their inaccessibility, they are usually not discovered until relatively late. Seventy-six percent of the tumors are reported to include metastases at the time of initial examination. Nodal disease is frequently bilateral because of the bilateral drainage of the posterior third of the tongue.

Approximately 25% of the patients with tongue cancers who present for MRI studies because of nodal disease have tumors in the posterior third of the tongue not visible or palpable by clinical examination. Tumors of the base of the tongue have a propensity to spread laterally into the glossopharyngeal sulcus and tonsillar bed regions and anteriorly into the vallecula and pre-epiglottic space. Therefore MRI investigations of the tongue and oropharynx fall into three categories:

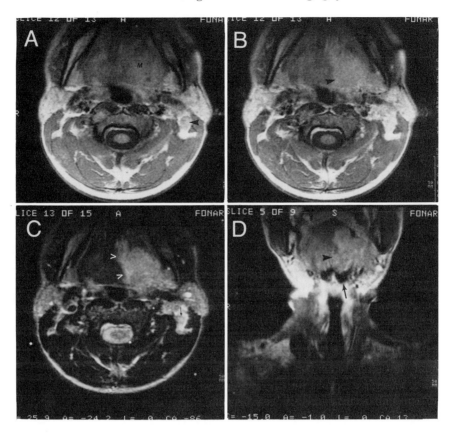

FIG 9–11.
Squamous carcinoma of the tongue base; MRI studies with and without gadolinium. **A**, axial T1-weighted image (SE 800/30) through the high tongue base reveals mass effect on the left (*M*) and associated adenopathy (*arrowhead*). **B**, similar level and pulse sequence following administration of gadolinium-DPTA reveals mild enhancement of the tongue base mass (*arrowheads*) with slightly decreased visualization of the lymph node. **C**, T2-weighted image (SE 2000/85) without gadolinium reveals high signal in the tongue base mass (*arrowheads*) and also increased signal in the region of the adenopathy (*arrow*) similar to that seen with gadolinium on the T1-weighted images. **D**, the coronal T1-weighted image is useful for defining the extent of the mass (*arrowhead*) and showing that is no extension to the supraglottic larynx. The vallecula is free of tumor (*arrow*).

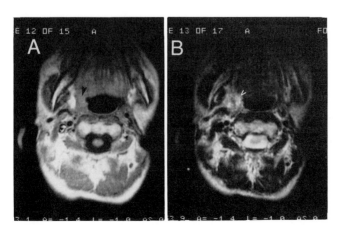

FIG 9–12.
Recurrent squamous carcinoma of the right tonsil. **A**, axial T1-weighted image (SE 649/22) reveals postsurgical changes in the left neck as well as right-sided tonsillar fullness (*arrowhead*). **B**, T2-weighted image (SE 2300/85) at the same level reveals an increased signal in the region of the tonsil (*arrowhead*) consistent with recurrent tumor, although edema or postbiopsy changes could appear the same.

1. Patients with known cancers in whom we wish to delineate the extent of the tumor and nodal metastases.

2. Patients presenting with atypical pain syndromes or nodal disease in whom we are searching for the primary tumor.

3. Patients with evidence of recurrent disease following treatment.

Many surgeons feel that total glossectomy is an option in only selected patients because the patient is left unable to swallow or manage secretions following total glossectomy. Laryngectomy is usually also required as part of this procedure, leaving the individual without a natural voice.

Therefore, limited conservational surgical resections of the tongue are performed when possible which require the preservation of one lingual artery and one hypoglossal nerve. These hemiglossectomies are only possible when the tumor has not crossed the midline or only minimally extends to the opposite side. Since most cancers of the tongue and floor of the mouth tend to extend along vascular pathways, this limitation proves crucial in many instances. Studies with MRI are thus directed to the tumor mass, its extent, and to the integrity of the midline.

In general, because MRI produces soft tissue detail regarding tongue and oropharynx that is superior to that of CT, MRI is considered the study of choice in this area. Lack of artifact from dental amalgam and beam hardening artifact from the mandible on MRI also eliminates two major shortcomings of CT in the examination of this area. Finally, the ability of MRI to view direct coronal and sagittal imaging planes is a distinct advantage in recognizing intrinsic tongue musculature and assessing tumor volume and spread for treatment planning.

LARYNX AND HYPOPHARYNX

Rarely does any radiologic imaging modality play a significant role in reaching a diagnosis of malignancy in the larynx and hypopharynx. These regions are so readily accessible to clinical examination that the combination of cytologic study and visual inspection usually strongly indicates the diagnosis of cancer. Therefore, the primary role of MRI is the same as that of CT in imaging the larynx and hypopharynx: to define the extent of the disease. While laryngoscopy can show mucosal surfaces and masses involving the lumen, deep extensions are difficult to detect at clinical examination alone; yet, in several areas, these extensions have profound implications of the management of disease. Both CT and now MRI to an even greater extent can define this important deep anatomy.[27-35]

Relatively T1-weighted images are ideal for the study of the larynx. T1-weighted sequences maximize the contrast between loose areolar tissue of the parapharyngeal and preepiglottic spaces, the neck, and most tumors. The higher signal intensity of squamous carcinoma on T2-weighted images is a disadvantage in studies of the larynx because the high-signal areolar tissue within the larynx becomes isointense with the tumor on these pulse sequences. The lower signal-to-noise ratio of the T2-weighted images also limits the use of thin slices and high-in-plane spatial resolution that are so valuable in the study of this region.

Axial and coronal imaging of the larynx will demonstrate the intrinsic musculature of the larynx as low-signal regions lying sandwiched between the bright signal of mucosa and submucosa glands, with bright signal of the loose areolar tissue separating the intrinsic muscle from the overlying thyroid cartilage. Infiltration of the intrinsic muscles or the adjacent bright-signal areolar tissue planes indicates deep infiltration and spreading tumor.

The space lying anterior to the epiglottis must consist of very loose areolar tissue in order for the epiglottis to invert during the act of swallowing. This loose areolar tissue creates extremely bright signal that is displaced by low signal when tumors infiltrate the region. In

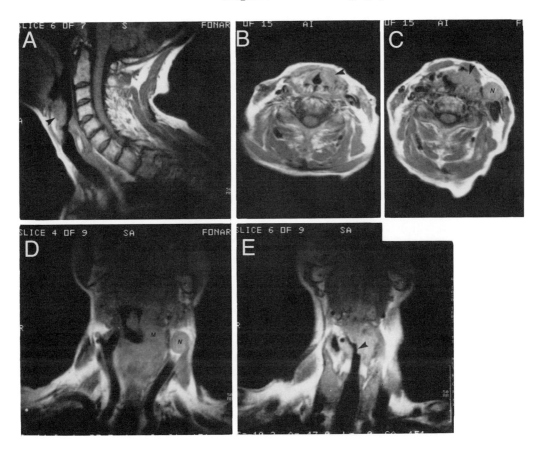

FIG 9–13.
Transglottic carcinoma in a 77-year-old woman. **A,** sagittal T1-weighted image (SE 480/30) reveals anterior lobulated soft tissue mass (*arrowhead*) narrowing the airway. **B,** axial T1-weighted image at the undersurface of the true vocal cords shows subglottic extension with additional involvement of the anterior soft tissue of the neck (*arrowhead*). **C,** axial T1-weighted image of the high false vocal cords shows involvement of the left paralaryngeal space and adjacent soft tissues (*arrowhead*). A large lymph node (*N*) is also present. **D,** coronal T1-weighted image (SE 600/30) of the posterior larynx reveals left-sided mass (*M*) and associated node (*N*). **E,** coronal T1-weighted images (SE 600/30) through the airway again shows left-sided soft tissue component with airway compromise (*arrowhead*).

the midline lie the low-signal ligaments that attach the epiglottis to the hyoid bone and thyrohyoid membrane, forming a barrier between the right and left sides of the larynx.[36] Tumor masses rarely extend from one side to the other unless they have crossed the midline along the mucosal surface.

The vertical spread of tumors is even more exacting, and surgeons feel quite comfortable with a 2- to 3-mm margin of tumor-free region adjacent to excisional planes because of the abrupt transition between the supraglottic and glottic lymphatics. Only in advanced lesions do the tumors spread down the inferior margin of the epiglottis to the anterior commissure and subglottic region or else from superior to inferior in the paralaryngeal space. Coronal and sagittal MR images with T1-weighted pulsing sequences readily demonstrate these spreads (Fig 9–13).

The primary function of the larynx is that of a sphincter rather than an organ for making sounds. This sphincter action requires a complicated system of coordinated muscular movements over cartilaginous plates and fascial planes. The embryology of the larynx itself is unique and bears careful attention when evaluating patients for voice-conservation surgery or precision radiation therapy. A horizontal cleavage plane of origin occurs at the level of the laryngeal ventricle, creating a supraglottic, glottic (true vocal cords) and subglottic region. The supraglottic larynx is embryologically part of the buccopharyngeal anlage, and its lymphatic drainage is shared with the tongue. The spread of tumors follows the lymphatic drainage and extends superiorly laterally and posteriorly to nodes in intimate association with the jugular vein at the level of the hyoid bone.

The true vocal cords and subglottic region act more like the trachea, with some of the lymphatic drainage being directly anterior from the anterior portion of the true vocal cords while the majority of the lymphatic drainage is posteriorly, inferiorly, and laterally. The lymphatic drainage of the lower subglottic space is circumferential in its pathways and communicates freely with the tracheal lymphatics.

The very early true cord tumor can be readily evaluated on indirect clinical examination and does not generally require an imaging study. The more advanced lesions that show extension to the anterior commissure regions above or below the vocal cord are quite a different matter. They require imaging techniques to show deep infiltration and full extent of the tumor.

Ideally the patient will undergo biopsy after the imaging examination. However, if a biopsy procedure has already taken place, the imaging study should be delayed 4 to 5 days or until edema subsides. The disruption of facial planes and edema resulting from a biopsy procedure can closely mimic tumor extension on MRI studies of this and other regions of the head and neck.

Important anatomic considerations to be delineated by MRI are cartilage invasion, vocal cord infiltration, pre-epiglottic space disease, and extension superiorly to the base of tongue or inferiorly to the subglottic space. The final decision whether to offer voice conservation surgery, radical surgery, or radiation therapy will depend on these factors.[37]

The loss of natural voice function resulting from a total laryngectomy can be devastating to many individuals. Less radical laryngeal resections that allow the preservation of natural speech and the protective sphincter mechanism of the larynx have been developed for certain smaller laryngeal tumors. Planning for any of these conservation laryngeal surgeries depends on an accurate preoperative knowledge of the precise extent of the disease within the larynx. Specifically, all techniques require an intact cricoid cartilage and at least one mobile arytenoid on which to construct the functional voice box. This essential information can be provided by CT and now MRI. To plan this type of operation, the direct coronal and direct sagittal imaging capabilities of MRI far surpass those of axial CT scanning in the ability to define critical information regarding the cranial-caudal extent of the tumors.

The recognition of tumor spread to other areas also markedly affects patient management. In the case of spread of the supraglottic tumor to involve the tongue base, a partial glossectomy may have to be performed in addition to the primary surgery. In other areas, extraorgan spread may render the tumor unresectable. Supraglottic cancers tend to spread superolaterally, while true cord tumors, and pyriform sinus and postcricoid region cancers tend to spread posteriolaterally and inferiorly (Fig 9–14).[38, 39] A shift of centering, or acquisition of extra slices, is necessary to show these nodal spreads. Finally, when cartilage invasion is present, cure with radiation therapy is often not possible. Therefore, the overall management of the patient must be reconsidered.

In comparison with CT, MRI consistently shows superior soft tissue definition. The use of direct coronal and sagittal imaging planes allows the visualization of intrinsic laryngeal muscular in addition to better definition of cranial-caudal tumor extension. Thus, MRI is now

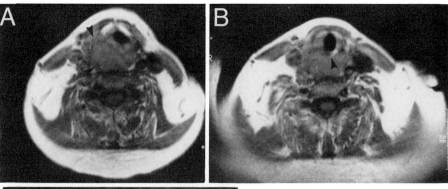

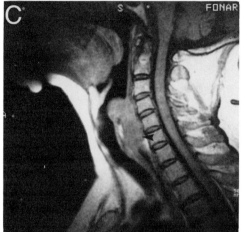

FIG 9–14.
Squamous cell carcinoma of the hypopharynx. **A,** axial sequence (SE 500/30) shows soft tissue mass (*arrowhead*) arising from the postcricoid region extending anteriorly. **B,** axial section through the level of the cricoid cartilage shows replacement of high-signal marrow, suggesting cartilage invasion by the tumor (*arrowhead*). **C,** sagittal view shows full cranial-caudal extent of the mass extending to the cervical esophagus (*arrowhead*).

the imaging study of choice for the evaluation of cancer of the larynx. The role of MRI can also be extended to replace CT scanning for the evaluation of the laryngeal airway and for the evaluation of benign lesions of the larynx.

CONCLUSIONS

Experience over the last 6 years indicates that MRI is now the imaging modality of choice in investigations of the nasopharynx, tongue, oropharynx, larynx, hypopharynx, and the majority of miscellaneous lesions of the neck.[40] Computed tomographic scanning can be used in the same regions; however, information obtained from CT is not as clearly demonstrated, and in some situations, such as malignancies of the tongue, the lesions may be missed entirely. Difficult clinical problem cases in which the two studies are complementary will still be present but will definitely be in the minority.

Aspiration cytology guided by MRI is now a reality through the use of specially developed MRI-compatible needles. Gadolinium-DTPA shows only limited promise for demonstration of head and neck cancer, although its final role remains to be defined.

REFERENCES

1. Lufkin R, Votruba J, Reicher M, et al: Solenoid surface coils in magnetic resonance imaging. *AJR* 1986; 146:409–412.
2. Lufkin R, Teresi L, Hanafee W: New needle for MRI guided aspiration cytology. *AJR* 1987; 149:380–382.
3. Lufkin R, Teresi L, Chui L, et al: A technique for MR guided needle placement in the head and neck. *AJR* 1988; 151:193–196.
4. Duckwiler G, Lufkin R, Teresi L, et al: Head and neck lesions: MR-guided aspiration biopsy. *Radiology* 1989; 170:519–522.
5. Robinson JD, Crawford S, Teresi L, et al: Gadolinium MR imaging in the head and neck. *Radiology* 1989; 172:165–170.
6. Teresi L, Lufkin R, Wortham D, et al: MRI of the normal intratemporal facial nerve. *AJR* 1987; 148:589–594.
7. Teresi L, Lufkin R, Hanafee W: MRI of the facial nerve: Anatomy and pathology. *Semin CT, US, MR* 1987; 8:240–255.
8. Teresi L, Lufkin R, Kolin E, et al: MRI of the intraparotid facial nerve. *AJNR* 1987; 8:253–259.
9. Teresi L, Lufkin R, Wortham D, et al: Parotid masses: Magnetic resonance imaging. *Radiology* 1987; 163:405–409.
10. Casselman JW, Mancuso AA: Major salivary gland masses: Comparison of MR imaging and CT. *Radiology* 1987; 165:183–189.
11. Mandelblatt SM, Braun IF, Davis PC, et al: Parotid masses: MR imaging. *Radiology* 1987; 163:411–414.
12. Rice DH, Becker T: Magnetic resonance imaging of the salivary glands. *Arch Otolaryngol Head Neck Surg* 1987; 113:78–80.
13. Mirich DR, McArdle CB, Kulkarni MV: Benign pleomorphic adenomas of the salivary glands: Surface coil MR imaging verus CT. *J Comput Assist Tomogr* 1987; 11:620–623.
14. Dillon WP, Mills CM, Kjos B, et al: Magnetic resonance imaging of the nasopharynx. *Radiology* 1984; 152:731.
15. Teresi LM, Lufkin RB, Vinuela F, et al: MR imaging of the nasopharynx and floor of the middle cranial fossa. Part I: Normal anatomy. *Radiology* 1987; 164:811–816.
16. Teresi LM, Lufkin RB, Vinuela F, et al: MR imaging of the nasopharynx and floor of the middle cranial fossa. Part II: Malignant tumors. *Radiology* 1987; 164:817–821.
17. Curtin HD: Separation of the masticator space from the parapharyngeal space. *Radiology* 1987; 163:195–204.
18. Cachin YU, Sancho-Garnier H, Micheau C, et al: Nodal metastases from carcinomas of the nasopharynx. *Otolaryngol Clin North AM* 1979; 12:145–154.
19. Mancuso AA, Maceri D, Rice D, et al: CT of cervical lymph node cancer. *AJR* 1981; 136:381–385.
20. Mancuso AA, Harnsberger HR, Muraki AS, et al: Computed tomography of cervical and retropharyngeal lymph nodes: Normal anatomy. *Radiology* 1983; 148:709–714.
21. Dooms GC, Hricak H, Crooks LE, et al: Magnetic resonance imaging of the lymph nodes: Comparison with CT. *Radiology* 1984; 153:719–728.
22. Dooms GC, Hricak H, Moseley MD, et al: Characterization of lymphadenopathy by magnetic resonance relaxation times: Preliminary results. *Radiology* 1985; 155:691–697.
23. Mancuso AA, Hanafee W: Elusive head and neck carcinomas beneath intract mucosa. *Laryngoscope* 1983; 93:133–139.
24. Unger JM: The oral cavity and tongue: Magnetic resonance imaging. *Radiology* 1985; 155:151–153.
25. Lufkin R, Hanafee W, Wortham D, et al: MRI of the tongue and oropharynx using surface coils. *Radiology* 1986; 161:69–75.
26. Batsakis JG: *Tumors of the Head and Neck: Clinical Pathological Consideration,* ed 2. Baltimore, Williams & Wilkins, 1979.
27. Stark DD, Moss AA, Gamsu G, et al: Magnetic resonance imaging of the neck. Part 1: Normal anatomy. *Radiology* 1983; 150:455.

28. Lufkin R, Hanafee W, Wortham D, et al: MRI of the larynx and hypopharynx using surface coils. *Radiology* 1986; 158:747–754.

29. Lufkin RB, Hanafee W: Application of surface coils to NMR anatomy of the larynx. *AJNR* 1985; 491–497.

30. Lufkin R, Larsson S, Hanafee W: NMR anatomy of the larynx and tongue. *Radiology* 1983; 148:173–175.

31. Glazer HS, Niemeyer HJ, Balfe D, et al: Neck neoplasms: MR imaging. Part II: Posttreatment evaluation. *Radiology* 1986; 160:349–354.

32. Glazer HS, Niemeyer JH, Balfe D, et al: Neck neoplasms: MR imaging. Part I: Initial evaluation. *Radiology* 1986; 160:343–348.

33. Stark DD, Moss AA, Gamsu G, et al: Magnetic resonance imaging of the neck. Part 2: Pathologic anatomy. *Radiology* 1983; 150:455.

34. McArdle CB, Bailey BJ, Amparo EG: Surface coil magnetic resonance imaging of the normal larynx. *Arch Otolaryngol Head Neck Surg* 1986; 112:616–622.

35. Castelijns JA, Gerritsen GJ, Kaiser MC, et al: MRI of normal or cancerous laryngeal cartilages: Histopathologic correlation. *Laryngoscope* 1987; 97:1085–1093.

36. Last RJ: *Anatomy: Regional and applied,* ed 6. New York, Churchill Livingstone, 1978.

37. Burstein FD, Calcaterra TC: Supraglottic laryngectomy: Series report and analysis of results. *Laryngoscope* 1985; 95:833–836.

38. Kirchner JA: Two hundred laryngeal cancers: Patterns of growth and spread as seen in serial section. *Laryngoscope* 1977; 87:474–482.

39. Larsson SV, Mancuso A, Hoover L, et al: Differentiation of pyriform sinus cancer from supraglottic laryngeal cancer by computed tomography. *Radiology* 1981; 141:427–432.

40. Lufkin R, Hanafee W: *MR Atlas of Head and Neck Anatomy.* New York, Raven Press, 1989.

Chapter 10

Magnetic Resonance Imaging of the Chest

Poonam Batra, M.D.

Magnetic resonance imaging (MRI) is a new imaging modality that demonstrates normal anatomy and defines disease processes in the chest.[1-4] The advantages of MRI are due largely to the availability of a wide range of soft tissue contrast and its ability to image vascular structures accurately without administration of contrast media. Direct multiplanar imaging capabilities and lack of ionizing radiation are other benefits. In this chapter MRI is discussed with regard to (1) the examination technique; (2) normal anatomy; (3) diseases in the mediastinum, hili, pulmonary parenchyma, and chest wall; (4) developing areas in thoracic MRI; and (5) disadvantages of MRI in the chest.

EXAMINATION TECHNIQUE

Permanent, resistive, and superconductive magnets have been used to acquire images of the chest. All our images were obtained on a 0.3-tesla (T) permanent magnet or electromagnet imaging system (Fonar, Melville, NY) by spin echo technique. The images were obtained with echo delay times (TE) of 18, 28, and 56 msec by the permanent magnet, or 30 and 60 msec with the electromagnet. The pulse sequence intervals [repetition time (TR)] were 300, 500, 1000, 2000, or 2500 msec. Each slice was 9.0 mm thick with a 3.0-mm gap between consecutive slices. In general, images were obtained in the axial plane in all patients. The T1-weighted (short TE, short TR) images were acquired in all cases with TEs of 18, 28, or 30 msec and TRs of 300 to 800 msec. Because gating images to the electrocardiogram (ECG) can greatly improve spatial resolution, this technique has now replaced ungated images with a short TR value (300 to 800 msec) in imaging of the chest.[5-7] Depending on the subject's heart rate, the TR value in ECG-gated sequence usually ranges between 700 and 1000 msec. However, adequate gating cannot be achieved in patients with marked cardiac arrhythmias, severe tachycardia, or low ECG voltage. The axial images obtained with gated/28 pulse

TABLE 10–1.

Technique for Magnetic Resonance Imaging of the Chest

Axial T1-weighted imaging	TE: 18, 28, or 30 msec TR: ECG gated or 300–800 msec
Axial T2-weighted imaging	TE: 56 or 84 msec TR: 1500–2000 msec or ECG gated
Add T1-weighted coronal or sagittal images as required	

sequence provided eight to nine images, while an SE 500/28 pulse sequence provided seven images. For imaging the chest in the axial plane, usually two contiguous sets of gated/28 or SE 500/28 were required to visualize thoracic structures from the lung apices to the level of the diaphragm. The T1-weighted, ECG-gated image sequence was followed by ungated T2-weighted images obtained in the axial plane with a TE of 56 or 60 msec and a TR of 1500 to 2000 msec. Depending on the site and nature of the abnormality, an additional T1-weighted, ECG-gated sequence in the coronal or sagittal plane was often obtained (Table 10–1). Both coronal and sagittal images were acquired with centering approximately 6 to 7 cm below the sternal notch. These images usually demonstrated the lungs from the apices to the level of the diaphragm. In general, gated/28 pulse sequences that provided eight to nine slices were sufficient to image the mediastinal structures from the descending aorta and azygos vein posteriorly to the anterior junction line anteriorly in the coronal plane. In the sagittal plane, eight to nine contiguous images would encompass all structures in the mediastinum and the right and left hili. All images were obtained while the volunteer or patient breathed quietly at normal tidal volume because of the length of time required to obtain the images. An ECG-gated sequence with a TE of 28 msec usually required 9 to 10 minutes to acquire, while a sequence of TE = 56 msec/TR = 1500 msec took 12 to 16 minutes depending on number of phase-encoding levels. The image quality was frequently poor in dyspneic patients. No respiratory gating was attempted. Respiratory gating at image acquisition (acquiring images only during the period of apnea) can improve image quality, but requires two to four times longer than ungated studies. The software techniques used to acquire images rapidly during breathholding are being developed currently to reduce respiratory motion artifacts.

In general, the most useful sequences are obtained with a TE of 28 msec and ECG gating or with a TR of 300 to 500 msec. These T1-weighted images provide the anatomic detail with optimum image contrast. Also a T2-weighted image with a SE 1500/56 sequence is often useful in providing additional information. The differential change of signal intensity in abnormal tissue on T1 and T2 image sequences facilitates the recognition and differentiation of abnormality from other tissues.[4] Furthermore, some diseases undergo similar signal shift even when present in different locations of the chest: for example, the signal intensity of

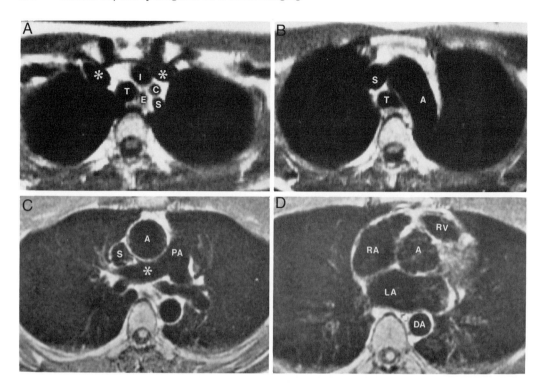

FIG 10–1.
Axial T1-weighted MR images from healthy volunteers. **A,** normal upper mediastinal anatomy at the level of origin of great arteries (SE 500/28). Brachiocephalic veins (*asterisks*), the innominate artery (*I*), carotid artery (*C*), subclavian artery (*S*), trachea (*T*), and esophagus (*E*) are visible. **B,** SE 500/28 image shows the superior vena cava (*S*), aortic arch (*A*), and trachea (*T*). **C,** SE gated/30 image shows main pulmonary artery (*PA*) to the left of aortic root (*A*). The right pulmonary artery (*asterisk*) is posterior to the superior vena cava (*S*) and aortic root. **D,** SE gated/30 image shows pulmonary veins draining into the left atrium (*LA*). Also visible are right atrium (*RA*), root of aorta (*A*), descending thoracic aorta (*DA*), and right ventricular outflow tract (*RV*).

parenchymal lung cancer is similar to the signal intensity of metastatic mediastinal adenopathy.

Because the inversion recovery technique requires longer data acquisition times and results in significantly less spatial resolution, it has not been found as attractive as the spin echo technique for chest imaging.[4]

NORMAL ANATOMY

Magnetic resonance imaging of the chest easily enables one to identify normal anatomic structures.[8–11] The normal anatomy of axial MR images is similar to that seen in computed tomography (CT) scans (Fig 10–1). Because of the paucity of signal from flowing blood, the vascular structures (devoid of signal) are distinguished easily from the bright signal of surrounding fat. Both systemic and pulmonary mediastinal vessels are well depicted on MR

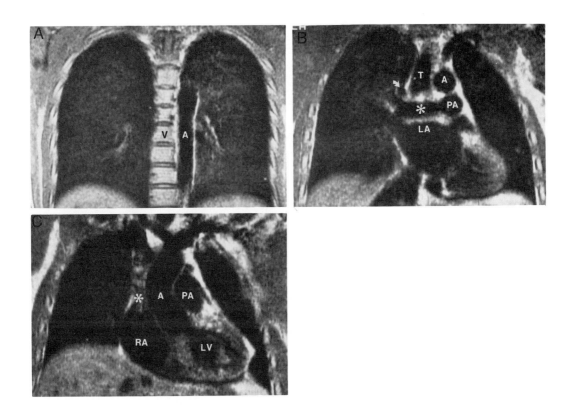

FIG 10–2.
Coronal MR images from healthy volunteers. **A,** SE gated/30 image shows the descending thoracic aorta (A) to the left of vertebral bodies (V). **B,** SE 500/28 image shows trachea (T), aorta (A), left pulmonary artery (PA), right pulmonary artery (*asterisk*), azygos vein (*arrow*), and left atrium (LA). **C,** SE 500/28 image shows the superior vena cava (*asterisk*) draining into right atrium (RA), ascending aorta (A), main pulmonary artery (PA), and left ventricle (LV).

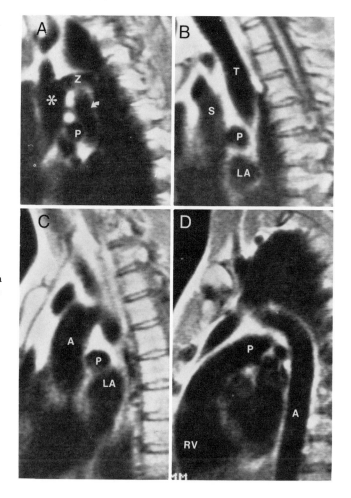

FIG 10–3.
Sagittal MR images (SE 500/28) from a healthy volunteer. **A,** an image to the right of midline shows the arch of the azygos vein (*Z*), superior vena cava (*asterisk*), right pulmonary artery (*P*), and posterior wall of bronchus intermedius (*arrow*). **B,** image through the trachea (*T*), superior vena cava (*S*), right pulmonary artery (*P*) and left atrium (*LA*). **C,** an image to the left of the midplane shows the ascending aorta (*A*), right pulmonary artery (*P*), and left atrium (*LA*). **D,** an image further left shows pulmonary artery (*P*), right ventricle (*RV*), and descending thoracic aorta (*A*).

images. The walls of these vessels rather than the interior are visible on MR images. The ascending aorta, aortic arch, descending aorta, and the great arteries arising from the aortic arch are well demonstrated (Fig 10–2). The mediastinal veins—including the subclavian veins, brachiocephalic veins, and vena cava—are visible. The ascending portion and the arch of the azygos vein is also frequently visible (Fig 10–3). The main pulmonary artery, the left and right pulmonary arteries, the right interlobar pulmonary artery, and the descending left pulmonary artery are seen routinely. The pulmonary arteries beyond the hili are not seen. Only the pulmonary veins close to the mediastinum and draining into the left atrium are visible.

The air-filled trachea and the main and lobar bronchi result in little or no MR signal but can be distinguished from other vessels by their appearance and location. Lungs, with their very low proton density, produce very little MR signal. However, minimal signal is frequently demonstrated in the posterior or dependent portions of the lung, which may be secondary to hypostatic congestion and minimal atelectasis in a supine patient.

Lymph nodes that are normal in size (less than 1 cm), when visible, appear less intense than the surrounding mediastinal fat. the thymus and esophagus can be seen on good quality spin echo images as regions of intermediate signal intensity, being more intense than trachea and mediastinal vessels but less intense than surrounding fat. On some slices the esophagus may contain air.

PATHOLOGIC STATES

Magnetic resonance imaging has proved useful in the diagnosis of a number of chest diseases. The diseases may be located in the mediastinum, hili, pulmonary parenchyma, pleura, or chest wall.

Mediastinal Abnormalities

Mediastinal masses consist of primary mediastinal tumors or metastatic lymphadenopathy and are easily distinguished from vessels and bronchi.[12-19] In all our patients the tumor tissue on T1-weighted images was less intense than mediastinal fat because of the longer T1 relaxation times for tumors than for mediastinal fat (Fig 10–4). The T1 values of masses averaged approximately 1500 msec, while the T1 values of surrounding mediastinal fat averaged slightly over 300 msec.[20] Because the T2 values of mediastinal masses and fat tend to overlap, mediastinal masses and fat will provide such an intense signal that the mass can be difficult or impossible to distinguish from the surrounding fat on T2-weighted images.

The anatomic relationship between tumor mass and mediastinal vessels has been well demonstrated by MRI. Also, MRI has demonstrated the displacement or compression of vessels and airways by the mass (Fig 10–5). Because the visible signal intensity of benign and malignant nodes is similar, signal intensity cannot be used to separate benign from malignant diseases. Ross and colleagues, who calculated the T1 and T2 values of benign and malignant diseases, also found that these values overlap and therefore cannot be used as criteria to distinguish benign from malignant mediastinal disease.[21] Although MRI was equivalent to CT scanning in providing anatomic detail and identifying diseases in the mediastinum, MRI had better inherent soft tissue contrast. Also, the streak artifacts that occur from the edges of pulsatile vascular structures, especially in contrast material-enhanced CT are not seen in MRI, which provides better images of small mediastinal vessels.

Vascular diseases of the mediastinum were easily identified by MRI without any exogenous contrast agents.[22] Aortic dissection, aneurysm, or coarctation can be defined.[23-25] In patients with superior vena cava obstruction or obstruction of the great veins, both the site of compression and site of obstruction can be demonstrated.[26, 27] Generally, however, venous collaterals are better defined with contrast-enhanced CT scanning. The sagittal or coronal planes are particularly useful for this purpose. The problem of wide mediastinum seen on chest radiographs because of tortuous or abnormal vessels can be accurately resolved by MRI.

Hilar Abnormality

The hilus consists of a bronchovascular bundle with relatively little signal arising from

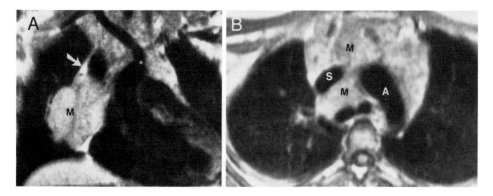

FIG 10–4.
Hodgkin's disease in a 20-year-old woman. **A,** coronal SE 500/28 image shows intermediate signal intensity mass (*M*) distinguishable from bright signal of fat (*arrow*) and minimal signal from vessels. **B,** axial SE 500/28 image shows an anterior mediastinal mass (*M*) displacing the superior vena cava (*S*) and aorta (*A*) posteriorly. Mass is also seen anterior to the carina (*M*).

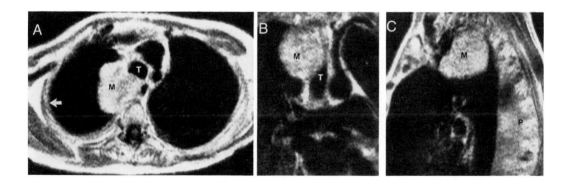

FIG 10–5.
Metastatic leiomyosarcoma in an 80-year-old woman. **A,** axial SE gated/28 image shows a mediastinal mass (*M*) displacing the trachea (*T*) and mediastinal vessels to the left. A right pleural effusion is also seen (*arrow*). **B,** coronal SE gated/28 image shows the mediastinal mass (*M*) compressing the trachea (*T*). **C,** sagittal SE gated/28 image shows the relationship of the mass (*M*) to the apex of the thoracic cage. Also note pleural effusion (*P*), which was found to be serosanguinous and malignant.

the lumen of bronchi, pulmonary arteries, or veins.[28] The lobar bronchi can be distinguished from the pulmonary vessels by their appearance and location in the hilus. The hilar masses appear as discrete areas of easily detectable signal (Fig 10–6). In a study of the appearance of normal hili,[29] small collections of fat and normal lymph nodes were visible. At three sites these collections were large and had the potential of being misinterpreted as enlarged hilar nodes (greater than 1 cm in size). These sites were, on the right side, at the level of bifurcation of the right pulmonary artery and at the origin of the middle lobe bronchus and, on the left

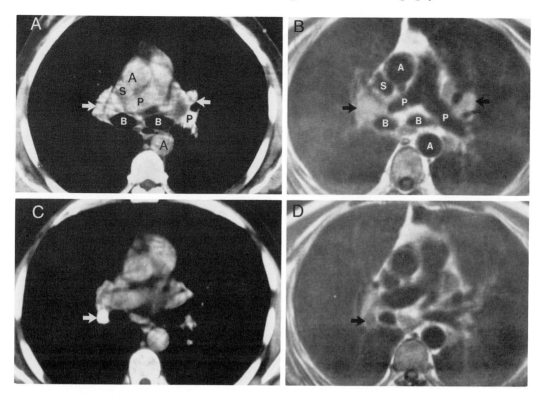

FIG 10–6.
Metastatic bronchogenic carcinoma in a 57-year-old man. **A,** contrast-enhanced CT scan shows right and left hilar masses (*arrows*) that are difficult to distinguish from right and left pulmonary arteries (*P*). Also note superior vena cava (*S*), ascending and descending aorta (*A*), and right and left main stem bronchi (*B*). **B,** axial SE 500/28 MR image easily distinguishes intermediate-signal-intensity right and left hilar masses (*arrow*) from right and left pulmonary artery (*P*). The superior vena cava (*S*), ascending and descending aorta (*A*), and right and left main stem bronchi (*B*) are well depicted. **C,** computed tomographic scan caudal to **A** shows a large focus of calcification in right hilus (*arrow*). **D,** axial SE 500/28 MR image at the same level as **C** shows the focus of calcification as a region of minimal signal difficult to interpret (*arrow*).

side, at the level of left upper lobe bronchus. In patients with a large hilar mass, the diagnostic information provided by both contrast-enhanced CT and MRI is the same. However, in patients who have a small hilar mass or have not been given contrast material, a confident differentiation of vessels from a mass is sometimes difficult. In fact, even following intravenous administration of contrast material, the degree of vascular opacification achieved is insufficient, in a significant number of cases, to define normal vasculature. In such cases MRI is definitely superior to CT in distinguishing hilar lesions from the bronchovascular bundles without the need of contrast medium. In patients whose hilar enlargement is secondary to a dilated vessel, MRI can clearly show the vascular nature of the mass (Fig 10–7).

Pulmonary Parenchymal Disease

At the present time pulmonary parenchymal disease is difficult to evaluate by MRI.

Because of the respiratory motion inherent in the long imaging times of MRI and its inferior spatial resolution, the resolving power of MRI is less than that of CT for small lung nodules less than 1 cm in size. Another difficulty with MRI is that calcification is not reliably identified. While on CT or plain radiography, calcification within a lung nodule is evidence of benignity, this distinction would be difficult to make when using only MRI. However, differentiation of a lung nodule from the end-on blood vessel would be easier to make with MRI than with CT because on MRI little signal would arise from the lumen of a blood vessel in which there is flowing blood. With MRI, nodules were best seen on images with a long repetition time (TR = 2000 msec) because of increased signal strength of the nodule and improved signal-to-noise ratio.[28] Large lung nodules are equally well seen on MRI or CT, but the configuration of the lung nodule—such as the smooth vs. spiculated margin—is better depicted by CT.[30] In addition, because segmental bronchi and fissures are not visualized on MRI, the exact

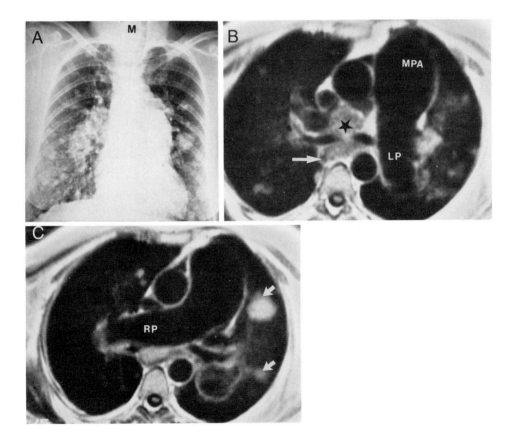

FIG 10–7.
Metastatic thyroid carcinoma in a 58-year-old woman. **A,** posteroanterior chest radiograph shows large thyroid mass (*M*), multiple metastatic lung nodules, and massive bilateral hilar enlargement. **B,** axial SE 500/18 MR image shows markedly enlarged main pulmonary artery (*MPA*) and left pulmonary artery (*LP*), precarinal (*star*) and subcarinal adenopathy (*arrow*), and poorly defined lung nodules. **C,** axial SE 500/18 MR image caudal to **B** shows a markedly enlarged right pulmonary artery (*RP*) and lung nodules (*arrow*). The markedly enlarged hili were secondary to pulmonary artery hypertension.

location of a primary lung lesion may be difficult to determine with MRI. This determination can easily be accomplished with CT and thus aid the bronchoscopist or surgeon.

Areas of consolidated lung produce signals that are easily seen against the normal signal void of pulmonary parenchyma. Several investigators have suggested that postobstructive pneumonitis and atelectasis can be distinguished from central tumor on MR images. They have reported that with short TR values (150 to 300 msec), tumors provide greater signal strength than distal pneumonitis. With long TR values (2,000 msec) the central mass appeared less intense than the peripheral consolidated lung.[31] In our experience the signals produced by tumors and lung disease with short and long TR values overlap, and their differentiation was not made consistently.

Mucus plugs have been shown within the bronchi in patients with cystic fibrosis.[32] Interstitial disease cannot be evaluated by MRI at the present time. In general, CT is superior for imaging parenchymal disease because of better spatial resolution and shorter scanning time.

Pleural Disease

Pleural effusion appears as a region of low signal intensity on T1-weighted images in the dependent portions of the thorax, while the signal intensity increases on T2-weighted images. However, in Cohen's experience the signal intensity of the pleural effusion was similar to that of masses.[4] This discrepancy may be related to variations in the lipid and/or protein content of the fluid. Calcification within the pleura, as seen in asbestosis, cannot be definitively identified with MRI. Pleural thickening or masses are seen as zones of intermediate signal intensity along the pleural surface (Fig 10–8). The relationship of pleural effusion and/or thickening to the dome of the diaphragm is better evaluated on coronal or sagittal planes.

Chest Wall Disease

The bony cortex of the ribs does not provide a MR signal, but the fat within the marrow produces a high signal that helps locate the position of the ribs. The cortical bone involvement of ribs by neoplasm cannot be assessed because calcium does not produce a MR signal. Larger metastasis to a rib is apparent as a soft tissue mass with intermediate signal strength, similar to that of muscle, which disrupts the normal tissue plane. Other investigators have found that bony metastases had decreased signal strength as compared with muscle.[1] This may be related to the presence of remaining mineralized bone at the metastatic site, creating a region of low signal intensity (long T1 of mineralized bone).

DEVELOPING AREAS IN MAGNETIC RESONANCE IMAGING OF THE CHEST

Magnetic resonance imaging has shown promise for demonstrating pulmonary emboli.[33–36] These appear as foci of increased signal in the pulmonary artery secondary to the thrombotic material itself, the alteration of flow in the region, or to both. At times, distinguishing areas of increased signal that represent slowly moving blood from those due to

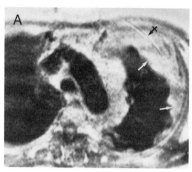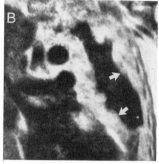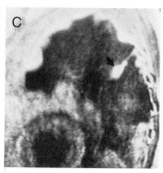

FIG 10–8.
Malignant mesothelioma in a 64-year-old woman. **A,** axial gated/28 image shows encasement of left lung by nodular pleural thickening (*white arrows*), which represents tumor. Note respiratory motion artifacts (*black arrow*) in this dyspneic patient. **B,** coronal gated/28 image shows the entire extent of tumor in left hemithorax (*arrow*). **C,** sagittal gated/28 image shows extension of tumor into oblique fissure (*arrow*).

thrombus could be problematic. Magnetic resonance imaging may also prove useful for evaluating blood flow.[37, 38]

The ability of MRI to detect hydrogen nuclei and to measure proton density could prove useful in quantitation of lung water and management of diseases characterized by pulmonary edema.

The ability of MRI to distinguish tumor from radiation fibrosis has been demonstrated. The relatively long T1 relaxation time and short T2 relaxation time of fibrosis is sufficiently characteristic and can be used to distinguish malignant tumors that demonstrate relatively long T1 and T2 relaxation times.[39]

Chemical shift imaging (hydrogen proton spectroscopy) allows discrimination of water protons and fat protons, but the utility of this technique for evaluating chest diseases remains to be determined.[40] Nuclear magnetic resonance spectroscopy of different nuclei is being investigated. Phosphorus-31 spectroscopy has been utilized to differentiate small-cell lung cancer from non-small-cell lung cancer in vitro.[41]

DISADVANTAGES OF MAGNETIC RESONANCE IMAGING IN THE CHEST

The disadvantages of MRI in chest imaging include the following: (1) motion degradation of the image often results because of long image-acquisition times; (2) patients with cardiac pacemakers cannot be imaged; (3) patients with surgical clips on major vessels following surgery, or those who are critically ill, claustrophobic, or very obese, are not suitable for MRI; and (4) calcification is not consistently identified with MRI.

CONCLUSION

Magnetic resonance imaging of the chest is most useful for the diagnosis of hilar masses and mediastinal vascular lesions. It is particularly useful for patients with hypersensitivity to contrast media or whose renal insufficiency makes administration of contrast media hazardous. Both MRI and CT scanning are comparable in the diagnosis of mediastinal mass or adenopathy, but the spatial resolution of CT is better than MRI. Computed tomography is markedly superior to MRI for imaging pulmonary parenchymal disease. At present, CT—with its better spatial resolution and shorter scanning time—remains the procedure of choice, following plain chest radiography, in evaluations of most chest diseases. Magnetic resonance image quality may improve with advances in technology that enable faster image acquisition time. In the future, physiologic changes and tissue characterization may be possible with MRI.

REFERENCES

1. Axel L, Kressel HY, Thickman D, et al: NMR imaging of the chest at 0.12T: Initial clinical experience with a resistive magnet. *AJR* 1983; 141:1157–1162.
2. Gamsu G, Webb WR, Sheldon P, et al: Nuclear magnetic resonance imaging of the thorax. *Radiology* 1983; 147:473–480.
3. Kundel HL, Kressel HY, Epstein D: The potential role of NMR imaging in thoracic disease. *Radiol Clin North Am* 1983; 21:801–808.
4. Cohen AM: Magnetic resonance imaging of the thorax. *Radiol Clin North Am* 1984; 22:829–846.
5. Mark AS, Winkler ML, Peltzer M, et al: Gated acquisition of MR images of the thorax: Advantages for the study of the hila and mediastinum. *Magn Reson Imaging* 1987; 5:57–63.
6. Ehman RL, McNamara MT, Pallack M, et al: Magnetic resonance imaging with respiratory gating: Techniques and advantages. *AJR* 1984; 143:1175–1182.
7. Runge VM, Clanton JA, Partain CL, et al: Respiratory gating in magnetic resonance imaging at 0.3 Tesla. *Radiology* 1984; 151:521–523.
8. Batra P, Brown K, Steckel RJ, et al: MR imaging of the thorax: A comparison of axial, coronal, and sagittal imaging planes. *J Comput Assist Tomogr* 1988; 12:75–81.
9. O'Donovan PB, Ross JS, Sivak ED, et al: Magnetic resonance imaging of the thorax: The advantages of coronal and sagittal planes. *AJR* 1984; 143:1183–1188.
10. Webb WR, Jensen BG, Gamsu G, et al: Coronal magnetic resonance imaging of the chest: Normal and abnormal. *Radiology* 1984; 153:729–735.
11. Webb WR, Jensen BG, Gamsu G, et al: Sagittal MR imaging of the chest: Normal and abnormal. *J Comput Assist Tomogr* 1985; 9:471–479.
12. Cohen AM, Creviston S, LiPuma JP, et al: NMR evaluation of hilar and mediastinal lymphadenopathy. *Radiology* 1983; 148:739–742.
13. Cohen AM, Creviston S, LiPuma JP, et al: Nuclear magnetic resonance imaging of the mediastinum and hili: Early impressions of its efficacy. *AJR* 1983; 141:1163–1169.
14. Gamsu G, Stark DD, Webb WR, et al: Magnetic resonance imaging of benign mediastinal masses. *Radiology* 1984; 151:709–713.
15. Batra P, Herrmann C, Mulder D: Mediastinal imaging in myasthenia gravis: Correlation of chest radiography, CT MR and surgical findings. *AJR* 1987; 148:515–519.
16. Batra P, Brown K, Steckel RJ: Diagnostic imaging techniques in mediastinal malignancies. *Am J Surg* 1988; 156:4–11.
17. Aronberg DJ, Glazer HS, Sagel SS: MRI and CT of the mediastinum: Comparisons, controversies, and pitfalls. *Radiol Clin North Am* 1985; 23:439–448.
18. Webb WR, Moore EH: Differentiation of volume averaging and mass on magnetic resonance images of the mediastinum. *Radiology* 1985; 155:413–416.
19. von Schulthess GK, McMurdo K, Tscholakoff D, et al: Mediastinal masses: MR imaging. *Radiology* 1986; 158:289–296.

20. Webb WR, Gamsu G, Stark DD, et al: Evaluation of magnetic resonance sequences in imaging mediastinal tumors. *AJR* 1984; 143:723–727.

21. Ross JS, O'Donovan PB, Novoa R, et al: Magnetic resonance of the chest: Initial experience with imaging and in vivo T1 and T2 calculations. *Radiology* 1984; 152:95–101.

22. Glazer HS, Gutierrez FR, Levitt RG, et al: The thoracic aorta studied by MR imaging. *Radiology* 1985; 157:149–155.

23. Kersting-Sommerhoff BA, Higgins CB, White RD, et al: Aortic dissection: Sensitivity and specificity of MR imaging. *Radiology* 1988; 166:651–655.

24. Dinsmore RE, Liberthson RR, Wismer GL, et al: Magnetic resonance imaging of thoracic aortic aneurysms: Comparison with other imaging methods. *AJR* 1986; 146:309–314.

25. von Schulthess GK, Higashino SM, Higgins SS, et al: Coarctation of the aorta: MR imaging. *Radiology* 1986; 158:469–474.

26. Weinreb JC, Mootz A, Cohen JM: MRI evaluation of mediastinal and thoracic inlet venous obstruction. *AJR* 1986; 6:679–684.

27. McMurdo KK, de Geer G, Webb WR, et al: Normal and occluded mediastinal veins: MR imaging. *Radiology* 1986; 159:33–38.

28. Muller NL, Gamsu G, Webb WR: Pulmonary nodules: Detection using magnetic resonance and computed tomography. *Radiology* 1985; 155:687–690.

29. Webb WR, Gamsu G, Stark DD, et al: Magnetic resonance imaging of the normal and abnormal pulmonary hila. *Radiology* 1984; 152:89–94.

30. Batra P, Brown K, Collins JD, et al: Evaluation of intrathoracic extent of lung cancer by plain chest radiography, computed tomography and magnetic resonance imaging. *Am Rev Respir Dis* 1988; 137:1456–1462.

31. Webb WR, Jensen BG, Sollitto R, et al: Bronchogenic carcinoma: Staging with MR compared with staging with CT and surgery. *Radiology* 1985; 156:117–124.

32. Gooding CA, Lallemand DP, Brasch RC: Nuclear magnetic resonance imaging of cystic fibrosis. *J Pediatr* 1984; 105:384–388.

33. Gamsu G, Hirji M, Moore EH, et al: Experimental pulmonary emboli detected using magnetic resonance. *Radiology* 1984; 153:467–470.

34. Moore EH, Gamsu G, Webb WR, et al: Pulmonary embolus: Detection and follow-up using magnetic resonance. *Radiology* 1984; 153:471–472.

35. Ovenfors C, Batra P: Diagnosis of peripheral pulmonary emboli by MR imaging: An experimental study in dogs. 1988; 6:487–491.

36. Thickman D, Kressel HY, Axel L: Demonstration of pulmonary embolism by magnetic resonance imaging. *AJR* 1984; 142:921–922.

37. Mills CM, Brant-Zawadzki M, Crooks LE, et al: Nuclear magnetic resonance: Principles of blood flow imaging. *AJR* 1984; 142:165–170.

38. Bradley WG, Waluch V, Laik S, et al: The appearance of rapidly flowing blood on magnetic resonance images. *AJR* 1984; 143:1167–1174.

39. Glazer HS, Levitt RG, Lee JKT, et al: Differentiation of radiation fibrosis from recurrent pulmonary neoplasm by magnetic resonance imaging. *AJR* 1984; 143:729–730.

40. Dixon WT: Simple proton spectroscopic imaging. *Radiology* 1984; 153:189–194.

41. Knop RH, Carney DN, Chen CW, et al: P31 NMR differentiation of small cell lung cancer (SCLC) and non-small cell cancer (NSLC) human tumor cell lines (abstract). Book of Abstracts, Society of Magnetic Resonance in Medicine, 1984, 13–14.

Chapter 11

Magnetic Resonance Imaging of the Cardiovascular System

Juan F. Lois, M.D.

Antoinette S. Gomes, M.D.

Magnetic resonance imaging (MRI) is a useful diagnostic technique in the clinical evaluation of patients with disease of the heart and great vessels. The different applications of MRI in the study of the cardiovascular system have been described in several large series.[1-3] Studies of the heart and great vessels can be performed rapidly, providing images with good spatial resolution. The ability of MRI to acquire images in multiple projections (such as coronal, sagittal, and oblique) without changes in patient positioning or image reformation from multiple axial scans as in computed tomography (CT) makes it an ideal tool for the evaluation of complex structures such as the heart and great vessels.[4-6] With electrocardiographic (ECG) gating, degradation of image quality resulting from cardiac motion can be significantly diminished, and the heart can be imaged in different phases of the contractile cycle. Thus, both anatomic and functional diagnostic information is available. The introduction of rapid imaging, as in cine MRI, makes it possible to differentiate normal and abnormal flow patterns, such as those occurring in valvular disease,[7] and because of the high temporal resolution, segmental cardiac contraction can be better evaluated.[8] Recently Sechtem and colleagues reported the use of cine MRI in the detection of shunt flow in patients with ventricular septal defects (VSD).[9] Currently two-dimensional (2D) Doppler echocardiography has been widely used in the study of the cardiovascular system. Although MRI will never be a bedside examination, as is 2D echocardiography, MRI is not operator dependent, can be performed through air or bone, and allows imaging with a large field of view. Other possibilities of MRI include myocardial tissue characterization[2] and MR spectroscopy, which may soon allow the acquisition of metabolic information from the human heart.[10]

NORMAL CARDIAC ANATOMY AND FUNCTION

In the study of the anatomic features of the heart and great vessels spin echo ECG-gated

MR imaging is most commonly used. On T1-weighted images the signal void of flowing blood is enhanced, and because of the shorter echo time (TE), the signal-to-noise and spatial resolution is higher. Axial images from the superior portion of the liver to the level of the origin of the great vessels are initially obtained and are frequently sufficient to demonstrate segmental cardiac anatomy.[11] If additional information is required, oblique images are obtained perpendicular or longitudinal to the areas of interest in the axial scan. Interleaved images are often needed to decrease the influence of partial voluming when imaging small or very thin structures. For assessment of cardiac size and function, systolic and diastolic dimensions are measured, preferably in short- and long-axis MR images. The left ventricular segmental wall thickness and cardiac chamber size may be evaluated in these projections and can be compared with measurements from echocardiography.[6] Ejection fraction measured from these images has good correlation with the results of left ventriculography.[12]

The normal left ventricle has an oval shape with the interventricular septum bulging slightly toward the right ventricle (Fig 11–1). The right ventricle is triangular in shape. The mitral and tricuspid valve leaflets are frequently seen. The aortic and pulmonary valves, on the other hand, are seldom visualized.

The pericardium appears as a linear low-signal structure and is often surrounded by epicardial and pericardial fat, which produce a bright signal.

ISCHEMIC HEART DISEASE

Ischemic heart disease is a major cause of morbidity and mortality. Complete evaluation usually requires invasive techniques such as coronary arteriography and contrast ventriculography. Noninvasive methods of measuring cardiac function include radionuclide blood pool scintigraphy and echocardiography; however, the resolution with these techniques is relatively poor, and some geometric assumptions are required.[8] Magnetic resonance imaging, on the other hand, has a wide field of view, requires no geometric assumptions, and produces a sharper edge definition.[3]

Old healed myocardial infarction appears on MRI as regions of signal intensity lower than that of healthy myocardium; it is associated with areas of wall thinning that coincide with the territory supplied by the occluded coronary artery branches.[13] The lower signal has been related to fibrosis, and McNamara and colleagues[13] suggest that when an area of wall thinning has a signal intensity similar to that of the surrounding myocardium it may represent residual viable tissue within the infarct zone. Extreme wall thinning and bulging occur at the site of left ventricular aneurysms.[14] Often areas of high MRI signal intensity are seen within left ventricular aneurysms. This has been attributed to slow flow of blood in the areas of akinesis or dyskinesis.[1, 15] With cine MRI, the areas of focal wall motion abnormalities can be identified and correlated with coronary artery occlusion.[8]

Experimental studies of acute myocardial infarction in animals have shown that significant increase in myocardial signal intensity and T1 and T2 relaxation times are present within a few hours following coronary artery occlusion. The best contrast between normal and infarcted myocardium has been obtained with more T2-weighted images.[16] The increase in signal and prolonged T2 relaxation have been attributed to the increase in water content at the infarct site,[17] loss of distinction between intracellular and extracellular water following destruction

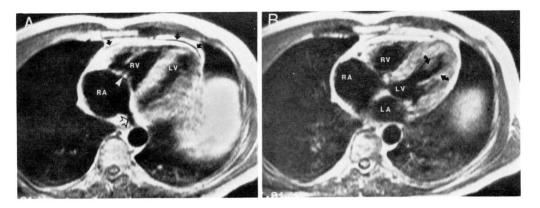

FIG 11–1.
Normal heart. **A,** axial MR image at the level of the mid-right ventricle (*RV*). The right ventricle has a triangular shape and a trabeculated inner surface. The *arrowhead* points to the tricuspid valve. The coronary sinus (*open arrow*) is seen draining into the right atrium (*RA*). The pericardium appears as a low-signal area separating the epicardial and pericardial fat (*solid arrows*). LV = left ventricle. **B,** axial MR image at the level of the mid-left ventricle. The left ventricle (*LV*) has an oval shape with a smooth inner surface. The papillary muscles are seen (*curved arrows*). LA = left atrium, RA = right atrium, RV = right ventricle.

of the cell wall,[18] reduced myocardial motion,[17] and in later stages to methemoglobin or other paramagnetic substances that accumulate in the infarcted area.[18]

In one recent study,[18] MR images from a group of patients with acute infarctions were contrasted with images from a group of healthy volunteers. In the patients, gated MR images showed focal areas of high signal intensity at the infarct site. The infarcted areas showed increased signal intensity relative to healthy myocardium on both the first and second echo images. However, the second echo image showed higher relative intensity. Gated MR images of healthy volunteers tended to show homogenous myocardial signal intensity; however, regions of higher signal intensity were noted in some cases.

The variation in signal intensity throughout the myocardium is not specific for myocardial infarction; in healthy patients variation may be secondary to respiratory or cardiac motion artifact. Another factor that may simulate myocardial infarction is flow signal appearing within the myocardium from spatial misregistration, as a result of the time disparity between the phase-encoding and the readout gradients.[19] Blood circulating slowly against the endocardium and partial voluming of the epicardial fat can also produce high signal in the myocardial wall.[18] In this series,[18] the increase in signal in infarcted areas as compared with normal myocardium increased significantly from the first to the second echo images, while the increase in signal in the myocardium of healthy volunteers decreased from the first to the second echo images. Thus, MRI has the potential for use in determining myocardial infarction size, but the sensitivity of MRI in identification of acute infarction is yet to be determined.

Frequently, mural thrombi are present within left ventricular aneurysms. On MRI, mural thrombi appear as structures of variable signal intensity with high to moderate signal, but they may be difficult to diagnose with MRI. As with 2D echocardiography, differentiation of thrombi from slow-flowing blood in the areas of wall motion abnormalities may be difficult because of flow artifacts produced by slow-flowing blood. Also, images in patients with left ventricular thrombi tend to be of lesser quality primarily because of respiratory artifacts.[20] In some cases the lesser quality is secondary to cardiac arrythmia, with consequent poor gating. Thrombus has been generally described as having intermediate signal intensity (similar to that of normal myocardium). When double echo imaging is performed, thrombi increase in contrast in the second echo image.[21] However, Zeitler and colleagues[15] have shown that the signal remains unchanged at the longer echo time. Additionally, the differential diagnosis of intracavitary thrombi and flow phenomena in the left ventricle is enhanced by a short repetition time and a second echo with a longer echo time. Imaging is best in the axial or coronal projection.[15]

The value of cine MRI in detecting regional wall motion abnormalities in ischemic heart disease is under current evaluation. Cine MRI used in conjunction with spin echo images has the potential to markedly improve noninvasive assessment of infarct size.[3, 8]

CORONARY ARTERIES AND CORONARY BYPASS GRAFTS

The proximal portions of the native right and left coronary arteries can often be seen on gated echo images of the heart. They appear as tubular structures with low internal signal or, in cross section, as round low-signal structures. Because of their tortuous course it is difficult to trace the normal coronary arteries on the surface of the heart.[22] At this time, stenosis of the native coronary arteries cannot be detected adequately with the resolution available.

Patent coronary artery bypass grafts (CABG) can be detected with MRI. They can be identified with T1-weighted spin echo technique as tubular longitudinal structures with low internal signal arising from the aorta and coursing toward the surface of the heart. They are frequently seen in cross section on axial images at the level of the pulmonary artery confluence and longitudinally on coronal-oblique images. Although resolution is not yet adequate to determine the presence of CABG stenosis, several studies reported that 84% to over 90% of patient vein grafts have been seen with MRI.[23, 24] Results have been lower for internal mammary grafts. Further experience and technological development are likely to result in improved visualization of grafts.

In a prospective study,[22] 84% of CABGs were identified, and in the same study 88% of the grafts were seen when the MR images were reviewed retrospectively. These results suggest that graft detection can be improved by knowing the numbers and locations of the grafts prior to the MRI examination. Grafts should not be confused with native coronary arteries. Such confusion is best avoided by identifying the graft at the origin from the aorta prior to following its course to the surface of the heart. Saphenous vein grafts originate higher than the native coronary arteries. On coronal views, saphenous vein grafts can be confused with the pericardial reflection, which also may show low signal. Postsurgical deformities in the retrosternal area and surgical clips can also produce artifacts.

CONGENITAL HEART DISEASE

Magnetic resonance imaging can be used to demonstrate a variety of congenital cardiac and vascular lesions.[3, 25–27] However, the majority of these abnormalities are clearly demonstrated with 2D ultrasound.

Visceroatrial Situs

Identification of the location of the inferior vena cava, of the coronary sinus entering the right atrium, and of the position of the liver and spleen allow determination of the abdominal situs. The visualization of the tracheal bifurcation into right and left main stem bronchi and establishment of their relationship with the pulmonary arteries allow determination of the thoracic situs and the presence of right and left thoracic isomerism. Often, coronal or sagittal-coronal views are needed for determination of situs by identifying the left atrial appendage, the left atrium, and the superior pulmonary veins as they enter the left atrium.

Ventricular Loop

By studying the relationship of the ventricles, the presence of a D or L loop can be determined. In axial scans the anatomic right ventricle is located anteriorly and has a triangular configuration with a trabeculated pattern. The left ventricle is located posteriorly, is oval in shape, and has a rather smooth wall with the two papillary muscles frequently identified (see Fig 11–1).

Great Vessels

The relationship of the great vessels is easily identified in axial projections. The position of both the ascending and descending aorta and of the main pulmonary artery together with the anatomic appearance of the ventricles allows for a complete segmental description of the congenital abnormalities present.

Atrial and Ventricular Septa

The ventricular septum can be studied in the axial and short-axis (sagittal-coronal) view. The membranous septum is normally very thin and because of partial voluming, the small membranous VSDs cannot be diagnosed with certainty with MRI unless seen in several images. The large-malalignment VSDs, as seen in the tetralogy of Fallot, are well outlined, and the relationship of the ventricular septum to the great vessels may be of significant help in the differential diagnosis. The atrial septum appears as a linear area of intermediate density surrounded by flow void in both atria. However, as with the membranous septum, the foramen ovale may erroneously appear interrupted on MR images in healthy patients because of partial voluming.

On the other hand, echocardiography has a much higher accuracy in the diagnosis of both atrial septal defect and VSD and is likely to remain the primary imaging modality in these patients.

In pulmonary atresia it is of particular importance to identify the presence of continuity between the right and left pulmonary arteries and to estimate the size of these vessels (Fig 11–2). This diagnosis of continuity is elusive at echocardiography and very often at angiography. In these cases MRI plays an important diagnostic role. Pulmonary arteries are usually best seen in the axial projection; however, demonstration of their size and the assessment of continuity may require both a sagittal-coronal view tailored to the patient's anatomy and interleaved axial scans.

Palliative shunts such as Blalock-Taussig, Glenn, or Fontan can be identified as structures with flow void connecting systemic arterial and pulmonary structures.

Pulmonary venous return is studied in both axial and coronal views. The course of the superior vena cava and inferior vena cava, and their relationship to both atria, can be outlined by obtaining axial images at multiple levels. A persistent left superior vena cava can be followed down to the coronary sinus; the "scimitar" syndrome can be diagnosed by the presence of an anomalous vein draining downward toward the inferior vena cava or portal vein systems. Anomalous pulmonary veins can sometimes be seen draining into the superior vena cava or right atrium.

CARDIAC MASSES

Until recently, echocardiography had been the primary imaging technique used in the evaluation of patients with suspected cardiac masses. However, the sensitivity and the specificity of 2D echocardiography is not 100%.[28] Magnetic resonance imaging, on the other hand, has been shown to provide high-quality images of the heart, cardiac tumor, thrombi, and paracardiac masses. When compared with echocardiography, MRI provides superior spatial and contrast resolution with a larger field of view. The heart can be imaged in several projections, thus facilitating determination of the size and extension of cardiac tumors. Involvement or compression of the great vessels and other mediastinal structures by tumor masses can also be determined. Magnetic resonance imaging is also useful in follow-up study of patients with cardiac tumors after therapy.[20] The tumors show variable signal intensity, very frequently similar to that of myocardium. It has been shown that MRI is particularly accurate in the evaluation of patients with suspected masses in the left atrium or involving the great vessels (Fig 11–3). Although it is likely that echocardiography will remain the primary imaging technique for the study of patients with suspected cardiac masses, MRI can be used in the instances when the echocardiogram is suboptimal or equivocal and when confirmation of the echocardiographic diagnosis is necessary.

ACQUIRED DISEASES OF THE AORTA

The contrast seen between flowing blood and the vessel wall on MR images makes MRI an ideal noninvasive modality for a study of the aorta.

Images are usually obtained using spin echo pulse sequences with ECG gating and a relatively short echo time (18 to 28 msec). Surface coils are used to enhance the image in infants and small children. The study is usually started in the axial projection centered at the sternal angle. Interleaved images are frequently needed. From these images sagittal-coronal oblique views are obtained with an electronic cursor positioned along the axis of the transverse aortic arch, thus imaging the aorta in a manner similar to the angiographic left anterior oblique view. Gross intracardiac anatomy, pericardial effusion, mediastinal and lung parenchymal anatomy, and the origins of the great vessels can be evaluated.

Normal Aorta

Flowing blood in the aorta appears as an area of signal void with the aortic wall—a thin, linear, parallel structure of higher signal. The aorta can be measured, and the width of the ascending aorta compared with the width of the descending aorta at the level of the diaphragm. The ratio of ascending aorta to the descending aorta in patients with a normal aorta is less than 1.8:1.[29]

Aortic Dissection

The presence of intimal flaps and of a true and false lumen in the aorta can be demonstrated by MRI. An intimal flap appears as an area of linear density with high MR signal located within the lumen of the aorta, frequently separating two areas of different signal that represent the different velocities of flowing blood in the true and false lumina.[29] (Fig 11–4). As with echocardiography, care must be taken in the diagnosis of aortic dissection when a clot is present within the false lumen. In some cases of concentric dissection of the aorta with clotted false lumen, it is very difficult to differentiate between a thickened aortic wall and a dissecting hematoma with a narrow false lumen and very slow flow or thrombus.[29] On MRI, calcifications appear as low signal and can be mistaken for irregularities of the aortic lumen, which is a relative disadvantage of MRI over CT scanning in this setting. Another problem in MRI of the aorta relates to the difficulty in differentiating between mural thrombus and slow-flowing blood, both of which may produce high signal intensity. To help in this differentiation the area in question may be imaged at different phases of the cardiac cycle, such as systole and diastole, or using a double echo sequence, or with gradient echo technique.

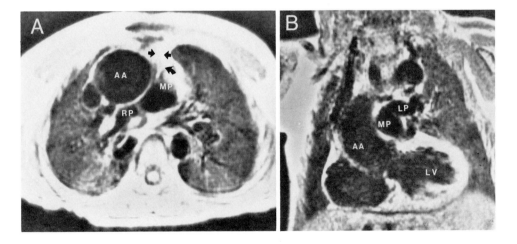

FIG 11–2.
Tetralogy of Fallot with pulmonary atresia. **A**, axial and **B**, coronal MR images show a dilated ascending aorta (*AA*) and atresia of the proximal main pulmonary artery (*MP*), which is not visualized (*straight arrows*). The distal main pulmonary artery is well developed but tapers proximally (*curved arrow*). There is continuity between the right (*RP*) and left (*LP*) pulmonary arteries, which are well developed and tortuous (*curved arrow*). LV = left ventricle.

FIG 11–3.
Left atrial myxoma. There is a rounded area of
intermediate signal within the left atrium (*arrowheads*)
that represents an atrial myxoma. *LA* = left atrium.

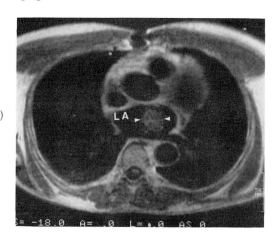

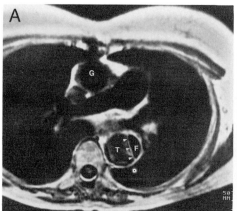

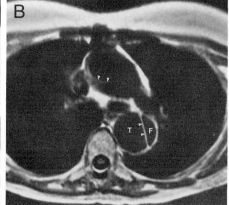

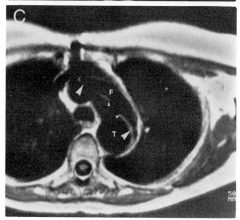

FIG 11–4.
Postoperative Debakey type I dissection of the aorta.
A, axial image at the level of the right pulmonary
artery shows the ascending aortic graft (*G*) and a
residual dissection in the descending aorta. The linear
high signal indicated by the *arrowheads* is an intimal
flap. Note the different signal between the true lumen
(*T*) and false (*F*) lumen, indicating different flow
velocity. **B,** axial image 1 cm higher shows the residual
intimal flap in both the ascending and descending
aorta (*arrowheads*). **C,** axial image at the level of the
aortic arch shows a large intimal flap extending into
both ascending and descending aorta (*large
arrowheads*) with a large defect within the intimal flap
(*small arrowheads*). T = true lumen, F = false
lumen.

On a double echo sequence, slow-flowing blood typically shows increased signal on a second echo as a result of even echo rephasing.[15]

Aneurysm of the Thoracic Aorta

Magnetic resonance imaging can clearly delineate the extension of the aneurysms of the thoracic aorta and their relationship to adjacent structures in the chest. Aneurysms appear as an area of dilation and irregularity with variable amounts of intramural thrombus (Fig 11–5). The aneurysm often contains flow artifacts that reflect the ectatic and turbulent flow present within the aneurysm. The location of the aneurysm with respect to the great vessels and mediastinal structures is frequently evident. Calcifications apear as low-signal curvilinear densities within the aortic wall. This appearance should not be confused with a separation of media and intima. In these instances a chest x-ray or a CT scan can be very helpful. In mycotic aneurysms the location, size, and presence of a soft tissue mass are clearly seen.

In general, MRI is sufficient for the preoperative evaluation of patients with aneurysms of the thoracic aorta, and arteriography can obviated in the majority of patients.

Aortitis

In patients with Takayasu's aortitis and other inflammatory diseases of the aorta, the aorta appears irregular with thickened walls and abnormal luminal changes. At this time the resolution with MRI is inadequate for the study of branch stenosis. In Takayasu's disease, involvement of the pulmonary artery can also be seen.

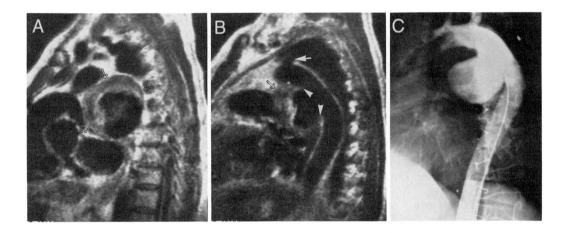

FIG 11–5.
A and **B**, atherosclerotic aneurysm of the thoracic aorta. Sagittal-coronal images show an 8-cm saccular aneurysm of the thoracic aorta (*open arrows*) with a broad neck (*arrowheads*) located distal to the left subclavian artery (*white arrow*). There is a large mural thrombus. Note the intermediate spiral-like signal within the aneurysm demonstrating circular and ectatic flow. **C**, aortogram confirms the presence of the aneurysm but gives very poor information regarding the mural thrombus or extension of the aneurysm.

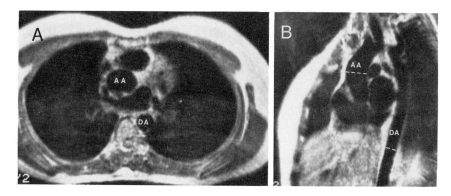

FIG 11–6.
Turner's syndrome in a 19-year-old patient. **A**, axial image at the level of the mid-ascending aorta (*AA*). *DA* = descending aorta. **B**, sagittal-coronal image at the level of the aortic arch. The midascending aorta (*AA*) is dilated. There is a ratio of 2.0:1 when compared with the descending aorta (*DA*) at the level of the diaphragm (normal ratio is 1.8:1).

Marfan's and Turner's Syndromes

In patients with Marfan's syndrome there is enlargement of the root of the ascending aorta and the sinuses of Valsalva. In patients with Turner's syndrome the aortic dilation, as shown in Figure 11–6, involves the midportion of the ascending aorta. These patients with congenital weakness of the media are at increased risk for aortic dissection and rupture. Furthermore, patients with Turner's syndrome are at an increased risk of aortic rupture with a lesser degree of aortic dilation than patients with aneurysm from other causes. Echocardiography is useful in evaluation of the lower portion of the ascending aorta; however, it is operator dependent and can give misleading echocardiographic measurements. Magnetic resonance imaging is now an accepted noninvasive method for follow-up study of these patients.

Traumatic Lesions

Traumatic lesions of the aorta may be lethal if not diagnosed early. Post-traumatic aortic tear, pseudoaneurysm formation, mediastinal bleeding, and lung contusion can be identified in patients with severe trauma. Aortic tears appear as areas of luminal irregularities, with a high signal band within the lumen representing the retracted torn aortic wall (Fig 11–7). We recommend MRI of the aorta in patients with a history of trauma in which the index of suspicion for an aortic rupture is relatively low. In these patients other causes of mediastinal widening can be readily diagnosed with MR imaging, thus obviating the need for arteriography. Patients in unstable condition or with a high index of suspicion of an aortic tear should undergo arteriography or CT examination.

Abdominal Aorta Aneurysms

Although aneurysms of the abdominal aorta can be easily seen with MRI (Fig 11–8).[30, 31]

the origin of the renal arteries is difficult to identify because of tortuosity of the abdominal aorta. Ultrasonography remains the primary imaging modality in these patients and, if required, arteriography to identify the relationship of the aneurysm and the major abdominal vessels.[31]

CONGENITAL ABNORMALITIES OF THE AORTIC ARCH

Magnetic resonance imaging has shown a high sensitivity in demonstrating anomalies of the aortic arch in older children and adults.[32, 33] Echocardiography has high sensitivity in

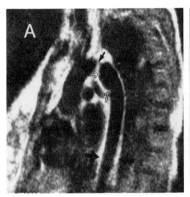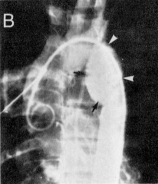

FIG 11–7.
Traumatic aortic tear. **A,** sagittal-coronal MR image at the level of the aortic arch shows a pseudoaneurysm at the aortic isthmus (*open arrows*) with a high-signal ledge at the area of the aortic rupture (*small solid arrow*) representing the proximal retracted walls of the torn aorta. There is also a periaortic hematoma (*large arrows*). **B,** thoracic aortogram confirmed the pseudoaneurysm (*arrows and arrowheads*). At surgery a complete transection of the aorta was found.

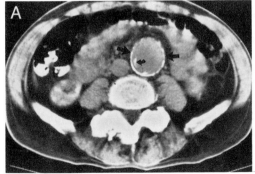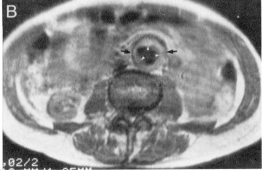

FIG 11–8.
Abdominal aortic aneurysm. **A,** CT scan at the level of the L-3 vertebral body shows a calcified abdominal aortic aneurysm (*straight arrows*). There are also calcifications within the mural thrombus (*curved arrow*). **B,** T1-weighted MR image at the same level shows the aneurysm. The mural thrombus and lumen are clearly defined (*arrowheads*). Calcifications appear as low signal (*arrows*).

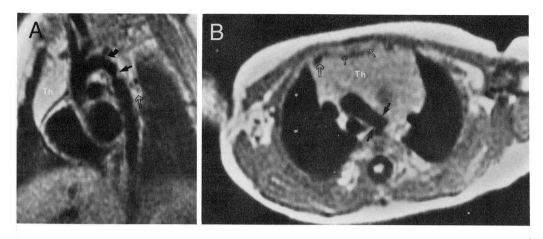

FIG 11–9.
Coarctation of the aorta. **A,** sagittal-coronal MR image shows a well-developed ascending aorta and a coarctation of the aorta (*straight arrow*) distal to the origin of the left subclavian artery (*curved arrow*). Collaterals are seen posteriorly (*open arrow*). Th = thymus. **B,** axial image at the level of the aortic arch shows tapering at the distal arch (*arrows*). There is a large internal mammary artery (*open arrows*) and a large mediastinal collateral, suggesting a high-grade coarctation.

neonates and infants but a lower sensitivity in older children. In adults, a complete echo-cardiographic study of the heart and great vessels may not be possible because of limitations in ultrasonic windows, the presence of calcified ribs, and chest deformities. Also, in patients with obstructive lung disease, intervening lung parenchyma may result in an inadequate study. On MRI the position of the ascending and descending aorta and the relationship of both aorta and pulmonary arteries are well demonstrated. The type of arch, the presence of diverticula, and the course of the descending aorta are demonstrated. Coarctation of the aorta can be seen in axial and sagittal-coronal views (Fig 11–9). In patients with a tortuous aortic arch, tortuosity may impede visualization of coarctation on the sagittal-oblique projection, but this difficulty can sometimes be overcome by interleaved scans or interleaved axial scans through the level of coarctation.[32]

Patent ductus arteriosus (PDA) less than 1 cm in diameter has been identified by utilizing interleaved axial and sagittal coronal MR images at the level of the aortic arch and main pulmonary artery.[29] However, PDA can be accurately demonstrated at echocardiography in a large proportion of infants and children with this anomaly.[32] The right aortic arch and the double aortic arch are easily identified on MR images. In truncus arteriosus and transposition of the great vessels, MRI may provide information regarding the relationship of the great vessels; the size of the pulmonary arteries; and, in cases of aortic pulmonary window, the echocardiographic diagnosis can be confirmed.

The use of MRI to visualize the aortic arch in children is recommended when the echocardiographic findings are inconclusive or clinical symptoms are severe enough to warrant catheterization. Because 2D echocardiography is less reliable, MRI plays a much more important role in the detection of aortic arch anomalies in adults. With the advent of newer techniques such as cine MRI and MR angiography, the role of MRI in the evaluation of the aorta is increasing.

REFERENCES

1. Higgins CB, Stark D, McNamara M, et al: Multiplane magnetic resonance imaging of the heart and major vessels: Studies in normal volunteers. *AJR* 1984; 142:661–667.
2. Herfkens RJ, Higgins CB, Hricak H, et al: Nuclear magnetic resonance imaging of atherosclerotic disease. *Radiology* 1983; 148:161–166.
3. Reed JD, Soulen RL: Cardiovascular MRI: Current role in patient management. *Radiol Clin North Am* 1988; 26:589–606.
4. Murphy WA, Gutierrez FR, Levitt RG, et al: Oblique views of the heart by magnetic resonance imaging. *Radiology* 1985; 154:225–226.
5. Feiglin DH, George CR, MacIntyre WJ, et al: Gated cardiac magnetic resonance structural imaging: Optimization by electronic axial rotation. *Radiology* 1985; 154:129–132.
6. Dinsmore RE, Wismer GL, Miller SW, et al: Magnetic resonance imaging of the heart using image planes oriented to cardiac axes: Experience with 100 cases. *AJR* 1985; 145:1177–1183.
7. Utz JA, Herfkens RJ, Heinsimer JA, et al: Valvular regurgitation: Dynamic MR imaging. *Radiology* 1988; 168:91–94.
8. Utz JA, Herfkens RJ, Heinsimer JA, et al: Cine MR determination of left ventricular ejection fraction. *AJR* 1987; 148:839–843.
9. Sechtem U, Pflugfelder P, Cassidy MC, et al: Ventricular septal defect: Visualization of shunt flow and determination of shunt size by cine MR imaging. *AJR* 1987; 149:689–692.
10. Bottomley PA, Herfkens RJ, Smith LS, et al: Altered phosphate metabolism in myocardial infarction: P-31 MR spectroscopy. *Radiology* 1987; 165:703–707.
11. Didier D, Higgins CB, Fisher MR, et al: Congenital heart disease: Gated MR imaging in 72 patients. *Radiology* 1986; 158:227–235.
12. Stratemeier EJ, Thompson R, Brady TJ, et al: Ejection fraction determination by MR imaging: Comparison with left ventricular angiography. *Radiology* 1986; 158:775–777.
13. McNamara MT, Higgins CB: Magnetic resonance imaging of chronic myocardial infarcts in man. *AJR* 1986; 146:315–320.
14. Higgins CB, Lanzer P, Stark D et al: Imaging by nuclear magnetic resonance in patients with chronic ischemic heart disease. *Circulation* 1984; 69:523–531.
15. Zeitler E, Kaiser W, Schuierer G, et al: Magnetic resonance imaging of aneurysms and thrombi. *Cardiovasc Intervent Radiol* 1986; 8:321–328.
16. Tscholakoff D, Higgins CG, McNamara MT, et al: Early phase myocardial infarction: Evaluation by MR imaging. *Radiology* 1986; 159:667–672.
17. Higgins CB, Herfkens R, Lipton MJ, et al: Nuclear magnetic resonance imaging of acute myocardial infarction in dogs: Alteration in magnetic relaxation times. *Am J Cardiol* 1983; 52:184–188.
18. Fisher MR, McNamara MT, Higgins CB: Acute myocardial infarction: MR evaluation in 29 patients. *AJR* 1987; 148:247–251.
19. von Schulthess GK, Fisher MR, Crooks LE, et al: Gated MR imaging of the heart: Intracardiac signals in patients and healthy subjects. *Radiology* 1985; 156:125–132.
20. Gomes AS, Lois JF, Child JS, et al: Cardiac tumors and thrombus: Evaluation with MR imaging. *AJR* 1987; 149:895–899.
21. Dooms GC, Higgins CB: MR imaging of cardiac thrombi. *J Comput Assist Tomogr* 1986; 10:415–420.
22. Gomes AS, Lois JF, Drinkwater DC, et al: Coronary artery bypass grafts: Visualization with MR imaging. *Radiology* 1987; 162:175–179.
23. White RD, Caputo GR, Mark AS, et al: Coronary artery bypass graft patency: Noninvasive evaluation with MR imaging. *Radiology* 1987; 164:681–686.
24. Love HG, Jenkins JPR, Foster CJ, et al: Coronary artery bypass graft patency as assessed by magnetic resonance imaging. *J Am Coll Cardiol* 1986; 7:147A.
25. Higgins CB, Byrd BF III, Farmer EW, et al: Magnetic resonance imaging in patients with congenital heart disease. *Circulation* 1984; 70:851–860.
26. Fletcher BD, Jacobstein MD, Nelson AD, et al: Gated magnetic resonance imaging of congenital cardiac malformations. *Radiology* 1984; 150:137–140.

27. Boxer RA, Singh S, LaCorte MA, et al: Nuclear magnetic resonance imaging in the evaluation and follow-up of children treated for coarctation of the aorta. *J Am Coll Cardiol* 1986; 7:1095–1098.

28. Come PC, Ryley MF, Markis JE, et al: Limitations of echocardiographic techniques in evaluation of left atrial masses. *Am J Cardiol* 1981; 48:947–953.

29. Lois JF, Gomes AS, Brown K, et al: Magnetic resonance imaging of the thoracic aorta. *Am J Cardiol* 1987; 60:352–358.

30. Lee JKT, Ling D, Heiken JP, et al: Magnetic resonance imaging of abdominal aortic aneurysms. *AJR* 1984; 143:1197–1202.

31. Amparo EG, Hoddick WK, Hricak H, et al: Comparison of magnetic resonance imaging and ultrasonography in the evaluation of abdominal aortic aneurysms. *Radiology* 1985; 154:451–456.

32. Gomes AS, Lois JF, George B, et al: Congenital abnormalities of the aortic arch: MR imaging. *Radiology* 1987; 165:691–695.

33. Amparo EG, Higgins CB, Shafton EP: Demonstration of coarctation of the aorta by magnetic resonance imaging. *AJR* 1984; 143:1192–1194.

Chapter 12

Magnetic Resonance Imaging of the Abdomen and Pelvis

Zoran L. Barbaric, M.D.

Lee C. Chiu, M.D.

LIVER

The liver is the largest parenchymal organ in the body and a frequent site for metastasis from a number of primary cancer sites. Metastases are the most frequent focal liver masses in patients with a known primary malignancy elsewhere. The most common focal liver mass in a patient with no known malignant disease is cavernous hemangioma (4% to 6% at autopsy), followed by focal fatty infiltration. The major emphasis in imaging the liver in a patient with a known primary malignant disease is differentiation between these entities. The acceptance of magnetic resonance imaging (MRI) of the liver will depend on how much better than computed tomography (CT) this imaging modality is in this particular task.

Computed tomography is a superb imaging modality for depiction of metastatic disease elsewhere in the abdomen, such as metastases to lymph nodes, kidneys, spleen, adrenals, retroperitoneum, and skeletal system. It is also good in differentiation of bowel from mass lesions and is thus far the best imaging modality for discovery of small pancreatic tumors. All this is done effectively and repetitively without significant variation from patient to patient, allowing standardization of the technique.[1] To be effective, MR must perform these tasks in a similar time frame and for a similar cost.

Pulse Sequences

Generally, T1-weighted and T2-weighted spin echo sequences are employed in imaging of the liver.[2] The T2 sequences that utilize motion suppression techniques are more effective in depicting the lesion. In general, T2-weighted sequences are preferred in high magnetic field imaging such as 1.5 tesla (T). A triple echo sequence of SE 2400/60, 120, 180 has been advocated by Stark et al. and reported to have 95% accuracy in differentiating cavernous hemangioma and liver carcinoma.[3, 4]

Techniques such as rapid imaging with suspended respiration,[5] dynamic MRI,[6] respiratory gating, or inversion recovery[7] are variations that may or may not become useful in the future of abdominal-pelvic imaging.

Are Magnetic Resonance Images Interpretable?

Motion artifacts and improper choice of pulse sequences severely impair the quality of MR images. The quality varies depending on the level of each patient's ability to lie still for the time necessary to complete the examination. The differences in quality from different machines also vary greatly. In general, if one can identify major hepatic veins and secondary branches of the portal system and the image is overall "grain" free, the signal-to-noise ratio is probably high and the image is considered good.

On heavily weighted T1 images, liver is usually more hyperintense (brighter) than the spleen. On T2-weighted images the liver becomes hypointense (darker) while the spleen becomes hyperintense (brighter). Also, one can judge whether there was enough T2 weighting by the appearance of the spinal fluid, which should become hyperintense (bright) on that pulse sequence. Tumors such as metastases and lymphoma tend to have signal intensities similar to that of spleen; therefore, the contrast difference between the spleen and the liver is a good indicator of what the contrast difference between liver and a tumor should be.

Paramagnetic Contrast Materials

Stable colloidal suspension of iron oxide administered intravenously several hours before the study may well become the method of choice for MRI of the liver. Colloidal particles are phagocytosed by the reticuloendothelial system of the healthy liver and are not retained in the area of metastases. Iron oxide, by increasing transverse relaxation, dramatically reduces signal intensity in the area of its distribution. Contrast difference between iron-laden liver and metastasis is greatly improved. Stark et al. report that the total number of detected lesions increased from 89 on precontrast images to 349 on postcontrast images (SE 500/28) in their series of 15 patients.[8] Smaller lesions were readily detected. The pharmaceutical compound is expected to be commercially available in several years.

Lipomatous Tumors

Angiomyolipoma and lipoma are rare benign tumors of the liver. Liver angiomyolipoma is associated with renal angiomyolipoma and tuberous sclerosis. Having high fat content, these tumors are easily detected on T1 spin echo sequences, where they appear hyperintense in comparison with the liver. In patients with tuberous sclerosis, other benign liver tumors may be present such as adenoma.

Cavernous Hemangioma

Cavernous hemangioma is a common benign tumor of the liver, with a reported incidence of 5% to 15%. On T1-weighted spin echo sequences it usually presents as a low-signal lesion compared with surrounding liver parenchyma.[9] Occasionally there will be a central nidus with an even lower signal intensity referred to as a "scar."

On T2-weighted images the mass becomes intensely bright (hyperintense) compared with almost any other focal liver mass (Fig 12–1). If present, the "scar," which has a high water content, also becomes hyperintense and blends with the rest of the tumor on T2-weighted

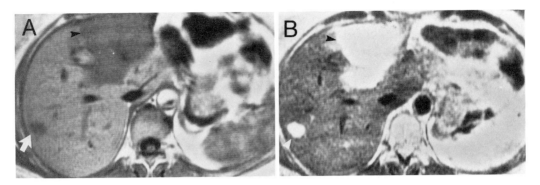

FIG 12–1.
Liver hemangiomas. Hemangiomas (*arrowheads*) are hypointense on T1-weighted sequences (**A**) (SE 18/300) and become very hyperintense on heavily T2-weighted sequences (**B**) (SE 85/2000, 0.3-T permanent magnet).

sequences. Diagnostic sensitivity and specificity are reported to be 84% and 85%, respectively, just on the basis of hyperintensity on T2-weighted images.

Tumor margins are sharply defined and rounded. When these criteria are computed together with the brightness on T2-weighted images, sensitivity and specificity improve to 90%.[10]

The modalities now competing for diagnostic accuracy are technetium-99m (^{99m}Tc) red blood cell imaging,[11] single photon emission CT,[9] dynamic CT, aspiration biopsy,[12] and selective angiography. Overall accuracy in the abdomen for these imaging modalities is shown on Table 12–1.

Differentiation between hemangioma and metastases from colon carcinoma is as high as 97.5% with MRI. Other metastases such as islet cell tumor and carcinoid are differentiated from hemangioma less frequently (61%).[13]

Although the MRI detection rate for cavernous hemangiomas is as high as 100%, other focal lesions may have similar features. It should be remembered that hepatic cysts, metastasis, hepatoma, and other focal liver masses may mimic the MRI findings of cavernous hemangioma and at times are indistinguishable.

Atypical appearance of cavernous hemangioma, such as less brightness or contour irregularity, may occur in the presence of hemorrhage and fibrosis.[14] Differentiation between hemangioma and hepatocellular carcinoma is reported as high as 94.6% on a 0.35-T instrument if T2 calculated values of the mass lesion are obtained using the two-point method.[15]

TABLE 12–1.

Overall Accuracy in the Diagnosis of Cavernous Hemangioma

Modality*	% Accuracy
Technetium-red blood cell imaging	90
MR imaging	90
CT scanning	53–89
US scanning	40

*MR = magnetic resonance, CT = computed tomography, US = ultrasound. For discussion, see text.

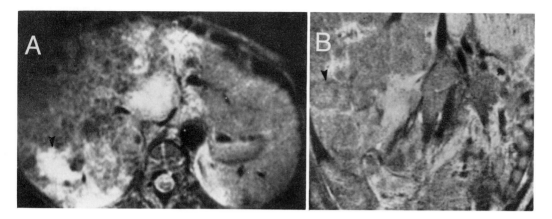

FIG 12–2.
Liver metastases from carcinoma of the colon. **A,** on a T2-weighted sequence (SE 100/2000), metastases (*arrowhead*) are irregular and give relatively high signal, which makes them bright. **B,** short inversion recovery technique using fat suppression may make metastases more readily visible as gray masses (*arrowhead*) within the liver.

Liver Metastases

Detection of metastasis to the liver may drastically alter the patient's prognosis and management. T1 and T2 relaxation times of liver metastases are significantly longer than those of the surrounding liver, allowing for contrast discrimination. By allowing either T1 or T2 tissue contrast to dominate the image, it should be possible to demonstrate metastatic disease in a high percentage of cases. On T1-weighted images the metastasis will be relatively hypointense (dark) in comparison with the surrounding liver tissues; on T2-weighted images it will appear as hyperintense (bright). The signal intensity (brightness) on a T2-weighted sequence is appreciably less than that for a cavernous hemangioma and more or less approaches the intensity exhibited by the spleen.

On low field strength magnets, both T1-weighted spin echo sequences are excellent for detection of the lesion if very short TE and TR are used. The signal-to-noise ratio is particularly good. The display of anatomic resolution and time necessary to complete the sequence outperforms T2-weighted spin echo sequences and inversion recovery sequences. On high field strength magnets, T2-weighted sequences have distinct advantage (Fig 12–2).

Internal architecture of a liver metastasis is often mixed with areas of necrosis, hemorrhage, and in some instances calcifications. Many metastases, particularly the larger ones, exhibit mixed signal intensities with the mass as compared to hemangioma or hepatic cyst.

Unfortunately at this point there is a discrepancy between the true value of MRI and CT scanning in evaluating focal liver masses. A recent study states that 95.4% of liver metastases may be imaged on the short T1 SE sequence.[16] Others do not find MRI superior to CT in the detection of liver metastasis.[17–20] What is certain is that more research is needed in this area, preferably on a multi-institutional level. The introduction of paramagnetic contrast material for the liver into everyday use is likely to establish MRI as the method of choice in the not too distant future.

Hepatocellular Carcinoma

Hepatoma has a high cure rate if detected and resected early when the tumor mass is less than 2 cm in diameter. The characteristic feature of the tumor is the fibrous capsule that surrounds the tumor, a finding not seen in metastasis, hemangioma, cysts, and so forth. The capsule is more pronounced as the tumor becomes larger. Fibrous tissue is relatively hypointense on both T1- and T2-weighted sequences and may be seen surrounding the tumor (ring sign). This capsule is apparently seen better with MRI (43%) than with CT (24%).[21]

Otherwise the tumor is isointense or slightly hyperintense to the liver on T1-weighted images and—as is the case with most liver masses—hyperintense on T2-weighted images[22] (Fig 12–3). Hepatocellular carcinoma may occasionally have an increased amount of fat, the presence of which may influence its appearance on MR images.

One of the frequent findings associated with hepatocellular carcinoma is extension of the tumor into the portal venous system. This may be demonstrated on MR images and becomes a useful differentiating feature.

Hepatic Cyst

Simple cyst of the liver does not occur as frequently as cysts in the kidney; nevertheless, it is a relatively common liver mass. In general these cysts are hypointense on T1-weighted sequences. Depending on the amount of protein in the fluid, the cyst may be very hyperintense on T2-weighted sequences and be indistinguishable from cavernous hemangioma on morphologic criteria alone (Fig 12–4). Both have a smooth, rounded appearance and are relatively homogeneous.

Hemorrhagic cyst of the liver may be hyperintense on both T1- and T2-weighted sequence.[23] There is a parallel with the hemorrhagic cysts of the kidney, numerous variations in signal intensities are possible.

Amebic Liver Abscess

Similar to most focal liver lesions, abscess is of lower signal intensity (darker) than the

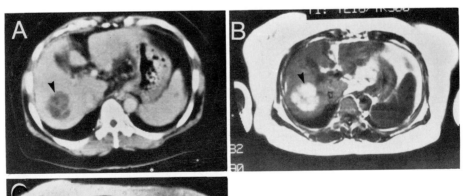

FIG 12–3.
Hepatoma after chemotherapy. On a CT scan with contrast material. (**A**) the liver mass (*arrowhead*) is nonenhancing. The combination of a very intense signal on T1-weighted sequence. (**B**) (SE 16/300) and rather low signal on T2-weighted sequence. (**C**) (SE 100/2000; 1.5-T superconducting magnet) suggests the presence of methemoglobin within the mass. (*Arrowheads* point to the hepatoma.)

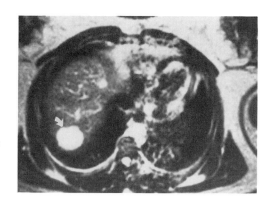

FIG 12–4.
Simple hepatic cyst (*arrow*) is hypointense on T1-weighted sequences and becomes hyperintense on T2-weighted sequence (SE 100/2000, 0.5-T superconducting magnet). The cyst may be difficult to differentiate from a hemangioma, which also may be smooth in appearance and give a very bright signal in this sequence.

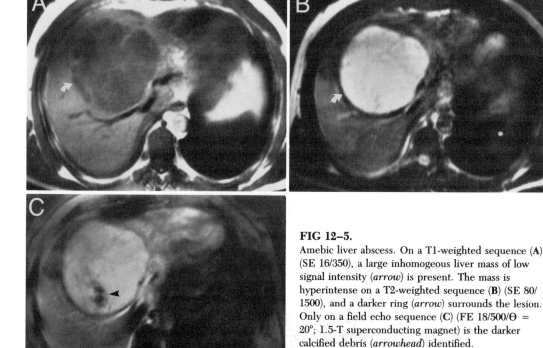

FIG 12–5.
Amebic liver abscess. On a T1-weighted sequence (**A**) (SE 16/350), a large inhomogeous liver mass of low signal intensity (*arrow*) is present. The mass is hyperintense on a T2-weighted sequence (**B**) (SE 80/1500), and a darker ring (*arrow*) surrounds the lesion. Only on a field echo sequence (**C**) (FE 18/500/Θ = 20°; 1.5-T superconducting magnet) is the darker calcified debris (*arrowhead*) identified.

liver on T1-weighted images and hyperintense (brighter) on T2-weighted studies (Fig 12–5). In the acute stage there may be edema surrounding the abscess. Within a period of several days, liquefaction within the abscess can be identified, and occasionally a fluid-fluid level. Irregularity of the inner wall and inhomogeneous appearance help distinguish it from simple cyst or hemangioma.[24–26]

In the healing stage, concentric dark and bright rings encircle the shrinking mass. These rings are quite common in the healing amebic abscess. The inner ring, which appears dark on T1- and T2-weighted images, likely represents collagen tissues. The surrounding area of hyperintensity representing edema of the normal tissues gradually disappears.[24–26]

Differential diagnosis includes metastases, bacterial liver abscess, and hematoma. Therefore, the concentric rings and internal architecture are nonspecific.[3]

An amebic empyema can be differentiated from a simple effusion as it is hyperintense (bright) on both T1- and T2-weighted sequences.

Fatty Infiltration

The liver will appear hyperintense as compared with the spleen on T1-weighted images.[27–30] Only moderate involvement can be detected. Spectroscopy may be the method of choice in the future. Focal fatty infiltration may present a diagnostic problem. The liver area involved is likely to be somewhat hyperintense on both T1- and T2-weighted images.

Hemosiderosis

Liver overload with iron may occur in conjunction with transfusional and idiopathic hemosiderosis. Low molecular weight iron, ferritin, hemosiderin, and hemoproteins are all found in increased quantities within the liver. Because some may act as a paramagnetic contrast medium, the liver may be quite hypointense (dark) on T1-weighted sequences[31, 32] (Fig 12–6).

Cirrhosis

Cirrhotic liver is usually small with an irregular surface and distorted intrahepatic vasculature. Cirrhotic liver, however, may still retain its normal configuration. Because there is abundance of fibrous tissues, the liver is predominantly hypointense (dark) on both T1- and T2-weighted sequences.[33–37] Regenerating hyperplastic nodules may be distinguished as somewhat hyperintense, rounded structures.[34–36]

Extrahepatic venous collaterals will be seen in the majority of patients.[3] These may be present in the splenic hilus and retrohepatic region, and anastomose with retroperitoneal vessels or extend anteriorly to the anterior abdominal wall or lower esophagus.

Ascites is common. The spleen may be enlarged.

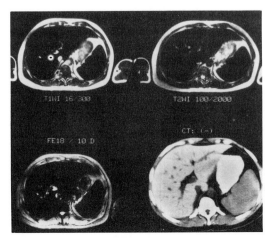

FIG 12–6.
Hemochromatosis. Both liver and spleen are exhibiting very low signal intensity on a T1-weighted sequence (*upper left*, SE 16/300), T2-weighted sequence (*upper right*, SE 100/2000), and field echo sequence (*lower left*, FE 18/400, 0.5-T superconducting magnet). CT scan (*lower right*) is given for comparison.

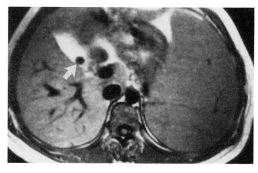

FIG 12–7.
Gallstone *(arrow)* and splenomegaly (SE 26/1066, 0.5-T superconducting magnet).

Budd-Chiari Syndrome

Venous outflow obstruction from the liver is most commonly caused by tumors arising from adrenal, liver, kidney, and retroperitoneum. The less common causes are congenital hepatic vein webs, polycythemia vera, and oral contraceptive use resulting in thrombosis. Primary tumors of the inferior vena cava are a rare cause.

The most prominent finding is the absence of hepatic veins on T1-weighted images (SE 300/18) and slitlike narrowing of the intrahepatic portion of the inferior vena cava.[38] A mass compressing the inferior vena cava or hepatic veins is usually present, and its origin can usually be determined. An intracaval web may be seen as the primary cause in rare instances.

Retroperitoneal collateral venous circulation develops in less than half of the patients. If the vena cava is involved, the azygos vein is likely to enlarge because it serves as a major collateral pathway. Intrahepatic collaterals may assume a pathognomonic "comma shape"[1] which, of course, is the characteristic ultrasound finding in this syndrome.

BILIARY TRACT AND PANCREAS

Normal Appearance

The gallbladder of a healthy patient is usually hypointense (dark) on T1-weighted images and hyperintense (bright) on T2-weighted images as compared with the liver. There is sufficient variability in signal intensity from the gallbladder, however, to address this topic very cautiously.[39]

Cholelithiasis

Gallstones have very low signal intensity and therefore can be detected under a dark form within the bright gallbladder on T2-weighed sequences more so than on T1-weighted sequences. Just what percentage of stones is detected by MRI is still not clear (Fig 12–7). Ultrasound obviously remains the imaging method of choice.

Cholecystitis

An inflamed gallbladder does not contain concentrated bile. On the contrary, the bile has been diluted by excretion of water (exudate) in the gallbladder, and the normal concentrating function of this organ is therefore reversed. It is not surprising that on a T1-weighted sequence (SE 500/56) the gallbladder may be more hypointense (darker) than the liver. Gallstones are no longer visible because they are also hypointense (dark) on this sequence and are not contrasted at all. Heavier T2-weighted pulse sequences are necessary under those conditions to bring out the contrast differences between the two structures.[40]

Chronic and acute cholecystitis are also difficult to separate from each other. Thickening of the gallbladder wall may be found in both instances. Pericystic fluid may also be present. In emphysematous cholecystitis one may expect a hypointense wall on T1- and T2-weighted sequences.

There are sufficient discrepancies, however, to conclude that more research is needed in this area before the more traditional imaging methods to replace MRI are even considered.

Biliary Dilatation

Both the intrahepatic and extrahepatic portions of the biliary system may be detected on MRI.[41] In general, bile will have low signal intensity on T1-weighted images and high signal intensity on T2, so that the dilated biliary tract may be distinguished from the venous or arterial system. One should recognize that bile signal intensity is variable and dependent on bile concentration, fasting, pressure within the biliary tract, and other factors. Ultrasound remains the imaging method of choice.

Cholangiocarcinoma

This uncommon tumor is potentially curable but difficult to diagnose preoperatively. Well-differentiated adenocarcinoma and scirrhous cholangiocarcinoma are two major subtypes. Both are isointense to the liver on T1-weighted images. On a T2-weighted sequence the adenocarcinomas have greater signal intensity than the liver, while the scirrhous type is generally almost isointense with the liver.[42] Nevertheless both types are detectable at about the same rate as they are on CT and ultrasound scanning (Fig 12–8). Ultrasound is somewhat more sensitive in the detection of biliary tract dilation. However, in the detection of portal vein invasion and establishment of its relationship to other major intrahepatic vessels, MRI may offer some advantages over CT. Extension into the liver and distant liver metastasis are also evident. Radiation therapy may decrease the signal intensity from the tumor, probably as a result of the cicatrization process in the healing stage.

PANCREAS

There is a paucity of literature concerning MR imaging of the pancreas.[43] The spatial resolution of CT is difficult to surpass, and peristaltic and other motion artifacts degrade MR images. Also, calcifications, such as occur in chronic pancreatitis or in certain tumors, may not be readily apparent. Nevertheless, on occasion, the pancreas may be exquisitely displayed on T1- and T2-weighted images. The smaller vascular structures surrounding the pancreas are much better seen on MR images than on CT scans. Anterior and posterior venous pancreaticoduodenal arcades are particularly well delineated.

Small pancreatic tumors are probably better examined by CT. Pancreatic pseudocysts and cystadenocarcinoma may show fluid levels of different signal intensity (Fig 12–9). Abscesses are seen as massive pancreatic enlargements with varying signal intensities.

Dilation of the pancreatic duct is detected on occasion. Post-traumatic hematoma of the second portion of the duodenum ("ring sign") may be beautifully demonstrated on T2 images.[44]

ADRENAL GLANDS

Adrenal masses are largely an incidental finding. The vast majority of adrenal masses are either nonfunctioning adrenal adenomas or metastases. In patients with primary malignancy elsewhere, one half of adrenal masses discovered during the work-up are metastases and the other half are benign and unimportant adenomas. The only method for differentiating between the two is either thin-needle aspiration biopsy or observable difference in the size of the adrenal mass in comparison with old examinations. All other adrenal masses are less common.

Detection

Adrenal glands are seen on most MRI studies almost equally well in both the coronal

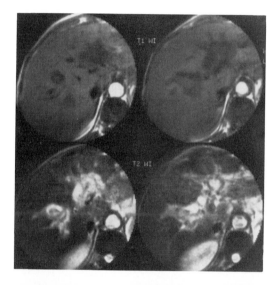

FIG 12–8.
Cholangiocarcinoma. Blood clots and tumor are seen in the dilated biliary ducts. T1-weighted sequence (*upper row*) and T2-weighted sequence (*lower row*, 0.5-T superconducting magnet).

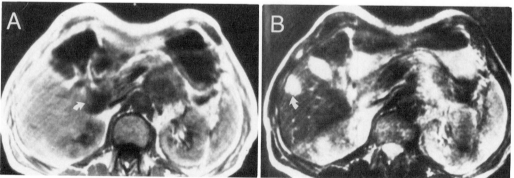

FIG 12–9.
Pancreas is perhaps the most elusive organ yet to be imaged by MRI. Moderate size pancreatic carcinoma is seen in the tail (*arrow*) and appears hypointense on a T1-weighted sequence (**A**) (SE 20/700). On T2-weighted sequences (**B**) (SE 80/2000, 0.3-T permanent magnet), the tumor has areas of high and medium signal intensities. A hyperintense liver metastasis is visible only on a T2-weighted sequence (*arrow*).

and transverse planes. Enlargement, abnormal contour, mass effect, and displacement of the adjacent organs are identical to what one expects to see on CT scans. MRI is equal to CT scanning in establishing the presence of adrenal masses for lesions larger than 1 cm.[45]

On T1- and T2-weighted sequences the adrenal glands are of a signal intensity similar to that of the liver.[46–48]

Calcification

Computed tomography is admittedly superior to MRI in the detection of minute adrenal calcification. Calcification is associated with a variety of benign and neoplastic conditions such as tuberculosis, adrenal cysts, Wolman's disease, Waterhouse-Frederick syndrome, neuro-blastoma, adenocarcinoma, and metastasis. Therefore, the presence or absence of calcification is of no practical value in trying to establish whether the mass is benign or malignant.

Hemorrhage and Necrosis

Both hemorrhage and necrosis may alter the signal characteristics of an adrenal mass. In general, hemorrhage is hyperintense on both T1- and T2-weighted sequences. Mixed, inhomogeneous signal is associated with tumor necrosis and is likely associated only with large neoplasms.

Nonfunctioning Adenoma vs. Adrenal Metastasis

Nonfunctioning adrenal adenoma tends to be isointense to the normal adrenal gland while adrenal metastasis tends to be hyperintense to the normal gland on T2-weighted imaging sequences.[49–51] Not all adenomas or metastases will behave in this way, however. The relative brightness exhibited by the mass may be measured as the signal intensity ratio between the lesion and some other tissues such as liver or retroperitoneal fat. In a recent report adrenal masses with a mass:liver intensity ratio of greater than 1.4 were metastases, while those less than 1.2 were adenomas.[50] Similarly, malignant masses had mass:fat intensity ratio greater than 0.8 while for adenomas the ratio was less than 0.6.[46] In both instances there was a gray zone where 21% and 31% of masses were indeterminate with respect to malignancy.

It is not surprising that the nonfunctioning adenomas may become hyperintense on T2-weighted sequences. Necrosis and hemorrhage of different degrees and varying ages may be found in the tumor, accounting for the aberrant behavior.[51]

Metastases may also be of relatively low signal intensity on T2-weighted sequences, contrary to what is expected.[8] This may significantly and adversely affect the specificity of MRI in differentiating between benign and malignant adrenal disease.

Pheochromocytoma

The diagnosis of pheochromocytoma is a clinical one. Extra-adrenal pheochromocytoma is present in 10% to 15% of patients and bilateral in 10% of the patients. The tumor is rarely malignant. Metastases in liver, lungs, lymph nodes, and bones may be functional. Elevated levels of serum catacholamines, urinary metanephrines, and vanillylmandelic acid (VMA) are found in a majority of the patients.

Pheochromocytoma is isointense to the liver on T1-sequences and markedly hyperintense on T2-weighted sequences.[52–56] Therefore the tumor, particularly the extra-adrenal tumor, is well contrasted against the background. Because 15% of pheochromocytomas are extra-adrenal (63% to 84% in Sipple's syndrome), MRI is the imaging method of choice.

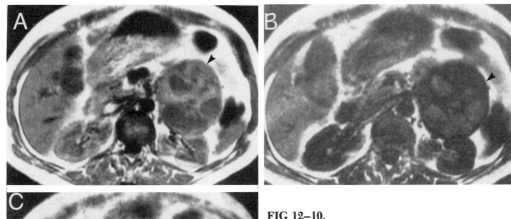

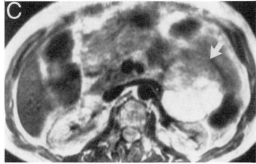

FIG 12–10.
Left adrenal pheochromocytoma exhibiting mixed signal intensities. On a T1-weighted sequence (**A**) the tumor (*arrowhead*) predominantly of low and medium signal intensity (SE 20/700). On inversion recovery (IR) sequence (**B**) the tumor (*arrowhead*) and the kidneys exhibit low signal intensity (IR 300/30/1651). Only parts of the tumor (*arrow*) are hyperintense on the T2-weighted sequence (**C**), indicating presence of tumor necrosis (SE 60/2000, 0.3T-permanent magnet).

Pheochromocytoma may produce mixed-intensity signal depending on intratumor hemorrhage, necrosis, and the presence of calcification (Fig 12–10).

Neuroblastoma

Neuroblastoma is a neural crest tumor originating from an adrenal (50%) or a sympathetic chain and is the most common solid malignant tumor in childhood. Both venous invasion and extension into the spinal canal are common. Ganglioneurinoma is a matured form of neuroblastoma. Distant metastases are present in 66% of patients at the time of diagnosis.

Ultrasound is the first examination of choice. Determination is made very rapidly if the palpable mass is solid or cystic (hydronephrosis, multicystic kidney, renal cyst).

In the presence of a solid abdominal mass and positive VMA test, imaging efforts are directed toward proper staging of the disease. Because vascular encasement and spinal cord involvement are crucial in determining surgical resectibility, MRI is the examination of choice.[56–58]

The tumor is hyperintense to the liver on T2-weighted images and about as intense as the liver on T1-weighted sequence. Internal architecture is usually uniform. Relatively low intensity calcifications are usually undetected by this imaging technique, although this is probably irrelevant.

Renal involvement, secondary hydronephrosis, lymph node enlargement, and bone metastases may all be identified.

Encasement of the great vessels is seen to greater advantage at MRI than on CT scanning because the vessels are so well depicted. Encasement of renal, celiac, and splenic veins as well that of the inferior vena cava have all been documented.

Finally, MRI is an excellent imaging modality for monitoring the effectiveness of therapy with regard to change in tumor size.

Cortical Hyperfunction

Primary hyperaldosteronism. Aldosteronomas are small tumors, frequently less than 1 cm in diameter, and should be searched for by CT as the primary imaging modality (Fig 12–11).[52]

Cushing's syndrome. Hyperfunctioning adrenal adenomas and adrenal carcinoma producing Cushing's syndrome are probably indistinguishable from nonfunctioning adrenal adenomas (Fig 12–12).[47–50] Adrenal carcinomas tend to grow large before the diagnosis is established. On occasion adrenal carcinoma may extend into the renal vein and inferior vena cava. About 50% of adrenal carcinomas are nonfunctioning and will not result in Cushing's syndrome.

Corticotropin (ACTH)-producing pheochromocytoma has also been described.[59] This tumor usually has a necrotic center and is hyperintense on T2-weighted MR sequences.

Secondary adrenal hyperplasia. Larger series are needed to determine the sensitivity and specificity of MRI in the detection of bilateral adrenal hyperplasia and macronodular hyperplasia secondary to ACTH-producing pituitary microadenomas.

Other Adrenal Masses

Myelolipoma is a benign neoplasm arising from the remnants of myeloproliferative tissues within the adrenal gland. The tumor consists of predominantly fatty tissues, and the signal intensities are similar to that of the surrounding retroperitoneal fat (Fig 12–13).

Adrenal cysts are usually hypointense on T1-weighted sequences, and hyperintense on T2-weighted sequences.

Summary: Imaging the Adrenal Glands

Magnetic resonance imaging is the modality of choice for evaluation of clinically suspected

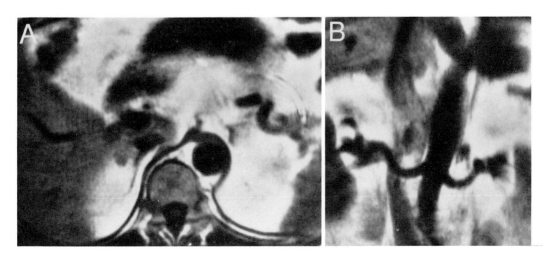

FIG 12–11.
Small aldosteronoma is seen in both axial (**A**) and coronal (**B**) imaging planes (SE 18/300, 0.3-T permanent magnet). These tumors are usually small, and CT may be the imaging modality of choice, considering its superior resolution. The first several centimeters of the renal arteries are well visualized and are unlikely to be involved with functionally significant atherosclerotic process.

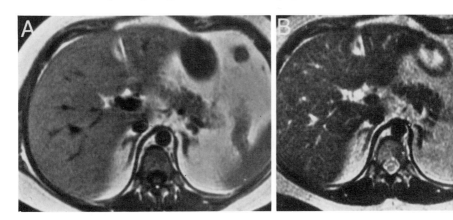

FIG 12–12.
Hyperfunctional cortical adenoma is detected in a patient with the symptoms of Cushing's syndrome. The tumor is of similar signal intensity to that of the adrenal gland on both T1-weighted (**A**) (SE 20/500) and T2-weighted sequences (**B**) (SE 80/2000, 0.3-T permanent magnet). At present, CT is considered superior in contrast resolution for detection of small tumors and focal nodular hyperplasia.

FIG 12–13.
Adrenal myelolipoma. Abundance of fat makes this benign tumor similar to the surrounding retroperitoneal fat (SE 18/300, 0.3-T permanent magnet). It remained unchanged in size for more than a year.

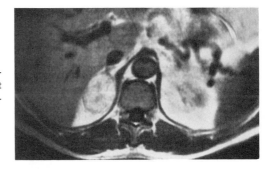

pheochromocytomas and for staging of neuroblastoma.

Magnetic resonance imaging is as good as CT in evaluating the presence of adrenal metastases in patients with primary malignancies elsewhere. Differentiating these from commonly present nonfunctioning adenomas may still require aspiration biopsy for definitive diagnosis. A very hyperintense mass on a T2-weighted sequence is more likely to be a metastasis, although there is an overlap.

Hyperfunctioning adrenal tumors and secondary hyperplasia are probably still best evaluated by CT. Aldosteronomas and Cushing's syndrome–producing adenomas are usually small, requiring the best resolution possible for their detection. Diffuse and macronodular hyperplasia is also difficult to detect even on CT.

Adrenal carcinoma, since it may extend into the major veins, is best staged using MRI.

RETROPERITONEUM

Lymph Nodes

Abdominal and pelvic lymph nodes are of medium signal intensity on T1-weighted SE sequences and are seen about as well as on CT.[60-63] On T2-weighted sequences lymph nodes become almost isointense to the surrounding fat and therefore are difficult to identify.

The most difficult aspect of lymph node MR imaging is differentiation between vessels and intestines.[63] Because bowel and nodes are frequently isointense, differentiation may on occasion be impossible, particularly in thin patients. Paramagnetic oral contrast material may eliminate this problem.

Vessels, particularly in the pelvis, may also be confused with the lymph nodes, principally because the signal intensity of the vessels may vary because of the "entry" phenomena. This problem may be solved by employing rapid single-slice gradient echo sequence over the area in question. The vessels become intensely bright on this sequence while the lymph nodes blend with the surrounding tissues, permitting differentiation.

Lymph nodes larger than 1 cm are considered abnormal. Coronal sections are quite useful because a very large area can be covered in a short period of time with very few slices, such as for repeated follow-up examinations after completion of therapy for diseases such as lymphoma and seminoma. Lack of radiation makes MRI a particularly attractive imaging modality for the latter group.

Inflammatory disease cannot be differentiated from malignant disease by the use of MRI.[61-63]

Oily lymphangiographic contrast material will render lymph nodes invisible, as the opacified lymph nodes become isointense with retroperitoneal fat. Under these circumstances CT is preferred over MRI.[64]

Primary Retroperitoneal Tumors

The most common primary retroperitoneal tumors are fibrosarcomas and liposarcomas. Liposarcomas may have high signal intensity on T1-weighted images because of an abundance of fatty tissue elements,[65, 66] although there are exceptions (Fig 12–14). Differentiation of fibrosarcomas from other tumors may be possible since a relatively high fibrous tissue component is likely to produce signal of low intensity on T2-weighted images.[67-69] Retroperitoneal hemangioma and hemangiopericytoma are hyperintense on T2-weighted sequences.[70]

Increased signal intensity may be found in the psoas muscle adjacent to a malignant tumor on T2-weighted sequences, a finding which may reflect the presence of edema.[71]

An obvious advantage of MRI is that it can provide imaging in different planes. This becomes particularly important in understanding the relation of the tumor to the great vessels prior to surgical removal of the tumor.

Retroperitoneal Fibrosis

Fibrous tissues are of low signal intensity both on T1- and T2-weighted sequences. Proliferation of fibrous tissues within the retroperitoneum may occur spontaneously or may be induced by various drugs. The cicatrizing process may produce ureteral and vascular occlusion and result in hydronephrosis. Collateral venous channels may develop and be detected on MR images. A leaking abdominal aortic aneurysm sometimes may result in retroperitoneal fibrosis.

Retroperitoneal Hematoma

Acute hemorrhage will present more or less as a mass lesion permeating along the retroperitoneal septations and fatty tissues. Occasionally on axial images sedimented blood is seen where distinct layers are clearly visible. Chronic blood accumulation will have an intense signal on T1- and T2-weighted sequences.[72]

Abscess

Inflammatory areas interspersed within the abscess cause an inhomogeneous intermediate signal, while gas appears dark on T1- and T2-weighted pulse sequences.[73] Abscess has relatively high signal intensity, somewhat less than fat, which increases on T2-weighted images.

Few retroperitoneal abscesses have been described, probably because these patients are usually too ill. They are often accompanied by intravenous poles, oxygen tanks, and respirators, which make the examination in the proximity of a strong magnet difficult.

Neurofibromatosis

Neurofibromas usually enlarge the neural foramen but may also be seen in the paraspinal and presacral regions. Masses of somewhat higher signal intensity than adjacent muscle are seen on T1-weighted images. On T2-weighted images neurofibromas become hyperintense as compared with the muscle and occasionally may show central areas of decreased signal intensity.[74]

ABDOMINAL VESSELS

The major drawbacks in abdominal vascular imaging with MRI are the "entry" phenomena

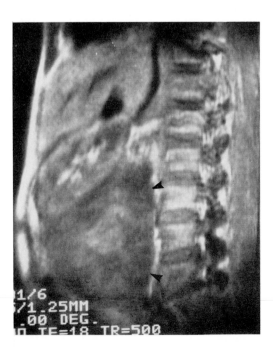

FIG 12–14.
Imaging in different planes may be useful on occasion. In this patient the tumor (*arrowheads*) is obviously displacing the kidney rather than originating from it. The cortex, as seen on this sagittal T1-weighted image (SE 18/500, 0.3-T permanent magnet), is intact and well contrasted with the adjacent mass. The tumor is a primary retroperitoneal liposarcoma. Unlike surrounding fat, it is relatively hypointense.

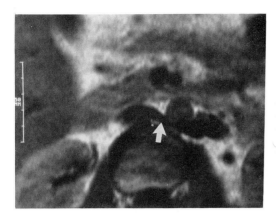

FIG 12–15.
Close-up view of a retroaortic left renal vein (*arrow*) in a patient with a testicular neoplasm. On CT the para-aortic component of this vessel was thought to represent an enlarged lymph node. Hypointense on a T1-weighted sequence, the vessel is easily distinguished from the lymph node, which is generally of medium signal intensity (SE 18/300, 0.3-T permanent magnet).

and turbulent flow in some vessels, which may give a false impression of intraluminal filling defect or narrowing. The outline of the major vessels is usually well seen on T1-weighted sequences if the patient is cooperative; unfortunately, this is also where the "entry" phenomena are the most pronounced. Slightly T2-weighted images (SE 1800/60) may show the vessels to better advantage, more consistently depicting hypointense lumen.[75] Image degradation resulting from longer acquisition time and motion artifacts is a disadvantage.

Projection gated subtraction angiography and other techniques are emerging.[76–78]

Venous System

Congenital anomalies such as left inferior vena cava, circumaortic venous ring, and retroaortic left renal vein are readily diagnosed and are unlikely to be confused with lymph node enlargement (Fig 12–15).[79]

Because the patient is relaxed and performs quiet breathing during the imaging process, the vena cava is not distended. For this reason the vena cava is not seen as readily in the coronal plane as the aorta.

Intracaval tumor-thrombus is usually associated with renal cell carcinoma or adrenal carcinoma, but can also be present in renal metastases and lymphoma. Their extension can be displayed accurately. Primary tumors of the vena cava are extremely rare. Spindle cell sarcoma may extend through the entire caval lumen and into both iliac veins (Fig 12–16).

Venous thrombus[80, 81] is of medium signal intensity on both T1- and T2-weighted (SE) images (Fig 12–17). Its signal intensity does not change appreciably with time. The venous thrombus may decrease in time as retraction and recanalization occur.

Abdominal Aorta

Identification of the size and extension of the abdominal aortic aneurysm and its relation to other major vessels can be accomplished with relative ease by MRI.[82–84] Renal and iliac artery stenosis are best detected by other imaging methods.

KIDNEYS

Renal Masses

Most renal masses larger than 3 cm are detected by MRI provided that image quality is

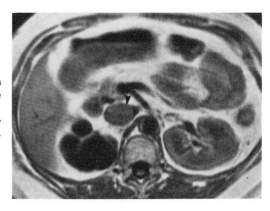

FIG 12–16.
The intraluminal filling defect in the inferior vena cava (*arrowhead*) is a spindle cell sarcoma extending from the iliac veins to the hepatic veins (SE 18/300, 0.3-T magnet). There is a grade IV hydronephrosis of the right kidney as a result of distal ureteral obstruction. "Entry" phenomena may mimic an intraluminal defect.

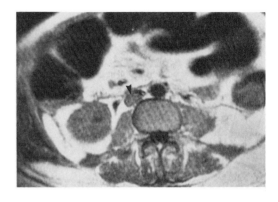

FIG 12–17.
Inferior vena cava thrombus. Most of the vessel lumen (*arrowhead*) is filled by a thrombus of medium signal intensity (SE 20/500, 0.3-T permanent magnet).

not adversely affected by motion artifacts. Lesions smaller than 3 cm in diameter are detected in 62% of cases.[85–87] For comparison purposes, the sensitivity for detection of lesions smaller than 3 cm in other imaging modalities is presented in Table 12–2.[88, 89]

Renal neoplasms have signal intensity similar to that of the renal cortex on both T1- and T2-weighted sequences, which is why smaller lesions are difficult to detect. On occasion a renal carcinoma may be hyperintense or even hypointense to renal cortex; however, the tumor is identified because of its mass effect, distortion of the renal outline, displacement of the collecting system, or impingement upon the renal sinus fat. It follows that CT currently is clearly the superior method for detection of small renal neoplasms.

While MRI lags behind CT in the detection of smaller lesions, staging is 82% correct

TABLE 12–2.
Overall Detection Accuracy for Renal Masses Less Than 3 cm

Modality	% Accuracy
CT scanning	94
US scanning	79
Angiography	74
Excretory urography	67
MR imaging	62

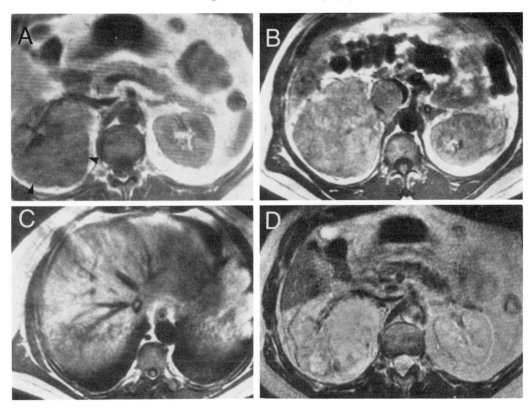

FIG 12–18.
Large right renal carcinoma (*arrowheads*) is present in the right kidney (**A**). On a T1-weighted sequence (SE 20/700) the signal intensity is almost equal to that of the renal cortex (**B**). On more cephalad image, extension into the vena cava is obvious (**C**). The cone of the tumor may be followed up to the hepatic vein confluence. On a T2-weighted sequence (SE 80/2000) the tumor and the kidneys become somewhat hyperintense and are of same signal intensity (**D**).

overall by MRI.[3] This relatively low number represents the inability of MRI to separate stage I from stage II disease which, however, does not have serious treatment implications as the treatment for these two stages is identical.

Magnetic resonance imaging is excellent in determining tumor extension into the renal vein, inferior vena cava (Fig 12–18), lumbar vein, contralateral renal vein, and right atrium.[90–92] It is also easy to differentiate enlarged lymph nodes from other retroperitoneal vessels such as the retrocaval left renal vein (Fig 12–19).

Extension of the renal carcinoma in the psoas is also easily depicted on T2-weighted sequences, where the muscle is hypointense and the tumor hyperintense. An arteriovenous malformation, which is sometimes associated with renal cell carcinoma, may be detected on occasion.[9]

Other Solid Renal Masses

Metastases, lymphoma, renal sarcomas, oncocytomas,[94, 95] and fibromas are indistinguishable from renal carcinomas on MR images.

Several histologic types of renal sarcomas are known to arise from the kidney. Of these, fibrosarcoma, and perhaps benign fibroma, may contain enough fibrous tissue to appear relatively hypointense on T2-weighted sequences.

Transitional cell carcinoma must attain considerable size before it can be detected by MRI. By that time the diagnosis is already evident. Again there are no distinguishing features.

Any solid and non-fatty tumor must therefore be considered malignant, and the purpose of imaging should be directed toward staging.

Only tumors containing large amounts of fatty tissue such as angiomyolipoma,[96, 97] lipoma, or hypernoma can be classified as benign. They appear isointense with the surrounding perinephric fat and in the case of angiomyolipoma may contain a large vascular component. Differential diagnosis includes hemorrhagic renal cysts, however. The solid nature of the tumor should be confirmed by ultrasound scanning.

Magnetic resonance imaging is the method of choice in further evaluation and staging of Wilms' tumor.[98–100] Variable signal intensities are seen on T1- and T2-weighted sequences depending on the presence of cystic components and hemorrhage. Vessels and intravascular extension are usually well depicted, and abnormal lymph nodes are detected. Computed tomography is almost as good as MRI except for the necessity of using intravenous contrast material. Since lung metastases are present in 10% of all patients at the time of diagnosis, CT scanning of the thorax is usually part of the imaging work-up.

Renal Cysts

Simple renal cysts are frequently encountered during abdominal MRI done for other purposes, and it is important to familiarize onself with their appearance. The most common appearance is that of a rounded mass with low signal intensity on T1-weighted sequence. On T2-weighted sequence the cyst fluid becomes hyperintense with the kidney tissue.[101, 102]

Renal cyst should be perfectly rounded, with smooth, thin wall. Thick walls, filling defects, or irregularity at the base should be considered signs of malignancy (Fig 12–20). If the cyst is not clearly seen because of motion artifacts, an ultrasonographic examination should be done. One should always remember the poor performance of MRI in demonstrating small deposits of calcium. Even moderate amounts of calcification within the cyst wall may

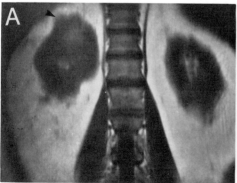
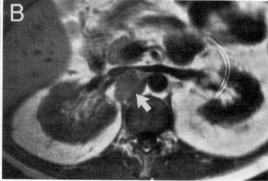

FIG 12–19.
Renal carcinoma of the upper pole of the right kidney was missed on an excretory urogram. Seen on a very posterior coronal section (**A**), this particular tumor (*arrowhead*) is relatively hypointense to the surrounding renal parenchyma. On axial T1-weighted image (**B**) (SE18/300, permanent magnet), the renal vein and inferior vena cava are uninvolved. However there is an enlarged retrocaval lymph node (*arrow*), presumably metastatic. Fluid is seen in hepatorenal angle.

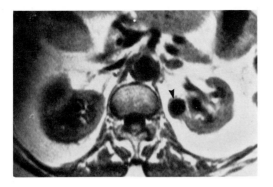

FIG 12–20.
Thick-walled renal cyst (*arrowhead*) is present at the medial aspect of the left kidney. Several peripelvic cysts are present in the right kidney (SE 18/300, 0.3-T magnet).

go unrecognized. Because anything more than a crescent of calcification within the wall should be regarded as a potential malignant cyst, CT scanning is superior to MRI in this respect.

Hemorrhagic renal cysts have varying appearances on MR images.[2] On T1-weighted sequences they may be either of low signal intensity (dark), medium signal intensity (gray and indistinguishable from renal cortex), or of high signal intensity (bright). On T2-weighted sequences all three signal intensities are possible. The signal intensity on any sequence largely depends on the length of time blood was present within the cyst.

Up to 30% of hemorrhagic renal cysts larger than 3 cm may contain renal carcinoma and should be further investigated by thin-needle aspiration. Hemorrhagic cysts smaller than 3 cm should be reexamined after 6 months to determine any change in size. In general, hemorrhagic cysts should be treated much the same as "hyperdense" cysts seen on CT scans.

Polycystic kidneys contain a variety of small and large cysts with a spectrum of different signal intensities both on T1- and T2-weighted sequences. Multiple hyperintense hemorrhagic cysts are frequently seen scattered throughout the kidney. Magnetic resonance imaging may be the only noninvasive means of detecting hydronephrosis in this group of patients.

Acquired cystic renal disease[103] associated with long-term renal dialysis is best seen by CT. Magnetic resonance imaging does not have the resolution necessary to adequately evaluate rather small cysts in what are small kidneys and to distinguish them from an occasional solid tumor.

Congenital Anomalies

Pelvic kidneys, horseshoe kidneys (Fig 12–21), and crossed-fused renal ectopia may be mistakenly diagnosed as a pelvic tumor even on ultrasound or nonenhanced CT scans. Frequently there is association with other pathologic processes such as obstruction, infection, and other congenital anomalies. Duplication of the collecting system, hypertrophied septum of Bertin, and renal dysmorphism may be detected by MRI.

Urolithiasis, Obstruction, and Inflammatory Diseases

The ability of MRI to discriminate renal calculus disease is nowhere near that of CT, projection radiography, or even ultrasound. This is one of the major drawbacks of MRI evaluation of the urinary tract system. In general a large calculus, because of its high calcium content, will be of low signal intensity both on T1- and T2-weighted sequences.

Dilation of the collecting system is readily apparent on MRI, but because the most common cause of obstruction is calculus disease, MRI is not the imaging method of choice.

Many other causes of obstruction may be very obvious on the MRI examination, particularly in patients with malignant masses, retroperitoneal lymphadenopathy, retroperitoneal fibrosis, and aortic aneurysm.

Inflammatory disease with mass effect such as abscess may appear as a complex renal cyst and may be indistinguishable from a solid renal tumor. In xantogranulomatous pyelonephritis, renal fascia is usually thickened, and perinephric space may be involved with inflammatory process. This disease is usually associated with renal calculi that may be difficult to recognize.

Renal Transplants

The ability of MRI to differentiate renal cortex and medulla did not do much to differentiate between parenchymal renal diseases on imaging basis alone (Fig 12–22). This is perhaps best illustrated in renal transplant patients, for whom the differential diagnosis between acute rejection, cyclosporine nephrotoxicity, and acute tubular necrosis is of considerable importance. The kidney in general responds by enlargement and loss of corticomedullary differentiation in most instances of rejection.[104–107] These findings are proportional to the severity of the process but, in addition to rejection, may also be seen in instances of

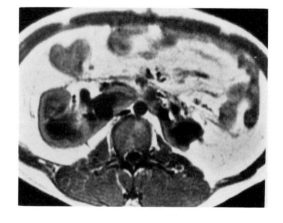

FIG 12–21.
Horseshoe kidney (SE 20/500, 0.3-T permanent magnet).

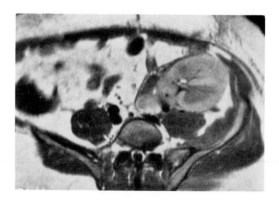

FIG 12–22.
Normal functioning renal allograft (SE 18/300, 0.3-T permanent magnet). Corticomedullary differention is evident. A collection of fluid producing several layers of different signal intensities is evident medial to the kidney. This most likely represents a small hematoma.

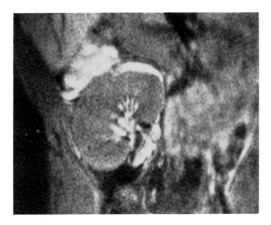

FIG 12–23.
In the process of rejection the renal transplant will enlarge, the cortex and medulla become indistinct from each other, and the renal sinus fat may become obliterated (SE 18/300, 0.3-T permanent magnet).

renal vein thrombosis, acute infection, acute tubular necrosis, and obstruction (Fig 12–23). Duplex ultrasound remains the method of choice for examination of these patients as a simpler, cheaper, and quicker alternative.[108–110]

Acute Renal Failure

General enlargement of the kidney is present and there is associated loss of corticomedullary differentiation on T1-weighted sequences. This finding is nonspecific and is seen in practically every parenchymal disease.

Physiologic Evaluation of the Kidneys

Paramagnetic contrast materials alter the local magnetic field and affect both T1 and T2 relaxation times of nearby hydrogen nuclei. In tissues in which they concentrate, the signal intensity (brightness) on T1-weighted images is generally increased and that on T2-weighted images is decreased.

Gadolinium-DTPA (diethylene triamine pentaacetic acid), a very stable chelate, is somewhat hyperosmollar and because of that must be administered intravenously rather slowly.[111, 112] The compound is excreted unchanged, principally by glomerular filtration. The recommended dose is 0.1 mmol/kg body weight. Following intravenous injection, healthy kidneys exhibit a rapid increase in brightness on T1-weighted sequences.

Sequential rapid imaging in 15-second intervals, through a preselected imaging plane, shows normal progression of the paramagnetic contrast through the cortex, medulla, and collecting system.[113, 114] The resemblance to ^{99m}Tc-DTPA nuclear medicine flow scan is striking except that the resolution is much better. For instance, in experimental animals, in the presence of renal ischemia the affected kidney does not become hyperintense (bright) as compared with the undiseased side.[112]

The true value of these substances in the evaluation of renal disease still remains the subject of much research. Approval has been granted by the U.S. Food and Drug Administration for neurologic imaging only at the time of this writing.

THE FEMALE PELVIS

In examining the female pelvis by MRI we have to remind ourselves what a powerful imaging modality ultrasound is, particulary in this region of the body.

Most ovarian tumors will be removed unless they are simple ovarian cysts. Most uterine lyomyomas are easily diagnosed by ultrasound. Perhaps the forte of MRI in evaluation of the female pelvis will be in staging various malignancies and evaluating a few congenital anomalies such as vaginal agenesis. At least in the short term this is likely to be so. At that time when MR becomes comparable to ultrasound in price, the priorities may and are likely to change.

Choice of Pulse Sequences

An examination of the female pelvis should begin by using a sagittal T2-weighted sequence. Axial T1-weighted sequences complement the study. To minimize motion, the patient's bladder should be only half full. Glucagon may be given intravenously to arrest peristaltic activity of the small and large bowel.

Normal Anatomy

Three distinct anatomic zones are identified on T2-weighted sequences. The innermost zone is hyperintense (*endometrium*); this is surrounded by a dark, hypointense area (*junctional zone*), and medium signal intensity muscular layer (*myometrium*).

The cervix may extend in the same direction as the uterine cavity or curve inferiorly. The size of the cervix is usually equal to that of the body of the uterus. In the cervical region, two (*endocervical canal, fibrous stroma*) and sometimes three zones are seen as well as the internal and external os. The cervix overall is hypointense (dark) as compared with the body of uterus, as it contains a large amount of connective tissues.

Vaginal fornices are seen in the majority of patients in the sagittal plane. The vaginal canal, vesicovaginal septum, rectovaginal septum, and levator ani are well seen in about 50% of cases. The broad ligaments, uterus, and vagina may also be clearly seen on axial or coronal T1-weighted images and/or on T2-weighted images.

Normal ovaries are identified in about 50% of cases. On T2-weighted images the ovaries are usually hyperintense (bright), and may be confused with fluid in the small or large bowel. On T1-weighted images the ovaries are of intermediate signal intensity (gray), and may also be difficult to differentiate from bowel loops.

Menstrual Cycle

Depending on the stage of the menstrual cycle, the endometrial zone may be very thin (*follicular phase*) or quite pronounced (*secretory phase*).[115–117] Following menopause the uterus is generally small and the endometrial zone may be sparse. On rare occasions follicles may be identified within the ovaries, but not nearly as well as with ultrasound.

Intrauterine Devices

Intrauterine devices may be seen and their location identified. Heating of the uterus, even in superconducting machines, does not occur.[118]

Positional Anomalies

Uterine anteversion, retroversion, retrodisplacement, retrocessment, and retroflection are easily seen on sagittal T2-weighted imaging sequences. If only axial or coronal sequences are used, an abnormally positioned uterus may simulate a mass.

Leiomyoma

Because of high fibrous tissue content and the occasional presence of calcification, leiomyomas are relatively hypointense on T1- and T2-weighted sequences.[119, 120] However, leiomyomas of varying signal intensities may be present, without any characteristic features (Fig 12–24). The relation of the tumor to the uterus and uterine cavity is easily determined. These tumors may be submucosal, subserosal, or endocervical. Their size and location can be determined with about the same accuracy as on ultrasound.

Endometrial Carcinoma

Endometrial carcinoma is the fourth most common malignancy in females. This is also the most common invasive malignancy of the female reproductive system. Because the endometrial cavity is so well visualized, particularly on T2-weighted sequences, endometrial carcinoma may be detected with MRI in 84% of the cases.[121, 122]

The uterus is usually enlarged and endometrial cavity expanded. Endometrial cavity is filled with high signal intensity endometrium or endometrial secretions. Endometrial carcinoma is seen as varying size nodules of intermediate (gray) signal intensity within the cavity (Fig 12–25).

Endometrial carcinoma cannot be differentiated from adenomatous hyperplasia or blood clots, which also may appear as intermediate signal intensity lesions within the endometrial cavity. Histologic diagnosis following curettage is therefore essential (Fig 12–26).

Correct staging may play a significant role in choosing appropriate therapy. Overall staging accuracy may reach 92% while accuracy in determining the depth of myometrial extension may reach 82%.[1]

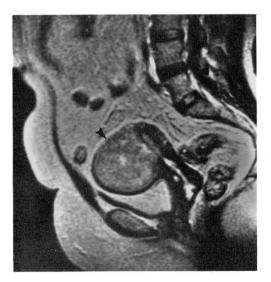

FIG 12–24.
Uterine leiomyoma (*arrowhead*). Sagittal T2-weighted image (SE 80/2000, 0.3-T permanent magnet). Because of high content of fibrous tissues and occasionally calcium deposits, these tumors are frequently hypointense.

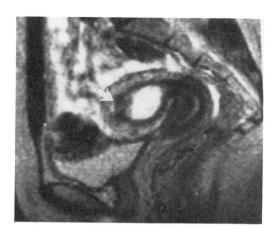

FIG 12–25.
Endometrial carcinoma presents as a mass of medium signal intensity within the bright endometrial (*arrow*) cavity on T2-weighted sequences (SE 80/2000, permanent magnet). Other entities may have a similar appearance, and the diagnosis is made histologically. MRI, however, may be useful in staging the disease.

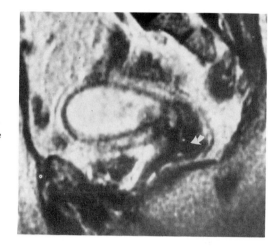

FIG 12–26.
Undifferentiated uterine carcinoma. On sagittal T2-weighted sequence (SE 80/2000, 0.3-T permanent magnet) an enlarged endometrial cavity is seen with a medium signal intensity intraluminal mass close to the cervix. The cervix (*arrow*) is of lower signal intensity than the myometrium, as it normally contains an abundant amount of connective tissues.

Cervical Carcinoma

The cervix is mostly connective tissue, with only 10% composed of smooth muscle. Therefore the cervix is mostly dark (hypointense) on MR images in contrast to relatively bright (hyperintense) cervical carcinoma (Fig 12–27). Parametrium, cardinal, and sacrouterine ligaments are seen. These structures contain vessels that frequently are somewhat varicose and exhibit a degree of stasis. These appear bright on T2-weighted image and should not be interpreted as an extension of cervical carcinoma. However, extension of the irregularly marginated tumor into the cardinal ligament is clearly seen.

An advantage of MRI is its capability to demonstrate the tumor mass and adjacent tissue planes directly.[123–125] Surrounding tissue edema may make the tumor appear larger than it really is.

The overall accuracy of MRI in the staging of cervical cancer is 81%; accuracy for determination of vaginal extension is 93%; that for parametrial extension is 88%.[1]

Ovarian Masses in General

Numerous pathologic processes may present as an ovarian mass. As is usual when there is a large choice of diagnostic possibilities, it is difficult to be specific about the diagnosis. Teratomas and endometrial cysts have certain appearances that are highly suggestive of the diagnosis. Many others, such as ovarian carcinoma, arrhenoblastoma, theca cell tumor, pseudomucinous cystadenoma and cystadenocarcinoma, fibroma, sarcoma, dysgerminoma, Brenner tumor (Fig 12–28), adenocarcinoma, or metastatic carcinoma to the ovary will be difficult to specifically diagnose by their general appearance on MR images. It will take time to accumulate the broad data needed to be more accurate in making specific preoperative diagnosis of an ovarian mass. Enlarged ovaries are those measuring more than 3 cm in their largest diameter.

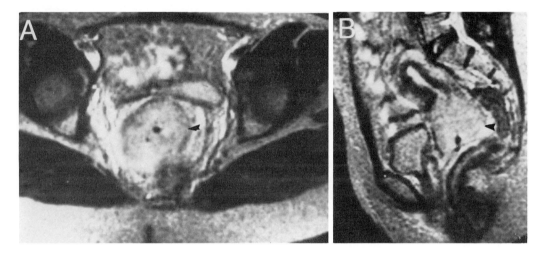

FIG 12–27.
Cervical carcinoma is seen as a mass (*arrowheads*) of medium signal intensity replacing an otherwise hypointense cervix (SE 100/2000, 0.5-T superconducting magnet). Sagittal (**A**) and transverse (**B**) images are shown.

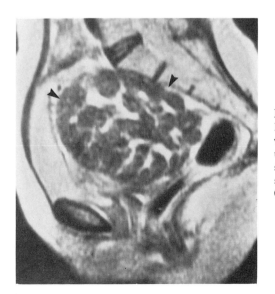

FIG 12–28.
Brenner tumor of the ovary (*arrowheads*). On a T1-weighted sequence (not shown) the tumor was of uniform medium signal intensity. On a T2-weighted sequence, areas of bright signal are present, interspaced with areas of low signal intensities (SE 80/2000, 0.3-T permanent magnet).

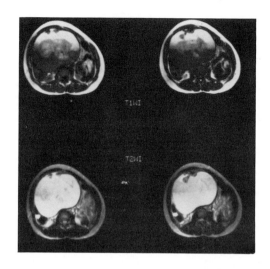

FIG 12–29.
Dermoid cyst. T1-weighted sequence (*upper row*, SE 16/650) demonstrates a fluid-fluid level within the cyst. Fluid level on the top is fatty and consequently isointense to the body fat. Floating debris may be seen within the cyst. Proteinaceous fluid on the bottom becomes hyperintense on T2-weighted sequence (*lower row*, SE 80/2000, 0.5-T superconducting magnet).

Ovarian Cystic Teratomas

Ovarian cystic teratomas are common ovarian tumors that account for about 20% of all ovarian neoplasms. Most contain yellowish, fatty liquid and solid components such as hair, teeth, and epithelial debris. As expected on a T1-weighted sequence, the fatty component is bright (hyperintense), on occasion even brighter than subcutaneous fat (Fig 12–29).

Floating or layering debris of intermediate signal intensity (gray) may occasionally be seen within the fat. This debris may change its position when the patient is turned onto the prone position. Nodular protrusions, sometimes bifurcating and resembling a palm tree, may also be seen within the fat. Togashi et al. recently described a pathognomonic atypical chemical shift artifact on a 1.5-T superconductive magnet in a majority of patients.[126]

Ovarian Cysts

Follicular ovarian cysts may be seen on a T2-weighted imaging sequence as very hyperintense (bright) structures. These cysts may be seen in all age groups, are nonseptated, solitary, and may become large.

Corpus luteum cysts may present as a pelvic mass of moderate size. Similar to most fluid-filled structures, the cyst is hypointense on T1-weighted images and hyperintense on T2-weighted images. Ovarian cysts may become infected and contain hemorrhagic fluid. Under those circumstances the MRI findings are variable.

Multilocular cysts are likely to be serous cystadenoma or mucinous cystadenoma.

Polycystic ovaries are enlarged and are seen to contain many predominantly larger cysts. These behave like other simple cysts and are hyperintense on T2-weighted images.[127]

Endometrial Cyst, Endometriosis, Fluid in Pouch of Douglas

The ovary is the most common site for ectopic endometrial implants. Endometrial cysts may be present in one or both ovaries and may contain aggregates of smaller cystic loculi. These cysts are usually hyperintense on T2-weighted images.[128]

Adhesions in the immediate surrounding areas may become abundant and cause loss of contour and outline of adjacent organs, such as the uterus and the bladder.

Endometrial implants of sufficiently large size in the peritoneal cavity, broad ligaments,

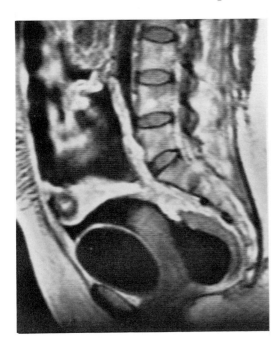

FIG 12–30.
Ascites seen extending around the uterus and into the
pouch of Douglas (SE 20/500, 0.3-T permanent
magnet).

or adjacent soft tissues may appear intensely bright on T2-weighted sequences. It appears
that MRI is more sensitive than ultrasound in depicting the location and extent of this disease.

In contrast, ascites or serous fluid in the pouch of Douglas is hypointense on T1-weighted
sequences (Fig 12–30).

Ovarian Carcinoma

Ovarian carcinoma comprises about 15% of all ovarian tumors. This tumor is frequently
bilateral; family history is elicited in 10% of cases. Ovarian carcinoma may be predominantly
cystic or solid. Papillary serous cystadenocarcinomas make up a high proportion of the cases
reported.

A mass lesion within the expected location is seen. Areas of degeneration, cysts, and
hemorrhage are detected.[129, 130] In advanced stages ascites is common and so are peritoneal
implants. These are difficult to detect on MR images if small in size. Distant metastases
involve the liver, lungs, bones, and lymph nodes. Locally, metastases are spread by infiltration
or continuity and may involve the tubes, broad ligament, uterus, bowel, and bladder.

VAGINA

T2-weighted sequences in transverse plane are optimal for evaluation of the vagina. The
muscular wall and the perivaginal venous plexus in relation to the urethra, bladder, and
rectum are well depicted by MRI.[131]

Vaginal Agenesis

Magnetic resonance imaging will clearly determine the presence or absence of the uterus and cervix. This alone may influence the type of corrective surgery needed. If functioning endometrial tissue is present, hematometra will develop after menarche; this, of course, is exquisitely demonstrated on T2-weighted spin echo sagittal sequences.[131, 132]

Vaginal Neoplasms

MR imaging appears to be the primary modality for staging vaginal neoplasms.[133]

Urethral Carcinoma (Female)

A single case report describes this carcinoma as a somewhat hyperintense mass (SE 2000/ 28) anterior to the vagina.[134] With the potential for demonstrating the spread of the tumor into the adjacent tissues and organs, MRI also offers the potential for accurate staging.

Female Incontinence

A rapid sagittal sequence obtained over a 10-second period during relaxation and straining may demonstrate the degree of urethral and bladder prolapse.[135]

URINARY BLADDER AND MALE PELVIS

Bladder Edema

In bladder edema, the thickened bladder wall is bright on a T2-weighted sequence.[136] In contrast, hypertrophied bladder wall, such as seen in outflow bladder obstruction, is hypointense on a T2-weighted sequence.

Carcinoma of the Bladder

The most exact method of examining the bladder is, of course, cystoscopy. The shortcoming of cystoscopic study is its inability to assess the extension of a neoplastic lesion through the thickness of the bladder wall or extension through the serosa beyond. Therefore, MRI within the bladder is expected to perform well in the staging of bladder carcinoma. Invasion of the outer muscular layer is probably better seen on T2-weighted images.[137, 138] T1-weighted images provide better contrast of the tumors within the bladder.

PROSTATE

Prostate and seminal vesicles are of uniform medium signal intensity on T1-weighted sequence. The outer zone becomes intensely bright on T2-weighted sequences (Fig 12–31).[139] Sometimes a third, inner, somewhat hyperintense periurethral zone may be seen.

Because the prostate is quite small, surface coil imaging could drastically improve resolution and therefore tumor detection and staging. The endorectal coil is being tested, apparently providing resolution that permits visualization of the ejaculatory ducts.[140]

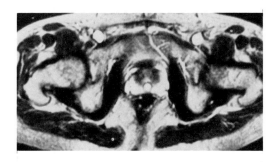

FIG 12–31.
Normal appearance of the prostate. On a T2-weighted sequence (SE 80/2000, 0.3-T permanent magnet) the posterior peripheral zone becomes hyperintense and well distinguished from the central zone. Since most of the prostatic carcinomas originate within the posterior zone they should become visible if their signal intensities differ.

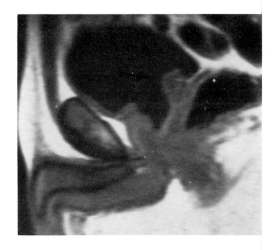

FIG 12–32.
Posttransurethral prostatectomy defect (*arrow*) is seen on a T1-weighted image (SE 18/300, 0.3-T permanent magnet).

Hypertrophy

Benign prostatic hypertrophy is seen as prostatic enlargement predominantly involving the inner zone. Postprostatectomy defect is seen following transurethral resection of the prostate (TURP) (Fig 12–32).

Carcinoma

Carcinoma of the prostate is the third most common carcinoma in the male, responsible for some 50,000 deaths a year. Carcinoma can be identified as a grayish area within the brightness of the posterior peripheral zone (Fig 12–33).[140–145]

Patients with stage B disease (cancer confined within the prostatic capsule) undergo radical prostatectomy, while patients with stage C (cancer extending through the capsule, or involving seminal vesicles) and above would undergo radiation therapy. Seminal vesicles that contain proteinaceous fluid turn intensely white on T2-weighted sequences and are of intermediate signal intensity if replaced by tumor.

A recent study[5] has demonstrated accuracy of 83% in differentiating stage B from stage C carcinomas, but only if multiple T1-weighted and multiple T2-weighted planes are used. This compares with an accuracy of 61% staged clinically, 65% by CT, and 61% by MRI using only images from the transverse T1-weighted plane.

Müllerian Duct Cyst

Müllerian duct cysts originate from fused müllerian ducts. Peak incidence is in the 3rd decade of life. The cyst may extend outside the prostate, compress upon the urethra and ejaculatory ducts, and could produce symptoms of outflow bladder obstruction, hematuria, pain, and infertility. Cystic fluid may be clear, mucoid, purulent, or hemorrhagic. The imaging of choice may be MRI as intraprostatic anatomy and the ability to obtain images in different planes can help localize the lesion more precisely.[146]

External Genitalia

Undescended testicle that cannot be palpated in the inguinal canal or detected by ultrasound should have a T2-weighted MRI study. Testicles are hyperintense on T2-weighted images and are therefore easily detected in the surrounding tissues.[147–150] In a recent study, 15 of 16 cases were correctly diagnosed. Lower signal intensity than normal in the contralateral testicle may indicate atrophy.

High-resolution imaging. In the superconducting imager the patient is positioned prone onto a 10-cm ring-type surface coil. This provides for high resolution and effectively eliminates motion artifacts.

Testicular tumors present as relatively gray and are within the bright testicle on T2-weighted sequence.[151] Ultrasound is still the examination of choice.

Hydrocele is seen as fluid collection of high signal intensity on T2-weighted sequences (Fig 12–34).

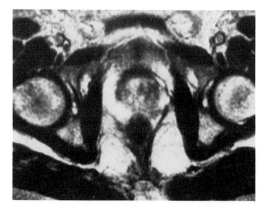

FIG 12–33.
Carcinoma of the prostate is seen as a relatively gray area within the bright posterior zone on this T2-weighted image (SE 80/2000, 0.3-T permanent magnet). Penetration through the capsule is more difficult to detect.

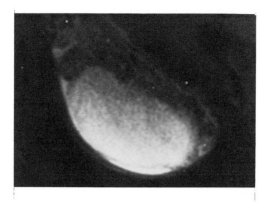

FIG 12–34.
A, small hydrocele is seen on this T2-weighted image (SE 80/2000, 0.3-T permanent magnet). The image was obtained with the use of a surface coil. The sagittal imaging plane allowed the testicle and the entire epididymis to be seen all at once.

REFERENCES

1. Chezmar JL, Rumanick WM, Megibow AJ, et al: Liver and abdominal screening in patients with cancer: CT versus MR imaging. *Radiology* 1988; 168:43–47.
2. Henkelman RM, Hardy P, Poon PY, et al: Optimal pulse sequence for imaging hepatic metastasis. *Radiology* 1986; 161:727–734.
3. Stark DD, Wittenberg J, Edelman RR, et al: Detection of hepatic metastasis: Analysis of pulse sequences performance in MR imaging. *Radiology* 1986; 159:365–370.
4. Stark DD, Wittenberg J, Middleton MS, et al: Liver metastasis: Detection by phase-contrast MR imaging. *Radiology* 1986; 158:327–332.
5. Edelman RR, Hahn PF, Buxton R, et al: Rapid MR imaging with suspended respiration: Clinical application in the liver. *Radiology* 1986; 161:125–131.
6. Ohtomo K, Itai Y, Yoshikawa K, et al: Hepatic tumors: Dynamic MR imaging. *Radiology* 1987; 163:27–31.
7. Bydder GM, Steiner RE, Blumgart LH, et al: MR imaging of the liver using short T1 inversion recovery sequences. *J Comput Assist Tomogr* 1985; 9:1084–1090.
8. Stark DD, Weissleder R, Elizondo G, et al: Superparamagnetic iron oxide: Clinical application as a contrast agent for MR imaging of the liver. *Radiology* 1988; 168:297–301.
9. Glazer GM, Aisen AM, Francis IR, et al: Hepatic cavernous hemangioma: Magnetic resonance imaging. *Radiology* 1985; 155:417–420.
10. Stark DD, Felder R, Wittenberg J, et al: MRI of cavernous hemangioma of the liver: Tissue specific characterization. *AJR* 1985; 145:213–222.
11. Brodski RI, Friedman AC, Maurer AH, et al: Hepatic cavernous hemangioma: Diagnosis with Tc99m-labeled red cells and single-photon emission CT. *AJR* 1987; 148:125–129.
12. Solbiaty L, Livraghi T, De Pra L, et al: Fine-needle biopsy of hepatic hemangioma with sonographic guidance. *AJR* 1985; 144:471–474.
13. Li KC, Glazer GM, Quint LE, et al: Distinction of hepatic cavernous hemangioma from hepatic metastases with MR imaging. *Radiology* 1988; 169:409–415.
14. Takayasu K, Moryama N, Shima Y, et al: Atypical radiographic findings in hepatic cavernous hemangioma: Correlation with histologic features. *AJR* 1986; 146:1149–1153.
15. Ohtomo K, Itai Y, Yoshikawa K, et al: Hepatocellular carcinoma and cavernous hemangioma: Differentiation with MR imaging. *Radiology* 1988; 168:621–623.
16. Stark DD, Wittenberg J, Butch RJ, et al: Hepatic metastases: Randomized, controlled comparison of detection with MR imaging and CT. *Radiology* 1987; 165:339–406.

17. Slizofski WJ: Focal hepatic mass screening: MR imaging or CT scanning? *Radiology* 1987; 163:830–831.

18. Bernandino ME: Focal hepatic mass screening: MR imaging or CT scanning? *Radiology* 1987; 162:282–283.

19. Reining JW, Dwyer AJ, Miller DL: Liver metastasis detection: Comparative sensitivities of MR imaging and CT scanning. *Radiology* 1987; 162:43–47.

20. Glazer GM, Aisen AM, Francis IR, et al: Evaluation of focal hepatic masses: A comparative study of MRI and CT. *Gastrointest Radiol* 1986; 11:263–268.

21. Itoh K, Nishimura K, Togashi K, et al: Hepatocellular carcinoma: MR imaging. *Radiology* 1987; 164:21–25.

22. Ebara M, Ohto M, Watanabe Y, et al: Diagnosis of small hepatocellular carcinoma: Correlation of MR imaging and tumor histological studies. *Radiology* 1986; 159:371–377.

23. Wilcox DM, Weinreb JC, Lesh P: MR imaging of hemorrhagic hepatic cyst in a patient with polycystic liver disease. *J Comput Assist Tomogr* 1985; 9:183–185.

24. Elizondo G, Weissleder R, Stark DD, et al: Amebic liver abscess: Diagnosis and treatment evaluation with MR imaging. *Radiology* 1987; 165:795–800.

25. Wall SD, Fisher MR, Amparo EG, et al: Magnetic resonance imaging in the evaluation of abscesses. *AJR* 1985; 144:1217–1221.

26. Ralls PW. Hemley DS, Colletti PM, et al: Amebic liver abscess: MR imaging. *Radiology* 1987; 165:801–804.

27. Heiken JP, Lee JKT, Dixon WT: Fatty infiltration of the liver: Evaluation by proton spectroscopic imaging. *Radiology* 1985; 157:707–710.

28. Itay Y, Ohtomo K, Kukubo T, et al: CT and MR imaging of fatty tumors of the liver. *J Comput Assist Tomogr* 1987; 11:253–257.

29. Ohtomo K, Itai Y, Furui S, et al: Hepatic tumors: Differentiation by transverse relaxation time (T2) of magnetic resonance imaging. *Radiology* 1985; 155:421–423.

30. Pope CF, Gore JC, Sostman HD, et al: Diffuse fatty infiltration of the liver by magnetic resonance. *Magn Reson Imaging* 1986; 4:267–271.

31. Stark DD, Moseley ME, Bacon BR, et al: Magnetic resonance imaging and spectroscopy of hepatic iron overload. *Radiology* 1985; 154:137–142.

32. Murphy FB, Bernardino ME: MR imaging of focal hemochromatosis. *J Comput Assist Tomogr* 1986; 10:1044–1046.

33. Stark DD, Goldberg HI, Moss AA, et al: Chronic liver disease: Evaluation by magnetic resonance. *Radiology* 1984; 150:149–151.

34. Itai Y, Ohnishi S, Ohtomo K, et al: Regenerating nodules of liver cirrhosis: MR imaging. *Radiology* 1987; 165:419–423.

35. Williams DM, Cho KJ, Aisen AM, et al: Portal hypertension evaluated by MR imaging. *Radiology* 1985; 157:703–706.

36. Schiebler ML, Kressel HY, Saul SH, et al: MR imaging of focal nodular hyperplasia of the liver. *J Comput Assist Tomogr* 1987; 11:651–656.

37. Itai Y, Ohnishi S, Ohtomo K, et al: Regenerating nodules of liver cirrhosis: MR imaging. *Radiology* 1987; 165:419–422.

38. Stark DD, Hahn PF, Trey C, et al: MRI of the Budd-Chiari syndrome. *AJR* 1986; 146:1141–1148.

39. Loflin TG, Simeone JF, Mueller PR, et al: Gallbladder bile in cholecystitis: In vitro MR evaluation. *Radiology* 1985; 157:457–459.

40. McCarthy S, Hricak H, Cohen M, et al: Cholecystitis: Detection with MR imaging. *Radiology* 1986; 158:333–336.

41. Dooms GC, Fisher MR, Higgins CB, et al: MR imaging of the dilated biliary tract. *Radiology* 1986; 158:337–341.

42. Dooms GC, Kerlan RK Jr, Hricak H: Cholangiocarcinoma: Imaging by MR. *Radiology* 1986; 159:89–94.

43. Stark DD, Moss AA, Goldberg HI, et al: Magnetic resonance and CT of the normal and diseased pancreas: A comparative study. *Radiology* 1984; 150:153–162.

44. Hahn PF, Stark DD, Vici LG, et al: Duodenal hematoma: The ring sign in MR imaging. *Radiology* 1986; 159:379–382.
45. Schultz CL, Haaga JR, Fletcher BD, et al: Magnetic resonance imaging of the adrenal glands: A comparison with computed tomography. *AJR* 1984; 143:1235–1240.
46. Chang A, Glazer HS, Lee JKT, et al: Adrenal gland: MR imaging. *Radiology* 1987; 163:123–128.
47. Glazer GM, Woolsey EJ, Borrello J, et al: Adrenal tissue characterization using MR imaging. *Radiology* 1986; 158:73–79.
48. White EM, Edelman RR, Stark DD: Surface coil MR imaging of abdominal viscera. Part II: The adrenal glands. *Radiology* 1985; 157:431–436.
49. Reining JW, Doppman JL, Dwyer AJ, et al: Distinction between adrenal adenomas and metastases using MR imaging. *J Comput Assist Tomogr* 1985; 9:898–901.
50. Reining JW, Doppman JL, Dwyer AJ, et al: Adrenal masses differentiated by MR. *Radiology* 1986; 158:81–84.
51. Baker ME, Spritzer C, Blinder R, et al: Benign adrenal lesions mimicking malignancy on MR imaging: Report of two cases. *Radiology* 1987; 163:669–671.
52. Glazer GM: MR imaging of the liver, kidneys and adrenal glands. *Radiology* 1988; 166:303–312.
53. Fink IJ, Reining JW, Dwyer AJ, et al: MR imaging of pheochromocytomas. *J Comput Assist Tomogr* 1985; 9:454–458.
54. Greenberg M, Moawad AH, Wieties BM, et al: Extraadrenal pheochromocytoma: Detection during pregnancy using MR imaging. *Radiology* 1986; 161:475–476.
55. Quint EL, Glazer GM, Francis IR, et al: Pheochromocytoma and paraganglioma: Comparison of MR imaging with CT and I-131 MIBG scintigraphy. *Radiology* 1987; 165:89–93.
56. Cohen MD, Weetman R, Provisor R, et al: Magnetic resonance imaging of neuroblastoma with a 0.15-T magnet. *AJR* 1984; 143:1241–1248.
57. Fletcher BD, Kopiwoda SY, Strandjord SE, et al: Abdominal neuroblastoma: Magnetic resonance imaging and tissue characterization. *Radiology* 1985; 155:699–703.
58. Dietrich RB, Kangarloo H: Retroperitoneal mass with intradural extension: Value of magnetic resonance imaging in neuroblastoma. *AJR* 1986; 146:251–254.
59. Doppman JL, Miller DL, Dwyer AJ, et al: Macronodular adrenal hyperplasia in Cushing disease. *Radiology* 1988; 166:347–352.
60. Dooms GC, Hricak H, Crooks LE, et al: Magnetic resonance imaging of the lymph nodes: Comparison with CT. *Radiology* 1984; 153:719–728.
61. Dooms GC, Hricak H, Moseley ME, et al: Characterization of lymphadenopathy by magnetic resonance relaxation times: Preliminary results. *Radiology* 1985; 155:691–697.
62. Lee JKT, Heiken JP, Ling D, et al: Magnetic resonance imaging of abdominal and pelvic lymphadenopathy. *Radiology* 1984; 153:181–188.
63. Dunlap HJ, Poon PY, Henkelman RM, et al: Magnetic resonance imaging in retroperitoneal lymphadenopathy. *J Can Assoc Radiol* 1987; 38:75–78.
64. Buckwalter KA, Ellis JH, Baker DE, et al: Pitfall in MR imaging of lymphadenopathy after lymphangiography. *Radiology* 1986; 161:831–832.
65. Dooms GC, Hricak H, Sollitto RA, et al: Lipomatous tumors and tumors with fatty component: MR imaging potential and comparison of MR and CT results. *Radiology* 1985; 157:479–483.
66. Dooms GC, Hricak H, Margulis AR, et al: MR imaging of fat. *Radiology* 1986; 158:51–54.
67. Totty WG, Murphy WA, Lee JKT: Soft-tissue tumors: MR imaging. *Radiology* 1986; 160:135–141.
68. Lee JKT, Glazer HS: Psoas muscle disorders: MR imaging. *Radiology* 1986; 160:683–687.
69. Weinreb JC, Cohen JM, Maravilla KR: Ileopsoas muscles: MR study of normal anatomy and disease. *Radiology* 1985; 156:435–440.
70. Kaplan AP, Williams, SM: Mucocutaneous and peripheral soft-tissue hemangiomas: MR imaging. *Radiology* 1987; 163:163–166.
71. Beltran J, Simon DC, Katz W, et al: Increased MR signal intensity in skeletal muscle adjacent to malignant tumors: Pathologic correlation and clinical relevance. *Radiology* 1987; 162:251–255.
72. Swensen SJ, Keller PL, Berquist TH, et al: Magnetic resonance imaging of hemorrhage. *AJR* 1985; 145:921–927.

73. Justich E, Amparo EG, Hricak H, et al: Infected aortoiliofemoral grafts: Magnetic resonance imaging. *Radiology:* 1985; 154:133–136.

74. Burk LD Jr, Brunberg JA, Kanal E, et al: Spinal and paraspinal neurofibromatosis: Surface coil MR imaging at 1.5T. *Radiology* 1987; 162:797–801.

75. Dumoulin CL, Hart HR Jr: Magnetic resonance angiography. *Radiology* 1986; 161:717–720.

76. Hale JD, Valk PE, Watts JC, et al: MR imaging of blood vessels using three-dimensional reconstruction: Methodology. *Radiology* 1985; 157:727–733.

77. von Schulthess GK, Higgins CB: Blood flow imaging with MR: Spin-phase phenomena. *Radiology* 1985; 157:687–695.

78. Meuli RA, Wedeen VJ, Geller SC, et al: MR gated subtraction angiography: Evaluation of lower extremities. *Radiology* 1986; 159:411–418.

79. Hricak H, Amparo E, Fisher MR, et al: Abdominal venous system: Assessment using MR. *Radiology* 1985; 156:415–422.

80. Erdman WA, Weinreb JC, Cohen JM, et al: Venous thrombosis: Clinical and experimental MR imaging. *Radiology* 1986; 161:233–238.

81. White EM, Edelman RR, Wedeen VJ, et al: Intravascular signal in MR imaging: Use of phase display for differentiation of blood-flow signal from intraluminal disease. *Radiology* 1986; 161:245–249.

82. Amparo EG, Hoddick WK, Hricak H, et al: Comparison of magnetic resonance imaging and ultrasound in the evaluation of abdominal aortic aneurysms. *Radiology* 1985; 154:451–456.

83. Amparo GE, Higgins CB, Hricak H, et al: Aortic dissection: Magnetic resonance imaging. *Radiology* 1985; 155:399–406.

84. Amparo EG, Higgins CB, Hoddick W, et al: Magnetic resonance imaging of aortic disease. *AJR* 1984; 143:1203–1209.

85. Fein AB, Lee JKT, Balfe DM, et al: Diagnosis and staging of renal cell carcinoma: A comparison of MR imaging and CT. *AJR* 1987; 148:749–753.

86. Patel SK, Stack CM, Taner DA: Magnetic resonance imaging in staging of renal cell carcinoma. *Radiographics* 1987; 7:703–728.

87. Hricak H, Theoni RF, Carroll PR, et al: Detection and staging of renal neoplasms: A reassessment of MR imaging. *Radiology* 1988; 166:643–649.

88. Amendola MA, Bree RL, Pollack HM, et al: Small renal carcinomas: Resolving a diagnostic dilemma. *Radiology* 1988; 166:637–641.

89. Lang EK: Angio-computed tomography and dynamic computed tomography in staging of renal cell carcinoma. *Radiology* 1984; 151:149–155.

90. Hricak H, Williams RA, Hedgcock MW: The value of NMR in depicting and staging renal malignancies. *Magn Reson Med* 1984; 94:172–173.

91. Hricak H, Demas BE, Williams RD, et al: Magnetic resonance imaging in the diagnosis and staging of renal and perirenal neoplasms. *Radiology* 1985; 154:709–715.

92. Choyke PL, Kressel HY, Pollack HM, et al: Focal renal masses: Magnetic resonance imaging. *Radiology* 1984; 152:471–477.

93. Selli C, Bartolozzi C, Lizzadro G, et al: Arteriovenous fistula associated with renal cell carcinoma: Demonstration by magnetic resonance imaging. *Urol Radiol* 1986; 8:190–192.

94. Remark RR, Berquist TH, Lieber MM, et al: Magnetic resonance imaging of renal oncocytoma. *Urology* 1988; 31:176–179.

95. Ball DS, Friedman AC, Hartman DS, et al: Scar sign of renal oncocytoma: Magnetic resonance imaging appearance and lack of specificity. *Urol Radiol* 1986; 8:46–48.

96. Bret PM, Bretagnolle M, Gaillard D, et al: Small, asymptomatic angiomyolipomas of the kidney. *Radiology* 1985; 154:7–10.

97. Vas W, Wolverson MK, Johnson F, et al: MRI of an angiomyolipoma. *Magn Reson Imaging* 1986; 4:485–486.

98. Kangarloo H, Dietrich RB, Erlich RM, et al: Magnetic resonance imaging of Wilms' tumor. *Radiology* 1987; 163:291–294.

99. Belt TG, Cohen MD, Smith JA, et al: MRI of Wilms tumor: Promise as the primary imaging method. *AJR* 1986; 146:955–961.

100. Dietrich RB, Kangarloo H: Kidneys in infants and children: Evaluation with MR. *Radiology* 1986; 159:215–221.
101. Marotti M, Hricak H, Fritzsche P, et al: Complex and simple renal cysts: Comparative evaluation with MR imaging. *Radiology* 1987; 162:679–684.
102. Brown JJ, van Sonnenberg E, Gerber KH, et al: Magnetic resonance relaxation times of percutaneously obtained normal and abnormal body fluids. *Radiology* 1985; 154:727–731.
103. Scanlon MH, Karasick SR: Acquired renal cystic disease and neoplasia: Complications of hemodialysis. *Radiology* 1983; 147:837–838.
104. Rholl KS, Lee JKT, Ling D, et al: Acute renal rejection versus acute tubular necrosis in a canine model: MR evaluation. *Radiology* 1986; 160:113–117.
105. Hricak H, Terrier F, Demas B: Renal allografts: Evaluation by MR imaging. *Radiology* 1986; 159:435–444.
106. Geisinger MA, Risius B, Jordan ML, et al: Magnetic resonance imaging of renal transplants. *AJR* 1986; 143:1229–1231.
107. Hricak H, Terrier F, Marotti M, et al: Posttransplant renal rejection: Comparison of quantitative scintigraphy, US, and MR imaging. *Radiology* 1987; 162:685–688.
108. Mitchell DG, Roza AM, Spritzer CE, et al: Acute renal allograft rejection: Difficulty in diagnosis of histologically mild cases by MR imaging. *J Comput Assist Tomogr* 1986; 11:655–663.
109. Halasz NA: Differential diagnosis of renal transplant rejection: Is MR imaging the answer? *AJR* 1986; 147:954–955.
110. Steinberg HV, Nelsson RC, Murphy FB, et al: Renal allograft rejection: Evaluation by Doppler US and MR imaging. *Radiology* 1987; 162:337–342.
111. Slutsky RA, Peterson T, Strich G, et al: Hemodynamic effects of rapid and slow infusions of manganese chloride and gadolinium-DPTA in dogs. *Radiology* 1985; 154:733–735.
112. Koenig SH, Spiller M, Brown RD III, et al: Magnetic field dependence (NMRD profile) of 1/T1 of rabbit kidney medulla and urine after intravenous injection of Gd (DTPA). *Invest Radiol* 1986; 21:697–704.
113. Kikins R, von Schulthess GK, Jäger P, et al: Normal and hydronephrotic kidney: Evaluation of renal function with contrast-enhanced MR imaging. *Radiology* 1987; 165:837–842.
114. Krestin GP, Friedman G, Steinbrich W, et al: Quantitative evaluation of renal function with rapid dynamic gadolinium-DTPA enhanced MRI. A comparison with radionuclide nephrography. *Soc Magn Reson Med* 1988; 643.
115. McCarthy S, Tauber CT, Gore J: Female pelvic anatomy: MR assessment of variations during the menstrual cycle and with use of oral contraceptives. *Radiology* 1986; 160:119–123.
116. Haynor DR, Mack LA, Soules MR, et al: Changing appearance of the normal uterus during the menstrual cycle. *Radiology* 1986; 161:459–462.
117. Demas B, Hricak H, Jaffe RB: Uterine MR imaging. Effects of hormonal stimulation. *Radiology* 1986; 159:123–126.
118. Mark AS, Hricak H: Intrauterine contraceptive devices: MR imaging. *Radiology* 1987; 162:311–314.
119. Hricak H, Tscholakoff D, Heinrichs L: Uterine leiomyomas: Correlation of MR, histopathologic findings and symptoms. *Radiology* 1986; 158:385–391.
120. Mintz MC, Thickman DI, Gussman D, et al: MR evaluation of uterine anomalies. *AJR* 1987; 148:287–290.
121. Hricak H, Stern JL, Fisher MR, et al: Endometrial carcinoma staging by MR imaging. *Radiology* 1987; 162:297–305.
122. Worthington JL, Balfe DM, Lee JKT, et al: Uterine neoplasms: MR imaging. *Radiology* 1986; 159:725–730.
123. Hricak H, Lacey CG, Sandles LG, et al: Invasive cervical carcinoma: Comparison of MR imaging and surgical findings. *Radiology* 1988; 166:623–631.
124. Togashi K, Nishimura K, Itoh K, et al: Uterine cervical cancer: Assessment with high-field MR imaging. *Radiology* 1986; 160:431–435.

125. Lee JKT: The role of MR imaging in staging of cervical carcinoma (editorial). *Radiology* 1988; 166:895–896.

126. Togashi K, Nishimura K, Itoh K, et al: Ovarian cystic teratomas: MR imaging. *Radiology* 1987; 162:669–673.

127. Mitchell DG, Gefter WB, Spritzer CE, et al: Polycystic ovaries: MR imaging. *Radiology* 1986; 160:425–429.

128. Nishimura K, Togashi K, Itoh K, et al: Endometrial cysts of the ovary: MR imaging. *Radiology* 1987; 162:315–318.

129. Dooms GC, Hricak H, Tscholakoff D: Adnexal structures: MR imaging. *Radiology* 1986; 158:639–646.

130. Mitchell DG, Mintz MC, Spritzer CE, et al: Adnexal masses: MR imaging observations at 1.5 T, with US and CT correlation. *Radiology* 1987; 162:319–324.

131. Togashi K, Nishimura K, Itoh K, et al: Vaginal agenesis: Classification by MR imaging. *Radiology* 1987; 162:675–677.

132. Hricak H, Chang YCF, Thurnher S: Vagina: Evaluation with MR imaging. Part I: Normal anatomy and congenital anomalies. *Radiology* 1988; 169:169–174.

133. Chang YCF, Hricak H, Thurnher S, et al: Vagina: Evaluation with MR imaging. Part II: Neoplasms. *Radiology* 1988; 169:175–179.

134. Fisher MR, Hricak H, Reinhold C, et al: Female urethral carcinoma: MR staging. *AJR* 1985; 144:603–604.

135. Yang A, Rosenshein NB, McLellan R, et al: Dynamic evaluation of pelvic prolapse using gradient echo fast scan and cinematic display. *Soc Magn Reson Med* 1988; 649.

136. Fisher MR, Hricak H, Crooks EL: Urinary bladder MR imaging. Part I: Normal and benign conditions. *Radiology* 1985; 157:467–470.

137. Fisher MR, Hricak H, Tanagho EA: Urinary bladder MR imaging. Part II: Neoplasm. *Radiology* 1985; 157:471–477.

138. Rholl SK, Lee JKT, Heiken JP, et al: Primary bladder carcinoma: Evaluation with MR imaging. *Radiology* 1987; 163:117–121.

139. Hricak H, Dooms GC, McNeal JE, et al: MR imaging of the prostate gland: Normal anatomy. *AJR* 1987; 148:51–58.

140. Schnall M, Kressel H, Pollak H, et al: Prostatic imaging with an endorectal probe (abstract). *Soc Magn Reson Med* 1988; 648.

141. Ling D, Lee JKT, Heiken JP, et al: Prostatic carcinoma and benign prostatic hyperplasia: Inability of MR imaging to distinguish between the two diseases. *Radiology* 1986; 158:103–107.

142. Hricak H, Williams RD, Spring DB, et al: Anatomy and pathology of the male pelvis by magnetic resonance imaging. *AJR* 1983; 141:1101–1110.

143. Hricak H, Dooms GC, Jeffrey RB, et al: Prostatic carcinoma staging by clinical assessment, CT, and MR imaging. *Radiology* 1987; 162:331–336.

144. Biondetti PR, Lee JKT, Lind D, et al: Clinical stage B prostate carcinoma: Staging with MR imaging. *Radiology* 1987; 162:325–329.

145. Mukamel E, deKernion JB, Hanna J, et al: Staging of localized prostate cancer. A clinical pathologic correlation. *J Urol* 1986; 136:1231–1233.

146. Thurnher S, Hricak H, Tanagho EA: Müllerian duct cyst: Diagnosis with MR imaging. *Radiology* 1988; 168:25–28.

147. Rholl KS, Lee JKT, Ling D, et al: MR imaging of the scrotum with a high-resolution surface coil. *Radiology* 1987; 163:99–103.

148. Baker LL, Hajek PC, Bukhard TK, et al: MR imaging of the scrotum: Normal anatomy. *Radiology* 1987; 163:89–92.

149. Fritzsche PJ, Hricak H, Kogan BA, et al: Undescended testicle: Value of MR imaging. *Radiology* 1987; 164:169–173.

150. Baker LL, Hajek PC, Burkhard TK, et al: Polyorchidism: Evaluation by MR. *AJR* 1987; 148:305–306.

151. Baker LL, Hajek PC, Burkhard TK, et al: MR imaging of the scrotum: Pathological conditions. *Radiology* 1987; 163:93–98.

Chapter 13 _____

Magnetic Resonance Imaging of Joints and Extremities

Leanne L. Seeger, M.D.

Lawrence W. Bassett, M.D.

Magnetic resonance imaging (MRI) has proved to be a powerful tool in the evaluation of a variety of musculoskeletal disorders.[1] Traumatic, inflammatory, neoplastic, and degenerative conditions of bone and soft-tissue can now be imaged without the use of ionizing radiation or the injection of radiographic contrast material, often with a sensitivity that far exceeds that of previous imaging modalities.

Advantageous features of MRI with respect to the musculoskeletal system include (1) the ability to directly image bone marrow, (2) an inherent high soft tissue contrast discrimination, and (3) direct multiplanar imaging. In addition, the use of surface coils has allowed acquisition of high-resolution images of the extremities and joints, providing detailed evaluation of anatomic subtleties not previously possible.

Musculoskeletal MRI examinations will yield the most information when tailored to specific clinical problems. In some situations, such as the evaluation of the knee for a meniscal tear or the hip for osteonecrosis, routine imaging protocols may be established. In other situations, however, the study must be modified for the specific patient and clinical problem. For cases of tumor or infection, selection of surface coil, imaging plane, and field-of-view will be determined by the type, size, and location of the suspected abnormality. It is therefore essential for the radiologist to be provided with an appropriate clinical history. Especially in cases of tumor or infection, radiographs should be reviewed prior to image acquisition to assure adequate coverage of the area of interest.

Although several normal musculoskeletal tissues have characteristic signal intensities with MRI, pathologic findings are often nonspecific (Table 13–1). It is often difficult or impossible to differentiate traumatic, inflammatory, and neoplastic disorders on the basis of their MRI appearance alone (Figs 13–1 and 13–2). In most cases, correlative imaging studies,[2] an appropriate clinical history, and/or physical and laboratory examination can assist one in arriving at the appropriate diagnosis.

Another warning relates to the choice of pulsing sequences, especially when evaluating fluid collections or marrow disorders. While it is tempting to use double echo imaging in order to decrease examination time, proton-density images impart a significant amount of T2

TABLE 13–1.

Tissue Signal Intensity on T1- and T2-Weighted Magnetic Resonance Images

Tissue	T1 Weighting	T2 Weighting
Cortical bone	Void	Void
Ligaments, tendons	Void	Void
Fibrocartilage	Void	Void
Normal fluid	Low	High
Tumor	Low to intermediate	High
Abnormal fluid (e.g., pus)	Intermediate	High
Hyaline cartilage	Intermediate	Intermediate
Muscle	Intermediate	Intermediate
Fat (marrow)	High	Intermediate to high

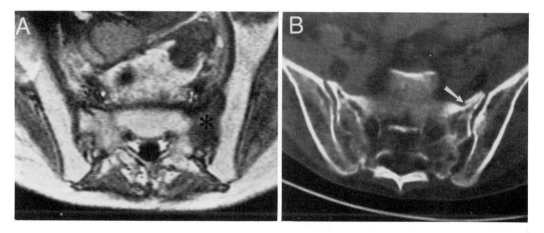

FIG 13–1.
Studies of a 72-year-old woman with breast carcinoma and sacral pain. **A,** T1-weighted MR image (SE 500/30) through the sacrum reveals a region of low signal intensity in the left sacral ala (*asterisk*). With T2-weighting, the signal intensity increased (not shown). **B,** computed tomographic scan through the region of abnormal marrow signal intensity shows a healing insufficiency fracture (*arrow*). There is no evidence of metastatic disease.

weighting to the image. As a result, it may be difficult to differentiate fat from fluid, and marrow abnormalities may be obscured.

Most of the images in this chapter were obtained with a 0.3-tesla imaging system. With the exception of the hip, all joint images were acquired with the use of a surface coil. Only spin echo images are shown, as widespread experience with newer imaging techniques in the extremities is limited.

BONE MARROW

Bone marrow T1- and T2-relaxation times vary with the age of the patient.[3] In the infant, hematopoietic (red) marrow occupies a large proportion of the marrow space. With increasing skeletal maturity, hematopoietic marrow is progressively replaced with fatty (yellow) marrow.

In the adult, most marrow infiltrative disorders are characterized in T1-weighted images by replacement of the normal high signal intensity marrow with intermediate to low signal

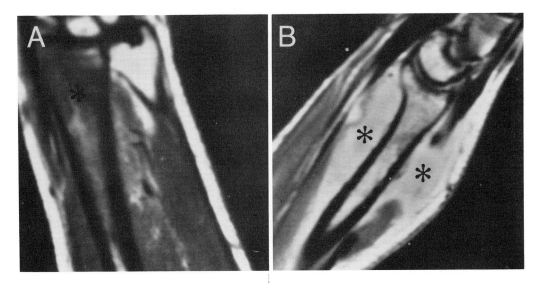

FIG 13–2.
Studies of a 32-year-old man referred for treatment of a distal radius lesion that had been diagnosed as sarcoma with MRI. **A,** coronal T1-weighted image (SE 800/30) demonstrates low signal intensity in the distal radius (*asterisk*). **B,** sagittal T2-weighted image (SE 2000/85). The signal intensity of the marrow increases, and there is a large adjacent soft-tissue mass (*asterisks*). Clinical information was needed for the correct diagnosis in this situation. The extremity was warm and erythematous, and the peripheral white cell count was markedly elevated. At surgery, this lesion represented infection rather than tumor.

intensity. The signal intensity of the lesion will increase in T2-weighted images. With trauma, the abnormal signal probably reflects edema or bleeding around the site of trauma.[4–6] In cases of neoplasm, abnormal marrow signal represents infiltration by tumor cells or edema. With infection, abnormal marrow signal may represent intraosseous abscesses and/or edema.[7, 8]

Diffuse marrow abnormalities may be difficult to identify with MRI, but can generally be recognized by consideration of the patient's age and through the use of both T1- and T2-weighted imaging. Diffuse tumor infiltration, such as leukemia, will manifest itself as abnormal low signal intensity on T1-weighted imaging, and high signal intensity on T2-weighting. Myelofibrosis displays low signal intensity in both T1- and T2-weighted images, because of the replacement of marrow by fibrous tissue, which has low signal intensity with all pulse sequences (Fig 13–3).

SOFT TISSUES

T1-weighted images are most useful for evaluation of normal anatomic relationships. Fat, which has a high signal intensity in T1-weighted images, is normally found within fascial planes and around neurovascular structures. Non-fatty masses located within tissues of high lipid content (e.g., subcutaneous fat) are best depicted in T1-weighted images. Tumors and infection have high signal intensity in T2-weighted images; therefore, T2-weighting is useful for depicting the extent of these lesions within muscle. Ill-defined regions of increased signal intensity may be seen within skeletal muscle adjacent to neoplasms and inflammatory processes. This increased signal is probably related to edema.[9] Hemorrhage into soft tissue will vary in signal characteristics according to the time between the onset of bleeding and image acquisition.

Injuries in ligaments and tendons are generally best depicted on MR images by imaging directly along the long axis of the structure of interest. T1-weighted images will show alterations in either signal intensity and/or configuration of the structure, and T2-weighted images display high signal intensity fluid at sites of tendon disruption.

MALIGNANT PRIMARY BONE TUMORS

Magnetic resonance imaging has proved to be a sensitive method for the detection of bone tumors and for determining their extent.[10–13] Multiplanar imaging allows optimal assessment of the relationship of the tumor to adjacent joints and neurovascular structures, making MRI an excellent imaging modality for planning surgery or radiation therapy.

Relaxation times for normal and abnormal marrow are clearly different, but there is too much overlap between benign and malignant processes for MRI to be useful in establishing a tissue diagnosis.[14] The specificity of MRI is poor, and radiographs continue to be the most important imaging tools for the differential diagnosis of bone tumors and for the determination of their aggressiveness. Radiography and computed tomography (CT) are preferable to MRI for demonstrating calcific or osseous deposits in tumor matrix, and for disclosing subtle cortical invasion by tumor. Should radiographs not be available, some of the same diagnostic information may be derived from the MR images. This includes location of the lesion within the skeleton (e.g., femur, humerus), location of the lesion within the bone (epiphysis, metaphysis, or diaphysis), and clinical data (sex and age). A limited tissue specificity can be derived from the comparison of true T1- and T2-weighted images. For example, lipoma will display high signal intensity equal to that of subcutaneous fat in both pulse sequences,[15] while fibrous tissue and calcification will have low signal with both T1- and T2-weighted imaging.[16] Benign

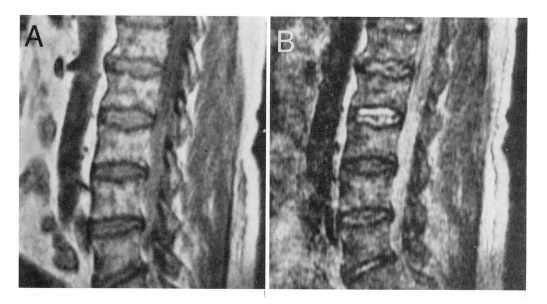

FIG 13–3.
Myelofibrosis in a 61-year-old man with aplastic anemia. **A**, sagittal T1-weighted image (SE 500/28). The bone marrow is diffusely inhomogeneous, and its signal intensity is abnormally low. **B**, sagittal T2-weighted image (SE 2000/84). The marrow signal intensity remains low and inhomogeneous. Bone biopsy revealed myelofibrosis.

mineralization cannot be differentiated from calcification or ossification associated with malignancy. The specific pattern of mineralization is again best depicted in radiographs.

The differential diagnosis of a primary malignant bone tumor should generally be established by radiography and/or biopsy prior to MRI. Cross-sectional imaging is then used to define the extent of tumor and its relationship to surrounding structures. In general, similar information is obtained with both CT and MRI, and often one of these cross-sectional studies will suffice.

Acquisition of MR images of bone tumors will often be dictated by the anticipated therapeutic approach to the lesion. When planning a limb salvage procedure, it is important to provide accurate measurements of the extent of tumor involvement with respect to both the end of the bone and surgical landmarks, and to assure that vital neurovascular structures are not invaded or encased by tumor. If a lesion is near a joint, extensive tumor infiltration into the synovium or joint capsule may preclude limb salvage; therefore, high-resolution images of the joint are essential. If disarticulation is planned, the periarticular soft tissues must be carefully evaluated for possible tumor extension.

BENIGN PRIMARY BONE TUMORS

Benign primary tumors of bone are a frequent incidental finding on MR images. If a question exists as to the cause of an unsuspected, abnormal focus of signal in the marrow, radiographs should be obtained. This is usually all that need be done to determine the benignity of the lesion.

OSSEOUS METASTATIC DISEASE

The high sensitivity of MRI for evaluating bone marrow makes it the ideal tool for detecting osseous metastatic disease and for determining its extent. This sensitivity stems from the fact that conventional studies [radiography, CT, and bone scanning with technetium-99m methylene diphosphonate (^{99m}Tc-MDP)] all rely on alterations in cortical and/or trabecular bone before disease can be detected. Osseous metastases are generally hematogenously spread, and the highly vascular bone marrow is the earliest site of involvement. Thus, MRI is the most sensitive imaging method for the early detection of osseous metastases.[17]

Magnetic resonance imaging is a useful adjunct in the evaluation of metastatic disease in the patient with a known primary tumor in three situations: (1) the symptomatic patient whose conventional studies do not show disease; (2) the asymptomatic patient with equivocal conventional studies; and (3) for planning radiation or surgical therapy for known lesions. The importance of acquiring both T1- and T2-weighted images must again be stressed. Several benign focal conditions will show low signal intensity on T1-weighted images, including bone islands and hemosiderin deposits related to multiple transfusions. Both of these entities will remain low in signal intensity with T2 weighting. Tumor deposits, on the other hand, will increase in signal intensity with T2-weighted imaging. With current imaging techniques, however, bone islands cannot reliably be differentiated from blastic metastases. Radiography or CT scanning may assist the diagnosis in this latter situation.

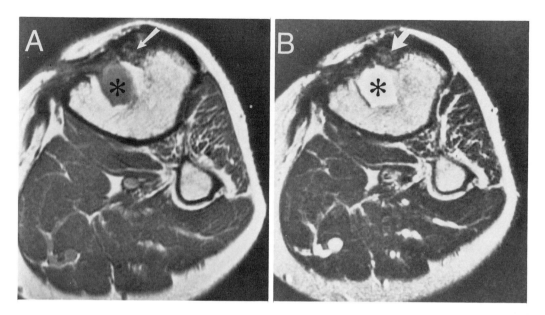

FIG 13–4.
Osteomyelitis in a 29-year-old man who had undergone removal of an intramedullary rod; he presented with cellulitis and a draining sinus near the anterior tibial tubercle. Imaging was requested to confirm the presence of a suspected rod tract infection. **A,** axial T1-weighted image (SE 500/30). The site of the previous intramedullary rod is evident (*arrow*). A well-defined region of low signal intensity is present in the marrow adjacent to but separate from the rod tract (*asterisk*) **B,** axial T2-weighted image (SE 2000/85). The signal intensity of the rod tract remains low, indicating healing with fibrous tissue (*arrow*). The adjacent marrow, however, now shows very high signal intensity (*asterisk*). At surgery, this represented the region of osteomyelitis.

INFECTION

Documentation of osteomyelitis in patients with cellulitis is a common diagnostic dilemma. The presence of osteomyelitis has a profound impact on patient management in terms of length of hospitalization, use of intravenous antibiotics, and health care costs. Radiographic changes of osteomyelitis are late, and occur only after there has been substantial bone destruction. Triple-phase ^{99m}Tc-MDP bone scanning has been used to differentiate cellulitis from osteomyelitis, but confusion can arise from increased uptake of the radionuclide on static images at sites of reactive periosteal new bone formation adjacent to foci of cellulitis, even when there is no actual bone marrow involvement.

The high sensitivity of MRI for demonstrating infiltrative disorders of bone marrow makes it an ideal method for determining the presence or absence of osteomyelitis.[7, 8] With marrow infection, both edema and inflammatory exudate will cause decreased marrow signal intensity with T1-weighted imaging and increased signal intensity with T2-weighting. With chronic osteomyelitis, a well-defined focus of abnormal signal intensity may be seen in the marrow, indicating an intraosseous abscess (Fig 13–4). Sinus tracts may be evident as well. Sclerotic reparative bone and fibrous tissue will have low signal intensity in both T1- and T2-weighted images. Normal bone marrow signal intensity excludes the diagnosis of osteomyelitis.

HIP

The most accurate noninvasive method for the early detection of osteonecrosis of the femoral head is MRI.[18-21] Although the MR appearance of ischemic necrosis is subject to some variability, in all cases, the abnormality is characterized in T1-weighted images by a decrease in the normal high-intensity signal of the bone marrow within the femoral head. The changes feature a ring or bandlike area of diminished signal, or a homogeneous or inhomogeneous focal region of diminished signal that includes the subarticular region of the femoral head (Fig 13–5).

Tissue changes accounting for the diminished signal have not yet been satisfactorily explained, nor have the pathophysiological mechanisms of the various MRI changes been proved. Replacement of marrow fat by histiocytic and fibrovascular connective tissues, combined with new bone proliferation, undoubtedly plays a contributing role.[22] With T2-weighted imaging, regions of necrotic bone (saponified marrow) will retain low signal intensity, while the signal intensity of surrounding areas of edema or fibrovascular repair tissue will increase. By imaging in the coronal plane, both hips may be evaluated simultaneously. This is effective in detecting asymptomatic disease in the contralateral hip.

Although normal bone marrow signal in T1-weighted images may exclude the diagnosis of osteonecrosis, it is prudent to acquire T2-weighted images routinely. This additional imaging sequence may assist in identifying other causes of hip pain (Fig 13–6).

Care must be taken not to confuse normal anatomic structures in the hip for disease (Fig 13–7). The fovia capitis femoris may be prominent in some individuals; its bilateral symmetry and typical location assist in its identification. The fused femoral head physis is usually evident as a horizontal low-signal band, and should not be mistaken for a fracture. Bands of low signal intensity extending from the dome of the femoral head to the medial femoral neck represent normal stress trabeculations. These too can be quite prominent.

Transient regional osteoporosis of the hip may be confused with osteonecrosis, both

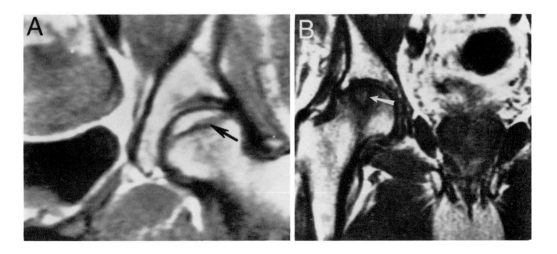

FIG 13–5.
Avascular necrosis of the femoral head in two different patients. Coronal T1-weighted images (SE 500/30). **A**, the ring, or band, of low signal intensity (*arrow*) in the femoral head represents avascular necrosis. **B**, the well-defined focus of low signal intensity in the femoral head represents avascular necrosis (*arrow*). The more extensive low signal that extends into the femoral neck increased with T2-weighting, and represents edema.

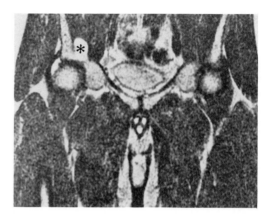

FIG 13–6.
Iliopectineal bursitis in a 30-year-old man with pain in
his right hip. Coronal T2-weighted image (SE 2000/85)
reveals high signal intensity in the iliopectineal bursa
(*asterisk*), implicating iliopectineal bursitis as the cause
of this patient's pain. The fluid collection was poorly
seen on the T1-weighted images.

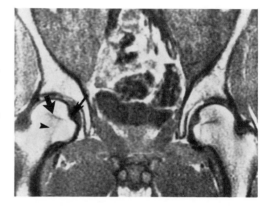

FIG 13–7.
Normal hips, coronal plane (SE 500/30). The fovea
capitis femoris (*thin arrow*) is the site of attachment of
the ligamentum teres femoris, and should not be
mistaken for a focus of osteonecrosis. Lines of low
signal intensity extending from the femoral neck to the
top of the femoral head (*arrowhead*) represent normal
stress trabeculation. Horizontally arranged trabeculae
at the site of the fused physis (*broad arrow*) cause a
band of low signal.

clinically and in MR images. In radiographs, transient osteoporosis is characterized by moderate to severe osteoporosis. The ^{99m}Tc-MDP scan typically shows intense accumulation of
the isotope in the femoral head. T1-weighted MR images may show decreased signal intensity
of the bone marrow of the head and neck. However, T2-weighted images show uniform high
signal intensity.[23, 24]

KNEE

Magnetic resonance imaging is well established as an accurate means of evaluating the
knee for internal derangement, and has replaced arthrography in many institutions.[25–28] Not
only can MRI confirm and localize clinically suspected disease, it can also determine the
presence of additional lesions.

A number of techniques have been suggested for use in routine MRI of the knee, and
the procedures used will depend on the imaging system employed. Generally, the majority
of significant abnormalities of the menisci and cruciate ligaments can be depicted with thin-
section sagittal imaging. When the patient is placed supine in the instrument and the leg

allowed to relax in a comfortable position, the knee will rotate externally approximately 20 degrees. This will align sagittal images along the long axis of the anterior cruciate ligament. If the collateral ligaments are of clinical concern, coronal imaging is needed. The patellofemoral joint is depicted best in the axial plane.

The menisci of the knee are composed of fibrocartilage, and are normally displayed as a homogeneous signal void with all pulsing sequences (Fig 13–8). In sagittal images, the meniscal mid-zones will have a "bow-tie" configuration. The anterior and posterior horns of both menisci should be well-circumscribed triangles. Occasionally, a normal meniscus will display an internal band or a triangle of intermediate signal intensity that conforms to the meniscal contour (Fig 13–9). The reason for this signal is poorly understood, but it is apparent that it does not represent a clinically significant pathologic process. The normal anterior cruciate ligament is imaged as a straight band of intermediate signal intensity that often shows striations (Fig 13–10). The normal posterior cruciate ligament is a gently curving signal void (Fig 13–11). On coronal images, the medial and lateral collateral ligaments can be seen as thin bands of signal void that blend imperceptibly with the cortex of the femur and the tibia and fibula.

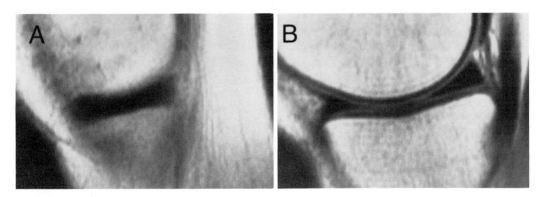

FIG 13–8.
Normal knee, sagittal plane (SE 800/30). With all pulse sequences, the menisci are homogeneous and devoid of signal. **A,** the midzone of the meniscus is in a "bow-tie" configuration. **B,** the anterior and posterior horns of the meniscus are triangular.

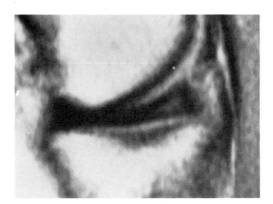

FIG 13–9.
Normal knee, sagittal plane (SE 800/30). Frequently, there is a focus of high signal within the meniscus that cannot be attributed to significant abnormality. The origin of this signal has not been determined with certainty. Unlike a meniscal tear, this signal does not extend to a meniscal surface.

FIG 13–10.
Normal anterior cruciate ligament, sagittal plane (SE 800/30). The anterior cruciate ligament (*arrows*) is a straight band of low-to-intermediate signal intensity. Internal striations are often present.

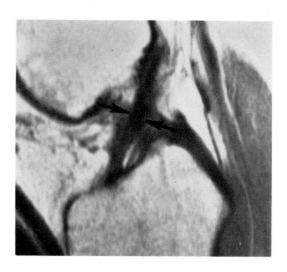

FIG 13–11.
Normal posterior cruciate ligament, sagittal plane (SE 800/30). With the patient's knee extended (as it is for MRI), the posterior cruciate ligament (*arrows*) is gently curved. Unlike the anterior cruciate ligament, the posterior cruciate ligament is imaged as a homogeneous signal void.

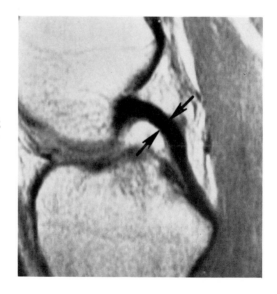

As with the hip, care must be taken not to mistake normal anatomic structures in and about the knee for abnormalities. Most potential pitfalls can be avoided by knowing the exact location of these normal structures. The transverse geniculate (intermeniscal) ligament connects the anterior horns of the medial and lateral menisci. Near its attachment, this ligament may be mistaken for a fragment torn from the anterior meniscal horn (Fig 13–12). Laterally, the popliteal tendon sheath creates a similar band of signal, which may mimic a vertical tear of the posterior horn of the lateral meniscus (Fig 13–13). The anterior and posterior meniscofemoral ligaments are found in the vicinity of the posterior cruciate ligament, and should not be confused for intra-articular loose bodies (Fig 13–14).

Meniscal tears are represented as linear foci of intermediate to high signal intensity that extend from the inner substance of the meniscus to its surface (Fig 13–15). In cases of extensive or complex tears, the meniscus may display diffusely abnormal signals. Degenerative changes

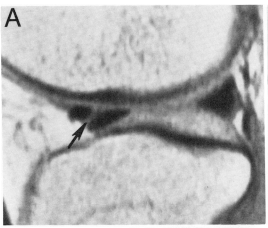

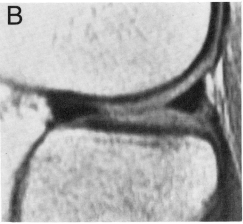

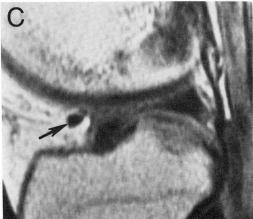

FIG 13–12.
Transverse geniculate ligament, sagittal plane (SE 800/30). **A,** the oblique band of increased signal intensity through the anterior horn of the meniscus (*arrow*) represents synovial tissue and/or fluid separating the ligament from the meniscus, and should not be mistaken for a tear. **B,** image immediately medial to **A.** The meniscus is normal. **C,** image immediately lateral to **A.** The ligament is now evident as a focus of low signal intensity (*arrow*) in the fat anterior to the meniscus. This band can be followed to its insertion on the opposite anterior meniscal horn.

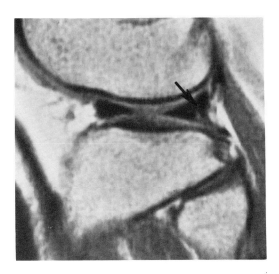

FIG 13–13.
Popliteal tendon sheath, sagittal plane (SE 800/30). This normal structure may mimic a tear of the posterior horn of the lateral meniscus.

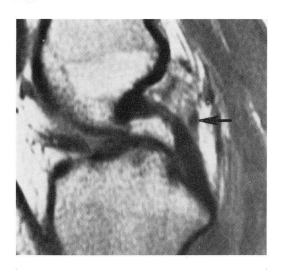

FIG 13–14.
Posterior meniscofemoral ligament, sagittal plane (SE 800/30). The ligament (*arrow*) is displayed as a round focus of low signal intensity behind the posterior cruciate ligament. This should not be mistaken for an intra-articular loose body.

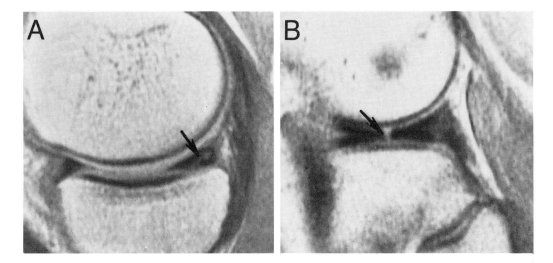

FIG 13–15.
Meniscal tears are evident as bands of intermediate signal intensity that extend to a meniscal surface. **A**, sagittal plane (SE 800/30). Tear of the posterior horn of the medial meniscus (*arrow*). **B**, sagittal plane (SE 800/30). Tear of the midzone of the lateral meniscus (*arrow*).

of the menisci are imaged as round foci of intermediate signal intensity within the substance of the menisci. Such degenerative foci may be an isolated finding, or they may be associated with a tear.

While MRI has not been shown to be highly sensitive for the evaluation of partial tears of the cruciate ligaments, complete ligament disruption is easily displayed. Complete disruption of the anterior cruciate ligament is evident either by failure to display the ligament on a series of contiguous or interleaved thin-section images, or by disruption along its normal smooth course (Fig 13–16).

When a collateral ligament is torn, MRI reveals abnormal signal intensity and disruption of the normally smooth course of the ligament (Fig 13–17). The adjacent soft-tissues may be thickened. Fluid, edema, or blood at the site of injury may be demonstrated on T2-weighted images.

Fluid collections in and about the knee are readily evident with MRI. In most instances, T2-weighted imaging is not needed for their depiction. Fluid collections may be intra-articular, or may be located within one or all of the many bursa about the knee. Knowledge of the location of the periarticular bursae will avoid confusion when an isolated bursal effusion (bursitis) is encountered.

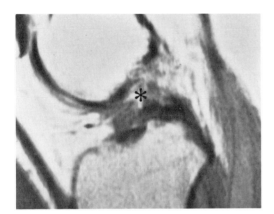

FIG 13–16.
Anterior cruciate ligament tear, sagittal plane (SE 800/30). The region of the anterior cruciate ligament (*asterisk*) displays inhomogeneous signal intensity, and the normally smooth course of the ligament has been disrupted.

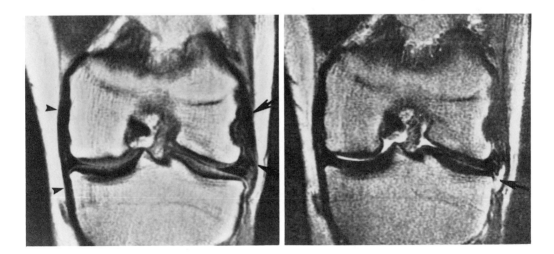

FIG 13–17.
Torn lateral collateral ligament. **A,** T1-weighted coronal image (SE 500/30). The lateral collateral ligament is diffusely thickened and shows abnormal intermediate signal intensity (*arrows*). The medial collateral ligament is normal (*arrowheads*). **B,** with T2-weighting (SE 2000/85), the fluid at the tibial insertion reveals the site of ligament rupture (*arrow*).

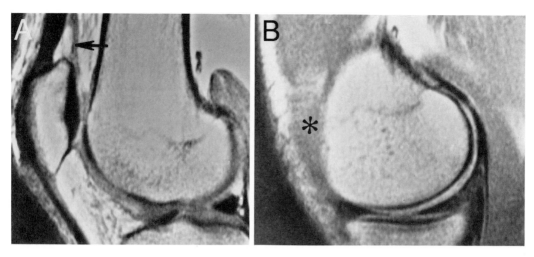

FIG 13–18.
Sagittal images of the knee (SE 800/30). **A**, no fluid is present in the suprapatellar bursa (*arrow*). **B**, image at the lateral aspect of the joint reveals a homogeneous region of intermediate signal intensity (*asterisk*), representing an effusion.

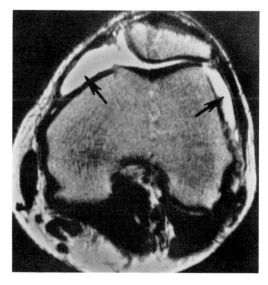

FIG 13–19.
T2-weighted axial image of the knee (SE 2000/85) demonstrating the distribution of a knee effusion. With the patient supine, fluid will first collect in the medial and lateral recesses (*arrows*). With larger effusions, the suprapatellar bursa will also be distended.

With sagittal imaging, small intra-articular effusions are best depicted on images near the medial or lateral aspect of the joint (Fig 13–18). This is because the medial and lateral recesses of the joint are the first to fill when the patient is supine (Fig 13–19). With larger effusions, the fluid may be seen to distend the suprapatellar bursa.

Synovial (ganglion) and meniscal cysts are readily displayed with MRI.[29] Because the optimal imaging plane will depend on the location of the cyst, knowledge of the presence and location of any palpable masses prior to imaging is extremely useful. Meniscal cysts are thought to result from pressure forcing intra-articular fluid through a chronic meniscal tear.

This increased pressure eventually causes herniation of the synovium into the soft tissues around the joint; the result is a fluid-fillet cyst that communicates with the joint by way of the meniscus. In cases of long-standing meniscal cysts, this communication may not be evident, but the adjacent meniscus should be abnormal. Ganglion cysts are thought to result from synovial herniation associated with a tendon sheath, and are therefore generally not associated with intra-articular abnormalities. In the vicinity of the knee, they are most often seen adjacent to the head of the fibula.

Magnetic resonance imaging is also extremely useful in depiciting osteochondritis dissecans (Fig 13–20). In this situation, important information to be derived from the image includes the extent of abnormal marrow, the integrity of the adjacent articular cartilage, and the presence or absence of intra-articular loose bodies.

Often, knowledge that a knee study is postoperative is not provided at the time of MR image acquisition and interpretation. This important clinical information may be evident on MR images by recognition of bands of low to intermediate signal intensity within the infrapatellar fat (Fig 13–21). This site is routinely used as a port for arthroscopic surgery. Artifact from tiny metal fragments may also be evident either in or around the joint, even when no internal fixation devices were utilized. These metallic fragments may be left by the arthroscope or other surgical instruments.

SHOULDER

Normal MRI anatomy of the shoulder has been described in detail[30–32] (Figs 13–22 through 13–24). Magnetic resonance imaging is now proving to be equal if not superior to previously available imaging modalities in the evaluation of a variety of common shoulder disorders, including impingement syndrome, glenohumeral instability, and osteonecrosis of the humeral head.[33–37]

Shoulder imaging requires the use of a surface coil and high-resolution techniques. The type of coil used will depend on the imaging system employed. Choice of imaging planes and pulse sequences will be determined by the type of abnormality suspected.

In its classic form, shoulder impingement syndrome implies inadequate space between

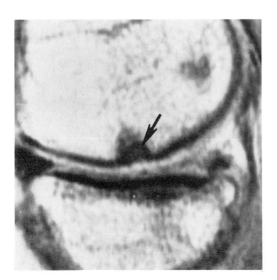

FIG 13–20.
Osteochondritis dessicans, sagittal plane (SE 500/30), in a 26-year-old man with knee pain. The subchondral focus of low signal intensity in the medial femoral condyle (*arrow*) represents osteochondritis dessicans. The adjacent articular cartilage is intact.

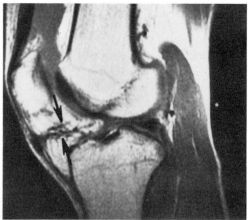

FIG 13–21.
Postoperative knee, sagittal plane (SE 800/30). The previous arthroscopic surgery is evident by the bands of low signal intensity in the infrapatellar fat (*arrows*).

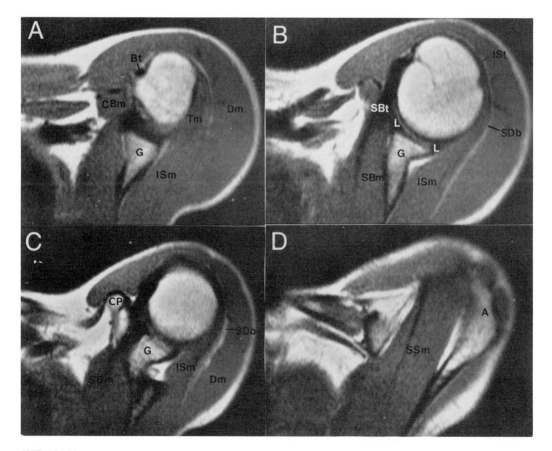

FIG 13–22.
Normal shoulder, axial plane (SE 500/30). Anterior is at the top of the image. **A,** level of the low humeral head. *Bt* = biceps tendon/groove, *CBm* = coracobrachialis muscle, *Dm* = deltoid muscle, *G* = bony glenoid, *ISm* = infraspinatus muscle, *Tm* = teres minor muscle. **B,** level of the mid humeral head. *ISt* = infraspinatus tendon, *L* = glenoid labrum, *SBm* = subscapularis muscle, *SBt* = subscapularis tendon, *SDb* = subdeltoid bursa. **C,** level of the coracoid process. *CP* = coracoid process. **D,** level of the supraspinatus muscle. *A* = acromion, *SSm* = supraspinatus muscle.

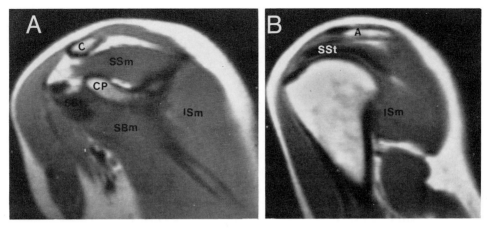

FIG 13–23.
Normal shoulder, sagittal plane (SE 500/30). Anterior is to the left of the image. **A**, medial to the humeral head. *C* = clavicle, *CP* = coracoid process, *ISm* = infraspinatus muscle, *SBm* = subscapularis muscle, *SBt* = subscapularis tendon, *SSm* = supraspinatus muscle. **B**, level of the mid humeral head. *A* = acromion, *SSt* = supraspinatus muscle.

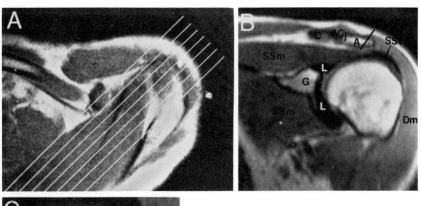

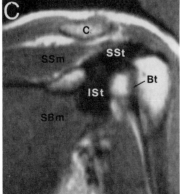

FIG 13–24.
Normal shoulder, frontal oblique plane (SE 500/30). **A**, axial image showing alignment of cursors for frontal oblique imaging. **B**, level of the mid acromioclavicular joint. *A* = acromion, *ACj* = acromioclavicular joint, *C* = clavicle, *Dm* = deltoid muscle, *G* = bony glenoid, *L* = glenoid labrum, *SAb* = subacromial bursa, *SBm* = subscapularis muscle, *SSm* = supraspinalus muscle; *SSt* = supraspinatus tendon. **C**, level of the anterior humeral head, through the bicipital groove. *Bt* = biceps tendon/groove, *ISt* = infraspinatus tendon.

the humeral head below and the structures of the coracoacromial arc above for normal movement of the subacromial bursa and supraspinatus tendon. Repeated mechanical trauma to these soft tissues leads to subacromial bursitis; supraspinatus tendinitis; and if unrelieved, tendon tear. Common offending structures include a congenitally low-lying acromion, spurs off the inferior aspect of the anterior acromion or acromioclavicular joint, or hypertrophy of the acromioclavicular joint capsule.[38] Prior to MRI, diagnostic imaging examinations had been ineffectual in the evaluation of early impingement syndrome, and the diagnosis was often delayed until the development of a full-thickness cuff tear. Now, however, MRI allows identification of not only the soft tissue damage resulting from this disorder but often of the specific offending structure. Diagnostic information is best obtained by imaging in the oblique plane along the long axis of the supraspinatus muscle. Both T1- and T2-weighted images should be acquired.

Subacromial bursitis is usually depicted in MR images as thickening of the normal bursal fat, and is thus high signal intensity in both T1- and T2-weighted images (Fig 13–25). Actually, this thickening probably represents hypertrophic synovitis, as the synovium both lies upon and is laden with fat. Less commonly, excessive fluid may be found in the bursa. In this situation, the fluid will be of low to intermediate signal intensity in T1-weighted images, and high signal intensity in T2-weighted images (Fig 13–26).

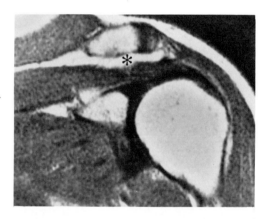

FIG 13–25.
Subacromial bursitis, frontal oblique plane (SE 500/30). The high signal intensity of the subacromial bursa is thickened (*asterisk*). The supraspinatus tendon is normal.

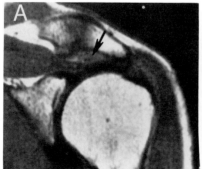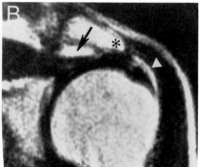

FIG 13–26.
Subacromial bursitis with effusion, frontal oblique plane. **A**, T1-weighted image (SE 500/30). Intermediate signal intensity is present in the region of the subacromial bursa immediately below the anterior acromion (*arrow*). **B**, with T2-weighting (SE 2000/85), the signal intensity increases, indicating the presence of fluid (*arrow*). Fluid is also present in the subdeltoid bursa (*arrowhead*). The bursal space between the fluid collections is not evident, because it is compressed by the anterolateral acromion (*asterisk*).

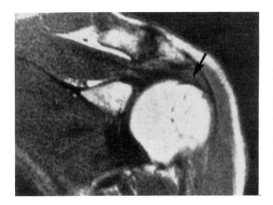

FIG 13–27.
Supraspinatus tendinitis, frontal oblique image (SE 500/30). The supraspinatus tendon shows diffuse abnormal intermediate signal intensity (*arrow*). The signal intensity in this region decreased with T2-weighting (not shown); therefore, this represents tendinitis rather than a tear.

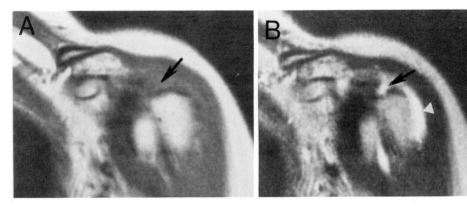

FIG 13–28.
Supraspinatus tendon tear. **A,** T1-weighted frontal oblique image (SE 500/30). There is abnormal intermediate signal intensity in the supraspinatus tendon (*arrow*). With only T1-weighted imaging, tendinitis cannot be differentiated from a tear. **B,** T2-weighted frontal oblique image (SE 2000/85). Fluid is now evident in the tear (*arrow*) and in the subdeltoid bursa (*arrowhead*).

Supraspinatus tendinitis is depicted in MR images as abnormal intermediate signal intensity within the tendon in T1-weighted images (Fig 13–27). With T2-weighted imaging, the abnormal area will either decrease or minimally increase in signal intensity. In the latter case, the signal intensity will not be as bright as that of fluid. A focal region within the tendon, which is of intermediate signal intensity in T1-weighted images and becomes very high in signal intensity with T2-weighting, indicates a tendon tear (Fig 13–28). Both T1 and T2 weighting are needed to avoid misdiagnosing ossific tendinitis for a tear. In the former condition, bone marrow within the tendinous ossification will display high signal intensity in both T1- and T2-weighted images.

Glenohumeral instability refers to dislocation or subluxation of the humeral head. Magnetic resonance imaging has proved to be useful in documentation of abnormalities resulting from glenohumeral instability, including attenuation or tear of the glenoid labrum (Fig 13–29), fractures of the boney glenoid rim or humeral head, and trauma to the subscapularis musculotendinous unit. Imaging can also help one to identify those patients with posterior or multidirectional instability by depicting abnormalities involving the posterior glenoid

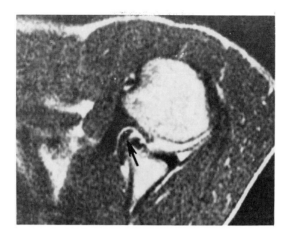

FIG 13–29.
Tear of the anterior glenoid labrum, axial plane, in a 16-year-old boy with a history of two episodes of anterior glenohumeral subluxation. On this T2-weighted image (SE 2000/85), the band of high signal intensity traversing the anterior labrum represents a tear *(arrow)*. The posterior labrum is normal in appearance.

labrum. Imaging to evaluate for glenohumeral instability should be done in the axial plane, with both T1 and T2 weighting. Comparison of the T1- and T2-weighted images will allow differentiation of fat from fluid in cases of capsule rupture or trauma to the subscapularis tendon or muscle.

The humeral head is the second most common site for osteonecrosis. The appearance of osteonecrosis of the head of the humerus may take on the same patterns as in the hip: bandlike, focal or diffuse regions of low signal intensity within the marrow. The key to the diagnosis of osteonecrosis in the humeral head is the appropriate choice of image plane. Images acquired in the sagittal plane with the arm internally rotated will show the earliest changes of osteonecrosis in the posterosuperior aspect of the humeral head. Images acquired in the coronal plane may be confusing as a result of partial volume averaging. In axial images, the normal inhomogeneous signal intensity of the humeral head metaphysis may be mistaken for osteonecrosis.

OTHER JOINTS

Magnetic resonance imaging has proved useful in the evaluation of ischemic necrosis of the talus and the carpal bones. Further clinical trials are needed to determine the role of MRI in the evaluation of other abnormalities of the ankle and wrist.

SUMMARY

As technology continues to improve, musculoskeletal applications of MRI will undoubtedly expand. Because most examinations must be tailored to the specific clinical problem, knowledge of the suspected clinical diagnosis and access to radiographs prior to image acquisition are often essential if the maximum amount of information is to be gleaned from each MRI examination.

REFERENCES

1. Ehman RL, Berquist TH, McLeod RA: MR imaging of the musculoskeletal system: A 5-year appraisal. *Radiology* 1988; 166:313–320.
2. Bohndorf K, Reiser M, Lochner B, et al: Magnetic resonance imaging of primary bone tumours and tumour-like lesions of bone. *Skeletal Radiol* 1986; 15:511–517.
3. Dooms GC, Fisher MR, Hricak H, et al: Bone marrow imaging: Magnetic resonance studies related to age and sex. *Radiology* 1985; 155:429–432.
4. Stafford SA, Rosenthal DI, Gebhardt MC, et al: MRI in stress fracture. *AJR* 1986; 147:553–556.
5. Yao L, Lee JK: Occult intraosseous fracture: Detection with MR imaging. *Radiology* 1988; 167:749–751.
6. Lee JK, Yao L: Stress fractures: MR imaging. *Radiology* 1988; 169:217–220.
7. Tang JS, Gold RH, Bassett LW, et al: Musculoskeletal infection of the extremities: Evaluation with MR imaging. *Radiology* 1988; 166:205–209.
8. Unger E, Moldofsky P, Gatenby R, et al: Diagnosis of osteomyelitis by MR imaging. *AJR* 1988; 150:605–610.
9. Beltran J, Simon DC, Katz W, et al: Increased MR signal intensity in skeletal muscle adjacent to malignant tumors: Pathologic correlation and clinical relevance. *Radiology* 1987; 162:251–255.
10. Richardson ML, Kilcoyne RF, Gillespy T III, et al: Magnetic resonance imaging of musculoskeletal neoplasms. *Radiol Clin North Am* 1986; 24:259–267.
11. Aisen AM, Martel W, Braunstein EM, et al: MRI and CT evaluation of primary bone and soft-tissue tumors. *AJR* 1986; 146:749–756.
12. Zimmer WD, Berquist TH, Mcleod RA, et al: Bone tumors: Magnetic resonance imaging versus computed tomography. *Radiology* 1985; 155:709–718.
13. Bloem JL, Bluemm RG, Taminiau AHM, et al: Magnetic resonance imaging of primary malignant bone tumors. *RadioGraphics* 1987; 7:425–445.
14. Pettersson H, Slone RM, Spainer S, et al: Musculoskeletal tumors: T1 and T2 relaxation times. *Radiology* 1988; 167:783–785.
15. Sundaram M, McGuire MH, Herbold DR, et al: High signal intensity soft tissue masses on T1 weighted pulsing sequences. *Skeletal Radiol* 1987; 16:30–36.
16. Sundaram M, McGuire MH, Schajowicz F: Soft-tissue masses: Histologic basis for decreased signal (short T2) on T2-weighted images. *Skeletal Radiol* 1987; 148:1247–1250.
17. Seeger LL, Bassett LW, Bertino F, et al: Magnetic resonance imaging for demonstrating undetected bone metastases (abstract). XVI International Congress of Radiology General Program 1985, p. 137.
18. Totty WG, Murphy WA, Ganz WI, et al: Magnetic resonance imaging of the normal and ischemic femoral head. *AJR* 1984; 143:1273–1280.
19. Markisz JA, Knowles RJR, Altchek DW, et al: Segmental patterns of avascular necrosis of the femoral heads: Early detection with MR imaging. *Radiology* 1987; 162:717–720.
20. Mitchell MD, Kundel HL, Steinberg ME, et al: Avascular necrosis of the hip: Comparison of MR, CT, and scintigraphy. *AJR* 1986; 147:67–71.
21. Mitchell DG, Rao VM, Dalinka MK, et al: Femoral head avascular necrosis: Correlation of MR imaging, radiographic staging, radionuclide imaging, and clinical findings. *Radiology* 1987; 162:709–715.
22. Bassett LW, Mirra JM, Cracchiolo A III, et al: Ischemic necrosis of the femoral head: Correlation of magnetic resonance imaging and histologic sections. *Clin Orthop* 1987; 223:181–187.
23. Bloem JL: Transient osteoporosis: MR imaging. *Radiology* 1988; 167:753–755.
24. Wilson AJ, Murphy WA, Hardy DC, et al: Transient osteoporosis: Transient bone marrow edema. *Radiology* 1988; 167:757–760.
25. Reicher MA, Rauschning W, Gold RH, et al: High-resolution MR imaging of the knee joint: Normal anatomy. *AJR* 1985; 145:895–902.
26. Reicher MA, Bassett LW, Gold RH: High-resolution magnetic resonance imaging of the knee joint: Pathologic correlations. *AJR* 1985; 145:903–909.

27. Li DK, Adams, ME, McConkey JP: Magnetic resonance imaging of the ligaments and menisci of the knee. *Radiol Clin North Am* 1986; 24:209–227.
28. Burk DL Jr, Kanal E, Brunberg JA, et al: 1.5 T surface-coil MRI of the knee. *AJR* 1986; 147:293–300.
29. Burk DL Jr, Dalinka MK, Kanal E, et al: Meniscal and ganglion cysts of the knee: MR evaluation. *AJR* 1988; 150:331–336.
30. Huber DJ, Sauter R, Mueller E, et al: MR imaging of the normal shoulder. *Radiology* 1986; 158:405–408.
31. Dominik HJ, Sauter R, Mueller E, et al: MR imaging of the normal shoulder. *Radiology* 1986; 158:405–408.
32. Seeger LL, Ruszkowski JT, Bassett LW, et al: MR imaging of the normal shoulder: Anatomic correlation. *AJR* 1987; 148:83–91.
33. Kneeland JB, Middleton WD, Carrera GF, et al: MR imaging of the shoulder: Diagnosis of rotator cuff tears. *AJR* 1987; 149:333–337.
34. Seeger LL, Gold RH, Bassett LW, et al: Shoulder impingement syndrome: MR findings in 53 shoulders. *AJR* 1988; 150:343–347.
35. Kieft GJ, Bloem JL, Rozing PM, et al: Rotator cuff impingement syndrome: MR imaging. *Radiology* 1988; 166:211–214.
36. Seeger LL, Gold RH, Bassett LW: MR imaging of shoulder instability. *Radiology* 1988; 168:695–697.
37. Kieft GJ, Bloem JL, Rozing PM, et al: MR imaging of recurrent anterior dislocation of the shoulder: Comparison with CT arthrography. *AJR* 1988; 150:1083–1087.
38. Neer CS II: Impingement lesions. *Clin Orthop* 1983; 173:70–77.

Chapter 14

General Pediatric Applications

M. Ines Boechat, M.D.

Theodore R. Hall, M.D.

Rosalind B. Dietrich, M.B., Ch.B.

Hooshang Kangarloo, M.D.

Magnetic resonance imaging (MRI) is the newest imaging modality available for diagnosis of diseases in children. Neither ionizing radiation nor administration of contrast media is required for MRI, and its imaging capability in several planes with good image resolution has made it especially attractive for use with this age group. While the exact role of MRI in pediatrics is still being defined, its importance in neuroimaging and in the evaluation of abdominal neoplasms has already been recognized (see Chapter 8).[1-3] Further progress with the use of rapid scanning techniques, improved instrumentation, and the development of receptor placed paramagnetic agents will undoubtedly enhance the utilization of MRI in pediatrics.

PATIENT PREPARATION, SEDATION, AND MONITORING

Patient cooperation is essential for a successful examination, as patients must remain immobile during the long image-acquisition times, which is a particular problem for children. It is worthwhile to spend a few minutes with the child and parents, explaining how the machine works and what is going to happen. The receptionist also gives the family a booklet about MRI, written in lay language, and questions are answered before the examination. Reassurance is very important and parents are encouraged to remain with the child during the examination, a positive way to decrease anxiety for all parties.

For children younger than 5 years of age, sedation is routinely utilized.[4] Children should be given nothing by mouth 3 to 4 hours before the examination, to prevent vomiting and subsequent aspiration. Children younger than 2 years of age receive chloral hydrate, 50 to 100 mg/kg body weight orally, 30 minutes before the examination. Older children are given intrarectal thiopental, 25 mg/kg, 5 to 10 minutes before the procedure. There are special cases that will require even deeper levels of sedation; the pediatric anesthesiologist is in

TABLE 14–1.

Results of Various Imaging Techniques in a 0.3-T Imager

Imaging Technique	Advantages	Disadvantages
Spin echo T1	Good visualization of anatomy	May not show abnormalities; relatively small number of slices
Spin echo T2	Good tissue contrast differentiation	Long imaging time (12 min); motion artifact
Multiple echo multiple repetition	Short imaging time (16 min); 15 slices; Good T1 and T2; Better than double echo; spin echo contiguity; slice profile; flow compensation	Motion artifact in upper abdomen due to scanning time
Inversion recovery	Extremely T1 weighted; good depiction of anatomy; Better tissue differentiation	Long imaging time (9 min); lower signal-to-noise ratio
Double echo	Good T2, same time as SE T2 (two images)	Poor T1 (proton density); poor visualization of abnormalities
Field echo	Short time (13 sec to 3 min); cine breath-holding; hemorrhage	Lower signal-to-noise ratio
Chemical shift	Fat-water differentiation; marrow abnormalities seen	Limited use

charge of drug administration and monitoring. An apnea monitor is used in all sedated patients. After the examination is completed, sedated children should be followed by a physician or a nurse until they are alert; a recovery room either in close proximity to the MRI suite or within the radiology department is the ideal solution.

PULSE SEQUENCES

Recent advances in MRI techniques have made available an impressive array of imaging choices to the radiologist. The MR signal intensity is a synthesis of the hydrogen concentration and the T1 and T2 relaxation values of the tissues. Depending on the imaging method used—spin echo, inversion recovery, short inversion recovery (STIR), complex rephasing incorporated surface probe (CRISP), different pulse sequences intervals, echo-delay times, and magnetic field strength—image contrast will greatly vary. Although some basic principles apply to all imaging units, each center has to develop its own parameters for optimal imaging of each part of the body. The advantages and disadvantages of the currently used imaging techniques for a 0.3-tesla permanent magnet system are listed in Table 14–1.

SURFACE COILS

Surface coils were developed to improve image quality. Solenoid surface coils have proved very useful in our experience.[5] They are made of several pairs of thin copper coils encased in foam, and flexible enough to be applied like a belt around the patient's body and secured with a fastening tape (such as Velcro). Several adjustable coils are available, ranging from 3 to 50 cm in diameter. The strong coupling of the surface coils results in improved signal-to-noise ratio when compared with images obtained with the standard body coil.[6]

CHEST IMAGING

Computed tomography (CT) is still the primary imaging modality for the chest when evaluating parenchymal lesions, because of its short scanning time and superior spatial resolution. However, MRI is very useful in the evaluation of the mediastinum (lymphoma, cystic hygroma, and other masses) (Fig 14–1).[7] The flow void due to normal blood flow seen in MR images of the pulmonary arteries is of great benefit in evaluating the pulmonary hili and is used in the detection of both hilar masses and vascular abnormalities. Cardiac imaging is accurate when electrocardiographic gating is used, delineating simple and complex intracardiac disease. Present indications for MRI include complex postoperative disease, evaluation of pulmonary arteries in pulmonary atresia, characterization of pulmonary venous anatomy, evaluation of the great vessels, and pericardiac structures.[8, 9]

ABDOMINAL IMAGING

Respiratory motion and bowel peristalsis are limiting factors in the evaluation of intraperitoneal abnormalities. There are no satisfactory contrast agents available for bowel opacification, and it may be difficult to distinguish between lymphadenopathy and overlying bowel. Magnetic resonance imaging plays a significant role in the evaluation of liver and retroperitoneal organs in children. Its most important role is in the diagnosis of abdominal neoplasms; evaluation of their extent; and, particularly, evaluation of tumor resectability.[10] When a child presents with an abdominal mass, the initial examination is plain radiography of the abdomen, followed by ultrasonography (US). If US shows a solid lesion that the physician suspects may be a neoplasm, then MRI is used to define the origin of the lesion. The examination should be tailored to define the tumor's extent and resectability. Magnetic resonance imaging is also an ideal modality for follow-up study of these patients. Table 14–2 illustrates the protocols used for body imaging at UCLA Medical Center.

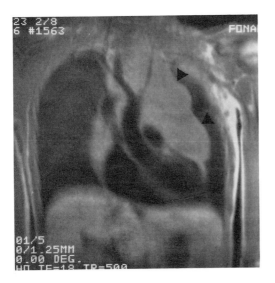

FIG 14–1.
Mediastinum. Lymphoma in a 12-year-old girl presents as a lobulated mass, of medium signal intensity (*arrowheads*) on a T1-weighted image (SE 500/18). (From Kangarloo H: Chest MRI in children. *Radiol Clin North Am* 1988; 26:263–275. Used with permission.)

TABLE 14–2.

Imaging Sequencing for Abdominal Magnetic Resonance Imaging

Anatomic Region	Coronal	Axial	Sagittal	Usual Sequence(s)	Additional Sequence
Chest					
Mediastinum	X	X	X	SE T1	
Rib cage		X		SE T1	
Shoulders		X		SE T1	
Sternum			X	SE T1	
Vertebrae	X		X	SE T1	Chemical shift
Parenchyma	X	X		SE T1	
Diaphragm	X			SE T1	
Abdomen					
Liver	X	X		SE T1, T2	Chemical shift
Adrenals	X			SE T1	SE T2
Kidneys	X			SE T1	IR
Pancreas		X		SE T1	
Aorta, inferior vena cava	X			SE T1	
Celiac artery, superior mesenteric artery		X		SE T1	
Pelvis					
Uterus			X	SE T1, T2 (MEMR)	
Ovaries		X		SE T1, T2 (MEMR)	
Sidewalls		X		SE T1 (MEMR)	

*X = plane selected for imaging different body parts; SE = spin echo; IR = inversion recovery; MEMR = multiple echo multiple repetition.

LIVER

Axial T1-weighted sequences are initially used in evaluating the liver and biliary tract. On these images, the organ parenchyma is well visualized, and structures such as the portal vein, the origin of celiac axis, and the superior mesenteric artery are clearly seen. The axial plane is also used for evaluation of the common bile duct.

Congenital anomalies of the hepatobiliary system, such as choledochal cyst and polycystic liver disease, are routinely evaluated by US scanning. Only when the US study proves inconclusive is MRI used to provide additional information. Magnetic resonance imaging plays an important role, however, in the visualization of congenital vascular anomalies of the liver, such as Budd-Chiari malformations and hemangiomas[11]; it sometimes plays a role in the evaluation of space-occupying lesions of the liver, such as cysts and abscesses. However, differentiation between various forms of liver cysts based on MRI appearance may be difficult, decreasing its diagnostic value. Generalized liver disease, such as cirrhosis and hemochromatosis, is also imaged well by MRI. Cirrhotic liver appears small with nonhomogeneous signal intensity, while hemochromatosis is seen as markedly lower signal intensity because of the deposition of iron and prolongation of T1 relaxation time.[12]

More useful than the ability of MRI to demonstrate generalized liver disease is its use in the visualization of vascular anatomy.[13] In children with severe liver disease who are candidates for palliative shunt procedures or liver transplantation, MRI can potentially obviate the need for angiography by demonstrating detailed vascular anatomy.

The most important role of MRI in the evaluation of liver disorders in children involves the diagnosis of hepatic neoplasms: defining the extent of disease and segmental anatomy, and therefore establishing the possibility of surgical resection.[1] It will also demonstrate thrombosis of portal and hepatic veins. Hepatoblastoma and hepatocarcinoma, the most common hepatic neoplasms seen in children, are well-evaluated by MRI (Fig 14–2). They appear as areas of low signal intensity on T1-weighted images and increased signal on T2-weighted sequences; characterization of tumor type is not always possible. Lymphoma, a much rarer lesion, also has lower signal intensity than the adjacent uninvolved liver on strongly T1-weighted sequences, but shows only slight increase of signal intensity on T2-weighted sequences. Vascular lesions such as hemangiomas and hemangioendotheliomas will have very high signal intensity on T2-weighted sequences, unless they are thrombosed. Our experience thus far indicates that MRI provides more information than CT in evaluating children with suspected liver tumors, particularly with regard to surgical resectability and tumor recurrence.[1]

PANCREAS, SPLEEN, MESENTERY

The pancreas is well-imaged on axial T1-weighted sequences.[14, 15] Although pancreatic lesions are rare in children, MRI can help in evaluating the size of the gland and in the detection of masses or pseudocysts. When obstruction of the common bile duct occurs secondary to a pancreatic neoplasm, stasis of bile within the dilated duct may be seen. More concentrated, old bile demonstrates higher signal intensity on T1-weighted images than does fresh bile (Fig 14–3).

Evaluation of the spleen is best accomplished using coronal T1-weighted images. Differentiation between benign and malignant splenomegaly on the basis of MR appearance only is not possible.[15]

Lesions infiltrating the mesentery, either tumors or inflammation (such as tuberculosis), are best imaged in the axial or sagittal planes. Thickened mesentery is best evaluated on T1-weighted sequences; it has a higher signal intensity than a gas-filled bowel loop but a signal intensity similar to that of the bowel wall. T2-weighted sequences have limited value because of image degradation secondary to the long imaging time.

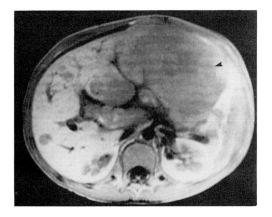

FIG 14–2.
Liver. Hepatocarcinoma in a 10-year-old boy with portal vein invasion and thrombosis. Magnetic resonance imaging study in the axial plane (SE 500/28) shows a large mass in the left lobe of the liver (*arrowheads*), with smaller lesions in the right lobe. (From Boechat MI, Kangarloo H, Gilsanz V: Hepatic masses in children. *Semin Roentgenol* 1988; 23:185–193. Used with permission.)

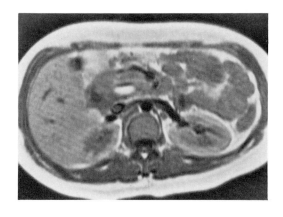

FIG 14–3.
Pancreas. Pancreatic lymphoma in a 16-year-old girl,
causing obstruction of the common bile duct and
layering of old/new bile, is well demonstrated in this
axial scan (SE 500/28)

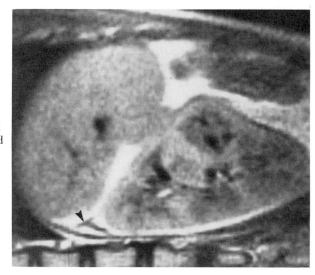

FIG 14–4.
Kidney. Normal appearance of kidney and adrenal
(*arrowhead*) in a 10-year-old girl. The T1-weighted
sequence (SE 600/30) in the coronal plane showed
detailed anatomy of both organs.

KIDNEYS

T1-weighted coronal images are the best to demonstrate the overall appearance of the
kidneys, their accurate length, and their relationship to adjacent organs (Fig 14–4).[16]
The cortex has higher signal intensity than the medulla, with clear corticomedullary
differentiation on T1-weighted images, especially when inversion recovery is used. The renal
artery and vein, the ureter, and the pelvicalyceal system all have low signal intensity. Renal
pyramids are relatively more prominent in neonates and young children; they become similar
to those seen in adult kidneys by about 12 years of age. Signal intensity from adipose tissue
(short T1 and long T2 relaxation times) is not visible in the renal hili of young children. It
progressively increases with age, when fat starts to accumulate in the region and is clearly
visible by puberty.

Congenital and acquired anomalies of the urinary tract are usually diagnosed by means
of US. When US findings are unclear, MRI study may be indicated. Because MRI is not
limited by bowel gas or bone, it can provide better topographic delineation of the abdomen,

enabling accurate diagnosis of congenital anomalies and, particularly, differentiation between renal agenesis and renal ectopia. The separation of the renal hilum by a band of lower signal intensity indicates a duplex collecting system. Anomalies related to fusion and location of the kidneys, such as cross fused ectopia and pelvic kidney, are well evaluated using coronal T1-weighted images, while a horseshoe kidney is best imaged on an axial T1-weighted sequence, which shows the isthmus (Fig 14–5). On coronal images, posterior images of the kidneys may not demonstrate the change in renal axis.

Ultrasonography is generally used to diagnose cystic diseases of the kidney, including multicystic disease, infantile polycystic disease, adult polycystic disease, and simple cysts. Magnetic resonance imaging plays an important role when evaluating associated complications, especially subacute hemorrhage, which appears as areas of high signal intensity on T1-weighted images (Fig 14–6). An uncomplicated simple cyst is seen as a low signal intensity mass displacing the remainder of the normal kidney. Hydronephrosis can also be diagnosed by MRI; the level of obstruction is best seen using coronal T1-weighted images. Early obstruction, without substantial dilation of the collecting system, is better diagnosed by means of T2-weighted images, as the hydronephrotic side shows higher signal intensity compared with the contralateral side, presumably because of the higher water content in the renal parenchyma.

Magnetic resonance imaging can be used in the diagnosis of both chronic and acute renal

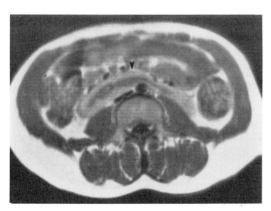

FIG 14–5.
Kidney. Horseshoe anomaly in a 11-year-old boy. The isthmus connecting the lower poles (*arrowhead*) is well seen in an axial T1-weighted image (SE 500/128). (From Dietrich RB, Kangarloo H: *Pediatric Body Imaging*, in Stark B (ed): *Magnetic Resonance Imaging*. St Louis, CV Mosby Co, 1988. Used with permission.)

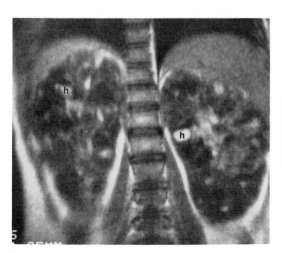

FIG 14–6.
Kidney. Juvenile polycystic disease in a 13-year-old girl. Magnetic resonance image in the coronal plane (SE 300/18) demonstrates the multiple cysts, some of them presenting subacute hemorrhage (*h*).

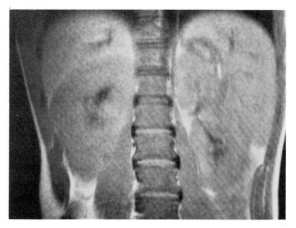

FIG 14–7.
Kidney. Lymphoma in a teen-age boy presents with bilateral nephromegaly and loss of corticomedullary differentiation in this coronal image (SE 500/28).

failure, but not their cause. Corticomedullary differentiation is absent in acute and chronic failure; renal size is normal in acute disease and small in chronic failure. Patients undergoing prolonged dialysis develop renal cysts and, rarely, tumors; periodic survey is recommended in this group of patients. However, MRI is useful in evaluating complications associated with renal biopsy, such as hydronephrosis and hemorrhage.

Several renal transplants patients were imaged with MRI and US for evaluation of rejection; the relatively poor results obtained with MRI may be related to the small number of parameters used in the evaluation of disease.[17] The ideal imaging procedure has not been determined yet, but US and renal nuclear scans are still the most widely used imaging modalities, especially with the introduction of Doppler.

Common renal neoplasms in children include Wilms' tumor and various forms of leukemia and lymphoma. Renal infiltration by lymphoma causes focal or generalized enlargement of the kidneys with low signal intensity and loss of corticomedullary differentiation in the involved portion (Fig 14–7). Involvement of the bone marrow in these patients can also be demonstrated by areas of lower signal intensity on T1-weighted images, a very useful sign in differentiating leukemia and lymphoma from Wilms' tumor.[18]

Wilms' tumor is the most common solid intra-abdominal neoplasm in children. Presentation is generally nonspecific, except for a palpable abdominal mass. Again, US is the initial imaging modality used to differentiate between cystic and solid lesions. If a solid lesion is visualized, a MRI examination in the coronal and axial planes is superior both to US and CT in diagnosing and defining the extent of Wilms' tumor, including vascular thrombosis by direct invasion of the renal vein and in the inferior vena cava (Fig 14–8).[19] It may also be possible to differentiate between classic Wilms' tumor and Wilms' tumor arising from nodular nephroblastomatosis. In the latter group of patients there are multicentric or diffuse tumors and tumor-like lesions; the contralateral kidney should be carefully examined because of the known increased incidence of bilateral lesions. Magnetic resonance imaging is also used for the evaluation of liver metastasis, tumor response to chemotherapy, and postsurgical follow-up studies.

ADRENAL GLANDS

With MRI, one can accurately evaluate normal and abnormal adrenal glands especially when T1-weighted coronal images are used (see Fig 14–4).[20] In neonates and young children, the adrenal gland is relatively large and may have convex borders, while in older children, it has straight or slightly concave borders. The signal intensity of the adrenal glands is slightly less than that of the renal cortex, similar to the overall signal intensity of the kidneys, and substantially less than that of perinephric fat. When the kidneys are absent or abnormally located, such as in those patients with renal agenesis, ectopia and so forth, the adrenal glands appear flat and platelike.

The most significant role of MRI in the evaluation of adrenal diseases in children is in the assessment of adrenal neoplasms.[21, 22] When the coronal plane is used, MRI may specifically demonstrate the characteristic configuration of pheochromocytoma and the extension of adrenal carcinoma into the renal vein, the inferior vena cava, and even the right atrium.

Neuroblastoma, the second most common solid neoplasm in childhood, occurs along the sympathetic chain in the nasopharynx, chest, abdomen and pelvis, or it may have unknown origin.[23] The most common location is in the abdomen, in the region of the adrenal glands.

Magnetic resonance imaging has a particularly important role in tumor staging of a child with neuroblastoma. Coronal T1-weighted images should be acquired initially to separate adrenal from paravertebral or renal neoplasm. By clearly visualizing the spine and the spinal cord, it is possible to evaluate intraspinal extension of a lesion confidently and obviate the need for invasive procedures, such as conventional or CT myelography (Fig 14–9). Neuroblastoma has a tendency to spread quite early to the retroperitoneal area, encasing and displacing arteries and veins. Demonstration of vascular anatomy is of paramount importance for evaluation of tumor resectability.[24] The aorta and the inferior vena cava are best seen on coronal T1-weighted images, whereas the superior mesenteric artery and the celiac axis are better visualized on the axial plane (Fig 14–10). Tumor metastasis to bone, bone marrow, and dura can also be evaluated with MRI. Compared with radionuclide bone scans, MRI appears to be more sensitive in detecting marrow and bone metastasis, although a nuclear medicine bone scan is better for screening. Magnetic resonance imaging is also more accurate than CT in evaluation of dural metastasis. Spine and long bones are best evaluated in the coronal plane and the brain dura in the sagittal plane. Again, MRI is the ideal imaging modality after chemotherapy and surgery.

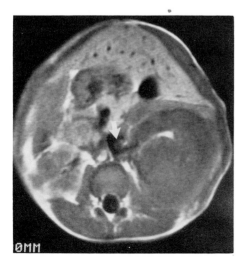

FIG 14–8.
Kidney. Four-year-old boy with Wilms' tumor. The large hypointense left renal mass extends through the renal vein into the inferior vena cava (*arrow*). The lesions are well demonstrated on this axial T1-weighted image (SE 500/18).

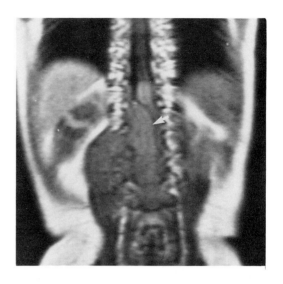

FIG 14–9.
Adrenal gland. Neuroblastoma in a 1-year-old girl, with invasion into the spinal canal (*arrow*) shown in the coronal plane (SE 500/28). The low-signal mass arises in the right paravertebral area and displaces the kidney laterally. (From Dietrich RB, Kangarloo H: Pediatric body imaging, in Stark B (ed): *Magnetic Resonance Imaging.* St Louis, CV Mosby Co, 1988. Used with permission.)

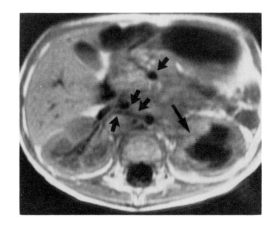

FIG 14–10.
Adrenal gland in a 5-year-old boy with a large neuroblastoma. Scan in the axial plane (SE 500/18) shows encasement of major vessels (*small arrows*) and left hydronephrosis (*arrow*).

PELVIS

A wide spectrum of pelvic and perineal lesions in children can be demonstrated with MRI. These include congenital anomalies such as hematometrocolpos (Fig 14–11), ectopic or absent gonads, pelvic kidney, cystic lesions (simple and hemorrhagic cysts, abscesses), and neoplasms (ovarian, from pelvic sidewalls and perineum).[18] Ultrasonography remains the screening modality of choice; MRI should be performed when the US study is equivocal or when the full extent of lesions must be assessed.

Selection of imaging planes and sequences is shown on Table 14–2. In summary, midline structures are evaluated in the sagittal plane, while paired structures are well seen in the axial plane. Short pulse sequences (T1-weighted) are routinely used; T2-weighted sequences are useful in the demonstration of ectopic gonads and in the exact definition of tumoral margins because of increased tissue contrast differentiation.

MUSCULOSKELETAL SYSTEM AND BONE MARROW

Although there are many similarities in the appearance of the joints in children and adults, some important differences should be noted (Fig 14–12). The growth plate (physis) produces a zone of low signal intensity and is wider in younger children. A line of low signal intensity may be identified at the site of the former growth plate in adolescents, even after radiographic evidence of closure. The ossified portion of the epiphysis contains marrow, thus having a higher signal intensity than the surrounding cartilaginous portion.

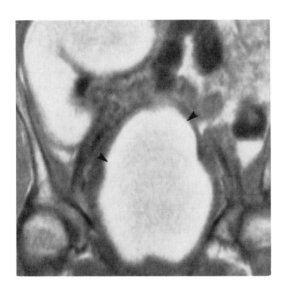

FIG 14–11.
Pelvis. Hematometrocolpos in a 14-year-old girl. Coronal T1-weighted MR image (SE 500/28) demonstrates dilation of the uterine cavity (*arrowheads*) and right fallopian tube with retained blood, which has high signal intensity because of the presence of methemaglobin.

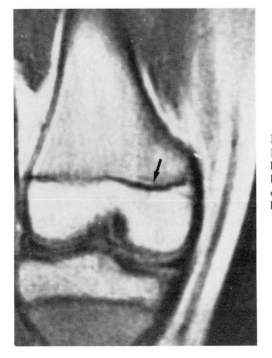

FIG 14–12.
Normal Knee. Coronal image (SE 468/40). There is higher signal intensity in the epiphysis than in the hematopoietic marrow areas of the metaphysis and diaphysis. The physis shows characteristic low signal band prior to closure (*arrow*).

Imaging of the musculoskeletal system is routinely done using spin echo pulse sequences; short TR, short TE (T1-weighted) sequences are the first to be performed, supplemented by long TR, long TE (T2-weighted) pulse sequences. Images in the coronal and sagittal planes are useful in the evaluation of extremities and spine, while imaging in the axial plane is indicated for pelvis and shoulder. When the spin echo technique is used, the MR signal intensity obtained may be high (marrow), low (bone cortex), or intermediate (cartilage and muscle) as a result of added signals from lipid and water protons. Chemical shift imaging, which is based in the subtraction of signals from fat and water, may be a useful technique when differentiating fatty from non-fatty marrow. Inversion recovery technique, which produces heavily T1-weighted images, has also been increasingly used in bone marrow evaluation.

Magnetic resonance imaging is the modality of choice for evaluation of the bone marrow in children. As the MR signal intensity of the bone marrow is related to the ratio of fat to other cells (in healthy children this ratio is around 50%), the signal is strong and uniform, particularly in the metaphysis and diaphysis. Results are not reliable when one is comparing signal intensity differences of the marrow between two patients or between two examinations on the same patient. Comparison with the signal intensity of an adjacent structure, such as muscle, provides more accurate information.[20] The marrow in a healthy pediatric subject has a uniform signal approximately three times more intense than that of adjacent muscle.

Marrow hyperplasia is characterized by low signal intensity because of decreased marrow fat; it is seen in the bones of patients with sickle cell anemia, hemophilia, and aplastic anemia. Anemic patients may show normal signal in the epiphysis and abnormal signal in the metaphysis and diaphysis, because most of the hematopoiesis occurs in these areas. Untreated aplastic anemia may show normal signal intensity because of overabundant fat. In the recovery phase, when there is marrow hypercellularity, the signal intensity decreases.

Leukemic patients will present with a nonuniform, patchy signal from the marrow; areas of low signal intensity on T1-weighted images become hyperintense on T2-weighted images.

Primary bone tumors, such as osteosarcoma and Ewing's sarcoma, are one of the most common indications for imaging of the musculoskeletal system by MRI. Soft tissue and marrow involvement are very well demonstrated, and coronal images provide good assessment of tumor extent, allowing preoperative planning.[25-28] T1-weighted images of children with osteosarcoma show a lesion with mixed signal intensity, the areas of low signal intensity representing mineralized tumor osteoid. On a T2-weighted sequence the lesion shows high signal intensity; this sequence also demonstrates soft tissue involvement and is usually obtained in the axial plane (Fig 14–13). Ewing's sarcoma will produce similar MR images, in different locations and age groups.

Metastatic bone disease may also be detected by MRI, although screening these patients with radionuclide bone scan is more desirable. Specific sites of high suspicion may then be selected for evaluation, because total body imaging by MRI is not technically feasible at this time.

Primary soft tissue neoplasms are also well imaged by MRI, depicting tumor size and extent, and depicting involvement of adjacent anatomic compartments, individual muscles, neurovascular structures, and joints.[29-31] Soft tissue lesions commonly evaluated by MRI include hemangiomas and lymphangiomas (which have low signal on T1 and high signal on T2), lipomas (high signal on T1 and T2), post-traumatic conditions such as scars and myositis (low signal on T1 and T2), and hematomas (acute and chronic hematomas have low signal on T1; subacute hematoma has high signal on T1).

Osteomyelitis may also be detected by MRI, although issues concerning the sensitivity of MRI vs. radionuclide bone scanning in osteomyelitis are still unsettled in the literature.

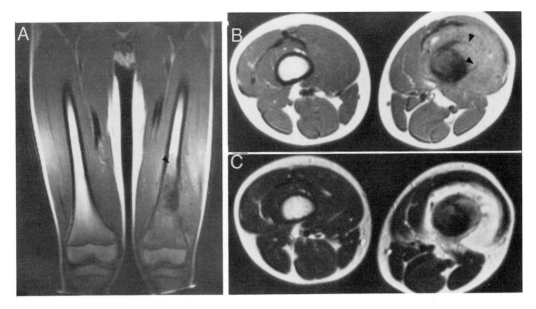

FIG 14–13.
Musculoskeletal. Osteosarcoma in a 7-year-old boy. **A,** coronal image (SE 500/30) is useful to demonstrate the extent of medullary invasion, as areas of decreased signal intensity (*arrowhead*) in contrast with the bright signal of fat in the undiseased marrow. **B,** axial image. This T1-weighted sequence showed periosteal rupture (*arrowheads*) and the soft-tissue component of this tumor. **C,** the T2-weighted image of the axial study again depicts marrow invasion, periosteal disrupture, and a soft-tissue component.

Magnetic resonance images may be useful when the bone scan and plain films are equivocal or show a normal appearance.

Aseptic necrosis is well imaged by MRI.[32] This modality also provides useful information concerning femoral head coverage and incongruity. Therefore, it may be employed when evaluating patients with congenital hip dislocation, slipped capital femoral epiphysis, and septic arthritis.[33]

REFERENCES

1. Boechat MI, Kangarloo H, Ortega J, et al: Primary liver tumors in children: Comparative study between MRI and CT. *Radiology* 1988; 169:727–732.
2. Dietrich RB, Kangarloo H, Lenarsky KY, et al: Neuroblastoma: The role of magnetic resonance imaging. *AJR* 1987; 148:937–942.
3. Kangarloo H, Dietrich RB, Ehrlich RM, et al: Magnetic resonance imaging of Wilms' tumor. *Urology* 1986; 28:203–207.
4. McArdle CB, Nicholas DA, Richardson CJ, et al: Monitoring of the neonate undergoing MR imaging: Technical considerations. *Radiology* 1986; 159:223–226.
5. Edelman RR, McFarland E, Stark D, et al: Surface coil MR imaging of abdominal viscera. Part 1: Theory, technique, and initial results. *Radiology* 1985; 157:425–430.
6. Lufkin MR, Votruba J, Reicher M, et al: Solenoid surface coils in magnetic resonance imaging. *AJR* 1986; 146:409–412.
7. Kangarloo H: Chest MRI in children. *Radiol Clin North Am* 1988; 26:263–275.
8. Fletcher B, Jacobstein M, Nelson A, et al: Gated magnetic resonance imaging of congenital cardiac malformations. *Radiology* 1984; 150:137–140.

9. Bisset III GS, Kirks DR, Strife JL: Vascular rings: Magnetic resonance imaging. *AJR* 1987; 149:251–256.

10. Boechat MI, Kangarloo H: MRI usurping CT's role in pediatric abdomen. *Diagn Imaging* 1988; 10:2:114–119.

11. Boechat MI, Kangarloo H, Gilsanz V: Hepatic masses in children. *Semin Roentgenol* 1988; 23:185–193.

12. Stark DD, Moseley ME, Bacon BR, et al: Magnetic resonance imaging and spectroscopy of hepatic iron overload. *Radiology* 1985; 154:137–142.

13. Weinreb JC, Cohen JM, Armstrong E, et al: Imaging the pediatric liver. MRI and CT. *AJR* 1986; 147:785–790.

14. Stark DD, Moss AA, Goldberg HI, et al: Magnetic resonance and CT of the normal and diseased pancreas: A comparative study. *Radiology* 1984; 150:153–162.

15. Haaga JR: Magnetic resonance imaging of the pancreas. *Radiol Clin North Am* 1984; 22:869–877.

16. Dietrich RB, Kangarloo H: Kidneys in infants and children: Evaluation with MR. *Radiology* 1986; 159:215–221.

17. Geisinger MA, Risius, B, Jordan ML, et al: Magnetic resonance imaging of renal transplants. *AJR* 1984; 143:1229–1234.

18. Dietrich RB, Kangarloo H: Pelvic abnormalities in children: Assessment with MR imaging. *Radiology* 1987; 163:367–372.

19. Kangarloo H, Dietrich RB, Taira T, et al: MR imaging of bone marrow in children. *J Comput Assist Tomogr* 1986; 10:205–209.

20. Kangarloo H, Dietrich RB, Ehrlich RM, et al: Magnetic resonance imaging of Wilms' tumor. *Urology* 1986; 28:203–207.

21. Schultz CL, Haaga JR, Fletcher BD, et al: Magnetic resonance imaging of the adrenal glands: A comparison with computed tomography. *AJR* 1984; 143:1235–1240.

22. Fink IJ, Reing JW, Dwyer AJ, et al: MR imaging of pheochromocytomas. *J Comput Assist Tomogr* 1985; 9:454–458.

23. Dietrich RB, Kangarloo H: Retroperitoneal mass with intradural extension: Value of magnetic resonance imaging in neuroblastoma. *AJR* 1986; 146:251–254.

24. Boechat MI, Ortega J, Hoffman AD, et al: Computed tomography in stage III neuroblastoma. *AJR* 1985; 145:1283–1287.

25. Brady TJ, Rozen BR, Pykert IL, et al: NMR imaging of leg tumors. *Radiology* 1983; 149:181–187.

26. Moon KL, Genant HK, Helms CA, et al: Musculoskeletal applications of nuclear magnetic resonance. *Radiology* 1983; 147:161–171.

27. Zimmer WD, Berquist TH, McLeod RA, et al: Bone tumors: Magnetic resonance imaging versus computed tomography. *Radiology* 1985; 155:709–718.

28. Totty WG, Murphy WA, Lee JKT: Soft tissue tumors: MR imaging. *Radiology* 1986; 160:135–141.

29. Aisen AM, Martel W, Braunstein EM, et al: MRI and CT evaluation of primary bone and soft tissue tumors. *AJR* 1986; 146:749–756.

30. Cohen MD, De Rosa GP, Kleiman M, et al: Magnetic resonance evaluation of disease of the soft tissues in children. *Pediatrics* 1987; 79:696–701.

31. Demas BE, Heelan RT, Lane J, et al: Soft tissue sarcomas of the extremities: Comparison of MR and CT in determining the extent of disease. *AJR* 1988; 150:615–620.

32. Bluemm RG, Falke THM, Ziegses de Plantes BG Jr, et al: Early Legg-Perthes disease (ischemic necrosis of the femoral head) demonstrated by magnetic resonance imaging. *Skeletal Radiol* 1985; 14:95–98.

33. Bissett GS III: Magnetic resonance imaging in pediatrics. *Clear Images* 1987; 1:6–17.

Index